THE COMPLETE GUI

Endurance Training

Jon Ackland

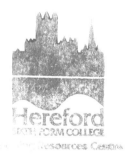

A & C Black • London

Published by A & C Black Publishers Ltd
37 Soho Square, London W1D 3QZ

Second edition 2003
Reprinted 2001
First edition 1999

Previously published as
The Power to Perform

Published by special arrangement with
Reed Books, a division of Reed Publishing (NZ) Ltd
39 Rawene Rd, Birkenhead, Auckland

ISBN 0 7136 6635 8

A CIP catalogue record for this book
is available from the British Library.

Acknowledgements
Cover photography © Martin Hughes / CORBIS

Typeset in 10½ on 12pt Palatino

A&C Black uses paper produced with elemental
chlorine-free pulp, harvested from managed
sustainable forests.

Printed and bound in Great Britain by
Biddles Ltd, Guildford and Kings Lynn

Dedication

This book is dedicated

- To my Mum and Dad (Maureen and Jim) and my sister (Jill) who have always supported and encouraged me. Thanks for all you have done for me throughout my life.

- To my wonderful partner, Kerri McMaster, who supported me tremendously in the writing of this book, and whose patience, wisdom and encouragement get me through life. A special thank you to Anne McMaster, whose constant support and care have helped me beyond words in the last few years.

- To my mentors and heroes, who unselfishly taught me what I needed to know about exercise and training. They are Gary Regtien, Jim Blair and the late Sam Johnson. The world would be a better place with a few more of you guys. Thanks for everything.

- Finally, to Arthur Lydiard, whose ideas revolutionised endurance training.

Contents

Foreword

It is very seldom that a book can simultaneously meet the learning and practical application needs of both athlete and coach. *The Complete Guide to Endurance Training* is one such book and has established the benchmark against which all training guides will be measured in future.

The guide is written in such a style that the diverse and complex issues of developing and preparing athletes for endurance sports are made perfectly understandable: training theory and practical programme design are clearly and concisely explained. Jon Ackland really knows the subject because he has been there.

Most impressive of all is the thorough attention to practical detail as the reader is guided through the steps of planning programmes that are designed to meet the needs of the athlete or the coach at their own level of development.

The Complete Guide to Endurance Training is essential reading for anyone involved in triathlon, Ironman, duathlon, distance running, cycle racing, mountain biking, rowing and all other forms of endurance activity.

Frank W. Dick O.B.E.
President, European Athletics Coaches Association
Author, *Sports Training Principles*

Preface

Why write a book on endurance training? After all, there are already plenty of books on endurance sports and training.

After working with thousands of endurance athletes over a number of years, I realised that too many were not asking themselves why they trained the way they did. Why did I do a long run yesterday? How fast should I ride tomorrow? Why begin speed-work this week and not next week? Why did I feel tired on an easy paddle? What should I do in the last week before a race?

I found these questions and others like them were not being asked often enough by athletes, if at all. Instead, when it came to their training programmes, many athletes were either guessing or blindly following what others were doing, or had done.

Endurance athletes, of course, have to train a lot. That comes with the territory. But many of the athletes I saw were training too often, too fast, and in a haphazard manner that frequently led to overtraining, injury and/or disappointment. Consistent success, it seemed, was elusive.

This was frustrating for the athlete and frustrating for me, because I knew there was a better way. And while I could help the athletes I saw in my role as an exercise/training consultant, I knew there were lots of others whom I couldn't see, but who with a little guidance could achieve a much higher level of performance than they had attained previously.

The Complete Guide to Endurance Training (previously published as *The Power to Perform*) focuses a great deal on the fundamentals. This does not mean, however, that the book lacks detail, or fails to address the 'nitty gritty' of endurance training. Far from it. There are enough 'McNuggets' of information in the following pages to feed even the hungriest mind!

The idea of writing a book is a simple one, of course. Actually writing it, and doing a good job, is far from simple. I knew from experience that this book had to be practical if busy, hard-working athletes and coaches were going to use it. Indeed, practicality was the guiding principle behind everything that went into the book, and the way it is presented. I hope this is apparent from page one.

Of course, no two athletes are the same! This book happily acknowledges your individuality not only by teaching you how to write your own programmes but also by providing you with the ability to create over 2000 individualised programmes tailored to your needs.

The Complete Guide to Endurance Training can be used whether you are 6 or 60, a champion or a weekend warrior, a sports scientist or someone who simply wants to get the best out of themselves.

Reading this book may take a little time, but it will, as they say, be time well spent. So, read on, train intelligently, 'put it in' when you have to, and have fun.

Jon Ackland
Auckland, New Zealand
September 1994

Preface to the second edition

How do you go about reaching your performance potential? How do you win an Olympic gold medal? How do you get the most out of yourself whether you're a beginner or a winner?

These are the questions that many athletes ask themselves and over my 20 years as a consultant on training for high performance, these are the questions I've needed to answer for the athletes I deal with each day. Initially working for the Institute of Sport and then in my own business at Performance Lab, we've worked at teaching people how to train and perform and have worked specifically on explaining **the diference between training and smart training**. Many athletes spend countless hours and tremendous energy working at improving their performance and many get despondent because they're not getting any better. To perform at your best you really need to know what you're doing, and that was the inspiration to write this book. There are certain key fundamentals to high performance, and easy manipulation of training components allows you to tailor make specific individualised training programmes for people of all talents and age. **Smart training** gives you better results for less effort using all the key training strategies employed by the best athletes and coaches in the world. There are ways of generating hugely improved performances if you know how to do it.

So here you have it. It's a few years since I wrote the book and that time has been very exciting. *The Complete Guide to Endurance Training* has become the 'Endurance Training Bible' in New Zealand and Australia and many outstanding performances have been attributed to the material contained in the book. There have been countless national champions, an Olympic champion, a number of world champions, many national records and even several world records. It has also helped many people new to the sports performance world access their potential abilities quickly. You'll find it very useful too.

Train hard, Train smart, Live long and perspire.

Jon Ackland
November 2002

The Complete Guide to Endurance Training has been specially adapted from the second edition of *The Power to Perform*. The publisher would like to acknowledge the assistance of Dr Sarah Rowell during this process. Sarah is a former Olympic marathon runner and international mountain and fell runner. After working for the National Coaching Foundation for nine years, she is now an independent sports science consultant.

Chapter 1

Understanding Your Training

Healthy or sick, rich or poor, famous or anonymous, we are all Time's obedient servants; each of us is obliged to admit that there are only so many hours in the day. Yet how many of us value time in the same way that we value money? Or diamonds? Or gold? Time is money, they say. But it's not. It's far more valuable, especially to an endurance athlete. Many hours of training have to be fitted in around education, work, family and the daily chores that make up a life. It is absolutely crucial, therefore, that training is as efficient as possible, with little or no wastage of time and/or effort.

For instance, ask yourself this question: Is all my training and effort giving me the best possible result in terms of fun, health and racing performance? I believe few athletes can honestly answer that question with an emphatic Yes! To avoid the twin demons of wasted time and wasted effort, it is necessary to design a training programme that is specific to your needs (competitive or otherwise). But before you do this you must know where you are going. What are your goals for the year? How are you going to achieve them? What was the aim of last month's training? Did you achieve it? What training have you got planned for tomorrow? Why? Until you can answer these questions, and many more like them, it is unlikely you will achieve the success you deserve from your efforts.

The key to realising your racing potential is understanding your training. In New Zealand we have a phrase, 'All the gears and no ideas'. Too many athletes could put this on their gravestone; much better to live under the banner 'Knowledge is power', for once you understand how to train effectively, not only will you improve, but you will enjoy yourself far more in the process. The most common misconception held by endurance athletes is that more is better. Too often this translates to 'garbage in, garbage out'. Generally, most endurance athletes need to train less – but more efficiently. For example, planning and analysing your training for ten minutes a week may be far more effective than doing another two hours of hard work. It's certainly more fun!

Thought should also be given to technique and equipment. Improvements in both these areas may yield far better results than simply doing more miles 'in the wrong position on the wrong bike'. A good example of this approach is the overweight athlete on an ultra-lightweight racing bike with aero helmet, disk wheels and a bad back, which forces him/her to ride in an upright position! A structured programme would not only bring better results and prevent injuries, but it might save the athlete several thousand dollars in equipment. Of course, good equipment can help you get the best out of yourself, and might even make training more enjoyable, but it's not the crucial factor. Efficient use of time and resources, that's the key.

♦ Make a plan ♦

The planning of each training week and month is vital if you want to achieve optimal performance. Many athletes put a lot of effort into training without carefully setting a programme that will bring improvement. After all, if you are going to dedicate considerable time and effort to your training, the least you can do is sit down and plan it! Right? Always aim to schedule 30 minutes planning time into your weekly training programme. Use this time to analyse what you have done and plan what you are going to do.

'Listen' to your body both during and after training. Did last week's speed session flatten you too much? Did you do too many miles? Let the way you feel and respond to different types of training guide you as you work out your programme. You alone will be the best judge of the type, volume and intensity of training that is best for you.

Monitor every aspect of training and note how it feels. This will give you a much better idea of how to pinpoint training errors and successes. And remember, bad performances and workouts can be just as beneficial if you learn from them. If you can continue to refine your training through analysis and planning, you will waste less time and perform far better.

As one top competitor has said, 'Champion athletes have two types of days – good days, and days where they learn something.' In other words, Train Smart!

♦ Basic training concepts ♦

1 *Specificity*
You race how you train. If you train slowly, you race slowly. If you train over short distances, you will only be able to race short distances. Training should simulate how you intend to race. The closer you get to race day, the stronger that simulation should be. Only by applying the principle of specificity will you be able to prepare your body properly for racing.

2 *Frequency*
To improve a certain aspect of your physical ability you will need to practise that aspect repeatedly. Crash training programmes normally result in you becoming injured or overtrained. Frequency also means consistency – a little often is much better than a lot seldom.

3 *Overload*
Workouts must overload your system if they are to promote the adaptation process. By adapting to greater and greater training workloads (stress) your ability in specific aspects of performance will improve.

4 *Recovery*
This is crucial. Recovery fosters improvement. An athlete who doesn't recover adequately from workouts will fail to improve, for it is during recovery, not training, that the adaptation to training (growth) occurs. Remember: training plus recovery equals improvement!

5 *Reversibility*
Training effects are reversible. If you don't train, or train less, you will (in the long term) lose fitness and performance.

6 *Flexibility*
Your training plan must be able to cope with unexpected developments at work, at home, and in your physical condition. You must also be able to adapt to different types of racing and racing conditions. A good training programme and athlete is flexible.

7 *Adaptability*
Training volumes and intensities must be increased gradually. Only then will your body

adapt to the increasing demands being placed upon it. Adaptation cannot be rushed!

8 *Maintenance*
During the off-season you should try and maintain some of the gains you made during the last competitive season. Do this by having an easy, low-intensity programme. Make it fun.

9 *Listen to your body*
Always listen to your body before, and during, training. A programme designed in advance cannot take into account the way you feel on any particular day. Some days you will be too tired to do the workout on your programme. On those days ignore the programme and take it easy. You are not a machine!

10 *Quality vs quantity*
The correct type of training, at the right intensity, for the right duration, will bring better results than simply doing high mileage for the sake of it. Don't get sucked in by the 'more is better' school of training. Think before you train.

11 *Goal setting*
Set achievable, realistic goals based on where you are at right now. These goals should cover the next few weeks (short-term goals), the next twelve months (intermediate goals) and your entire sporting career (long-term goals). If you don't achieve a goal, don't get despondent. Sit down and see if you can learn something about your preparation, your racing tactics or your goal-setting strategy. Good athletes don't have good days and bad days, they have good days and learning days.

12 *Trainability*
Training improvements do not occur consistently over time. There will be periods when you improve a lot, and there will be times when you don't seem to be making any progress at all. Improvements tend to be greatest early on in a training programme. The cumulative fatigue that results from high mileage can make you feel like you are on a performance plateau during high mileage phases. The answer? Hang in there and be patient!

13 *Warming up, warming down*
Try and warm up before every workout, especially before speedwork or other high-intensity sessions. This will reduce the risk of injury and improve the quality of the workout. Warm-downs will help flush out by-products in the muscles. This promotes faster recovery and means you will be better prepared for your next workout.

14 *Technique*
A good technique will make you a better athlete. Take the time to refine your technique.

◆ The components of training ◆

By understanding and controlling the following training components you will train and compete more effectively.

1 *Intensity*
Intensity is the effort or energy required for a particular form of training. The intensity of the workout must be sufficiently stressful to allow adaptation to overload to occur.

2 *Duration*
This is the length of time it takes to complete a workout.

3 *Volume*
Volume is a measure (miles/km, hours/minutes) of how much work you perform

during a workout. Intensity and volume are inversely related – the more intense the workout, the lower the volume of the workout.

4 *Rest periods*

Rest periods are the length of time between periods of training, for example between intervals or sprints or workouts. The length of the rest period depends on the relationship between the intensity/volume of the workout and the athlete's tolerance to training.

5 *Repetitions*

Repetitions (reps) are the number of times a specific form of training is completed during a workout, for example 3 × 1 km. Repetitions are generally associated with speedwork and shorter duration intervals. They are generally grouped into sets.

♦ How long will it take to ♦ be the best you can?

Generally, it will take at least two to five years to get close to your peak in a sport. Further increases can still occur after this (and probably will), but the increments of performance improvement will be smaller. When this starts happening, the only way to get better is to train smarter! Remember too that talent plays a large part in all endeavours; not everybody will reach the top in their chosen sport (you can thank your parents for that!). And if you are not one of these chosen few, then you need to set your sights on your own targets, personal bests, and having fun.

The fun aspect cannot be emphasised enough. If you are not going to be an Olympic champion, and perhaps even if you are, try and keep your sport in perspective. In particular, don't turn it into another job! Also, don't try to hurry your rate of improvement.

Champions are not made overnight, even if the media would sometimes like you to believe this is so. One athlete, after a journalist implied his success was awfully sudden, replied: 'Yeah, it's only taken me ten years to become an overnight sensation!'

Here are ten variables that can influence your sporting development.

1 Talent (doing a sport that suits your physical and mental make-up)
2 Coaching
3 Log book use, analysis and refinement of training (very important)
4 Technique (skill acquisition)
5 Training specificity
6 Training frequency
7 Commitment and mental approach to the sport
8 Knowledge and experience in training and racing
9 Having a training programme that suits you
10 Equipment (generally one of the least important)

♦ Length of training ♦ build-up

Many athletes, both elite and novice, believe it only takes a few weeks to get fully fit for a race. Unfortunately, it is not that easy if you want to perform to your potential (and we usually do). If base training – the foundation of your fitness – is not done adequately, then the quality of your speedwork and racing will suffer accordingly. Having said that, starting specific training too soon can also pose a few problems, mainly to do with boredom and loss of enthusiasm. Don't get too keen too soon. Many athletes who do huge mileages during winter never make it to the startline come summer. In this respect, training is just like good comedy – timing is everything!

Assuming you already have a reasonable level of conditioning, here are some approximate guidelines on how long it will take you to prepare (base, speedwork, taper) for a number of different events. Speedwork generally starts four to eight weeks before the race.

Event	Preparation time (weeks)
Ironman triathlon	16–20
Mountain bike	12
Olympic/sprint triathlon	12
Cycle race 60–100 km	12
Cycle race 160 + km, tour	16–20
Rowing	12
Marathon	16–20
10 km race	12
Multisport	12–20

◆ Why base, speed, peak? ◆

Figure 1.1 (*see* below) shows the performance pyramids of two athletes. The athlete on the left's (competitor 1) training history is less than the athlete's on the right (competitor 2).

This results in competitor 1 achieving a lower peak performance than competitor 2.

There is a logical and natural progression in training for a sport. The height of an athlete's performance pyramid is largely determined by his/her training history for a specific sport. The greater that history, the greater the base (training preparation). This is because an experienced athlete is better able to cope with larger base training volumes (they've done it all before) than the novice athlete. For an athlete, a big base provides a better tolerance to training, a faster recovery from training, and the ability to handle more speedwork. All these factors add up to a potentially higher peak in performance, although other factors such as talent, specificity of training, and so on, can greatly influence just how well an athlete performs. Nevertheless, there is no doubt that the greater the training history, the better an athlete is likely to do.

If you haven't got time to train fully and are interested in just completing an event, the following table (*see* page 6) shows the minimum number of days you should plan to train each week to finish the event comfortably.

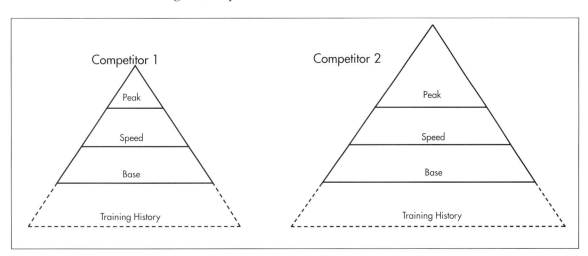

Figure 1.1 Why 'Base, Speed, Peak'?

Minimum number of training days per week required to train for an event

Sport	Minimum no. of training days
Cycle/mountain biking	
40 km (1 hr)	2
80 km (2.5 hrs)	3
160 km (5.5 hrs)	3–4
Tour (12 hrs over 2 days)	5–6
Triathlon	
Sprint	3
Standard	3–4
Half-Ironman	4–5
Ironman	5–6
Rowing	3–6
Running	
10 km	2–4
Half-marathon	4–5
Marathon	5–6

♦ The energy systems ♦

The body uses two main energy systems, one of which breaks down into two further parts. These systems are:

1 The **Anaerobic** energy system, which breaks down into the alactic (immediate) and lactic (non-oxidative) sub-systems.

2 The **Aerobic** energy system (oxidative).

The anaerobic system is used during high-intensity exercise where energy demands exceed aerobic metabolism. In other words, this system is used when you are exercising without oxygen, in sprinting, for example. The *anaerobic alactic* system is used during very high intensity exercise (maximum effort under ten to twenty seconds) and supplies immediate energy. It does not require oxygen to function (anaerobic) and no lactic acid is produced (alactic). The *anaerobic lactic* system does not require oxygen to function (anaerobic). It does, however, produce lactic acid as a major by-product of energy production (lactic). The anaerobic lactic system is used in moderately intense activity lasting between ten seconds and two to three minutes. It is used when oxygen is in short supply or when there is a complete lack of oxygen.

The aerobic energy system takes in, transports and uses oxygen. It requires the presence of oxygen to function. It is the main source of energy for events lasting longer than three to four minutes. The aerobic energy system is used for moderate intensity exercise and is developed and maintained through cardiovascular exercise, such as cycling, running, swimming, kayaking and rowing. Cardiovascular exercise stimulates the cardiovascular system (heart and blood vessels) and is, quite simply, any exercise that increases heart rate. It is also called cardiorespiratory exercise because it improves the ability of the heart and lungs to deliver oxygen to the working muscles.

♦ The distance vs duration ♦ debate

Many athletes and coaches preach duration rather than distance when quantifying training. The reasoning behind this is that by training for duration rather than distance, you can avoid having to push yourself over a specific distance when you are tired. You simply train more slowly when tired, and still complete your workout. This may help prevent injury and overtraining.

There is, however, an argument for the use of distance. After all, if you are going to race over a specific distance, you have to cover it no matter how long it takes – no excuses! For this reason, particularly when training for longer races, it is sometimes better to use distance for your training.

I believe that both duration and distance should be used, for this provides more information (but don't become one of those 'crazies' who have to beat their previous time over the distance every time!). For example, when you do a workout over a set distance don't look at your stopwatch. At all! Afterwards, however, total time or lap times can be compared against distance. You can then evaluate your workout and condition by considering the following:

- if you complete the distance in the usual time at the usual heart rate, things are good;
- if you complete the distance in a faster time at the same or lower heart rate, things are even better – you are getting fitter;
- if you complete the distance in a faster time but at a higher heart rate, you are exercising too hard;
- if you complete the distance in a slower time at the same heart rate or a higher heart rate, you are too tired.

By combining distance and duration you can gain a lot more information on training than you can by just exercising to a set distance or duration. The question should not be whether to use distance or duration to quantify your training, but what is the most effective way to train. The answer then becomes simple: a combination of distance and duration is best.

♦ Planning for adventures ♦ and simulating race conditions

During base work and the off-season particularly, plan exciting training sessions. Be adventurous rather than sticking to the same old training routes. And take friends with you so training also becomes a social occasion. This can help keep you fresh and enthusiastic.

During the speed phase you should start simulating race conditions, intensities and environments. If you can train on the course you will race on, do so. But don't train on the course every day as boredom can set in! Training on the course will help you to handle the course conditions better, improve pace judgement and make you aware of any special considerations that the course may require in racing.

Chapter 2

The Principles of Training

Training should be simple to understand and enjoyable to do. If it is both these things, then you are well on the way to success. Indeed, training should be looked on as a personal adventure that is fun, challenging and rewarding. Perhaps above all else, training should let you look through 'the window of your potential' and see that the only limits you have are those you place on yourself.

◆ Training volumes vs ◆ intensities vs performance

Volume is the amount of training completed; intensity is the effort required for a particular form of training. Volume increases and decreases during training depending on where you are at in your build-up. Intensity, on the other hand, increases throughout your build-up, gradually in base but more rapidly during speedwork. Volumes of intensity increase and decrease.

Performance increases in a similar pattern to intensity but remains low for a longer period of time and has a more gradual increase. During speedwork, performance begins to improve more rapidly and is at its peak rate of increase during the taper period (and to a lesser degree during compensation weeks at the end of mesocycles – more about this later). This means that despite all your hard training in base, you won't see the real benefits until very late in build-up. Figure 2.1 illustrates the changes in these three factors during a training programme.

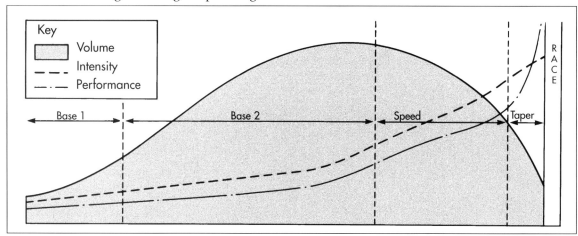

Figure 2.1 Volume vs intensity vs performance

◆ Training seasons and ◆ periodisation

Training is a form of stress. If it is done correctly, you adapt to that stress and become stronger. If it is done incorrectly, training wears you down and you can become 'weaker' – sick, injured, demotivated or over-trained. When you are any one of these things, you won't get the best out of yourself.

It is essential, therefore, that training is organised, in the true sense of the word. This means it balances work (stress) and recovery (active recovery or rest) – the two key ingredients of any good training programme. To help you achieve this balance, training is broken down into different phases. This process is called periodisation. Although top Olympic athletes sometimes work off a four-year training plan (e.g. Finland's Lasse Viren – double gold medallist at the 1972 and 1976 Olympics), for most athletes, the longest and most logical training period is a year. A year can be broken down into three seasons. These are:

1 Off-season (transition)
2 Pre-season (preparatory)
3 In-season (competitive)

Figures 2.2 (below) and 2.3 (*see* page 10) give examples of how a year can be broken down into three seasons based around race events.

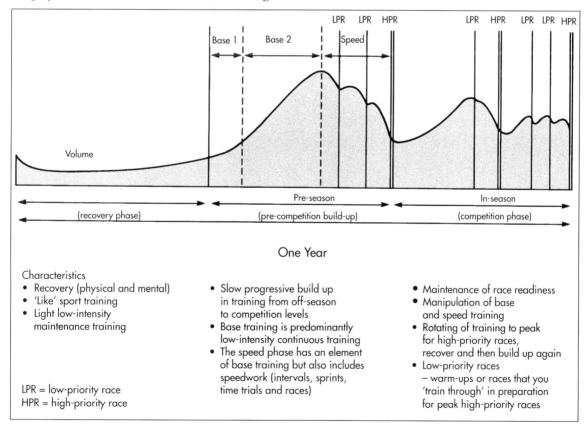

| | | | LPR LPR HPR | LPR HPR LPR LPR HPR |

Volume

Base 1 Base 2 Speed

Pre-season
(recovery phase) (pre-competition build-up)

In-season
(competition phase)

One Year

Characteristics
- Recovery (physical and mental)
- 'Like' sport training
- Light low-intensity maintenance training

- Slow progressive build up in training from off-season to competition levels
- Base training is predominantly low-intensity continuous training
- The speed phase has an element of base training but also includes speedwork (intervals, sprints, time trials and races)

- Maintenance of race readiness
- Manipulation of base and speed training
- Rotating of training to peak for high-priority races, recover and then build up again
- Low-priority races – warm-ups or races that you 'train through' in preparation for peak high-priority races

LPR = low-priority race
HPR = high-priority race

Figure 2.2 The training seasons

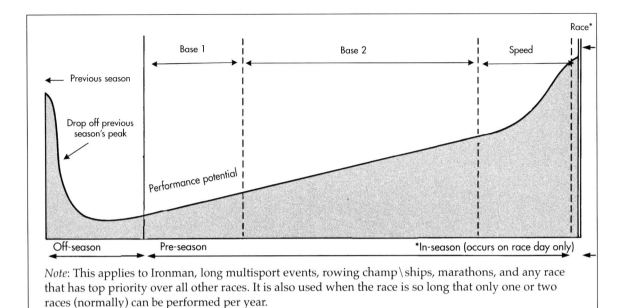

Note: This applies to Ironman, long multisport events, rowing champ\ships, marathons, and any race that has top priority over all other races. It is also used when the race is so long that only one or two races (normally) can be performed per year.

Figure 2.3 Seasons and periodisation for an endurance athlete aiming to peak once for a major event in a year

Pre-season – preparatory phase (generally twelve to sixteen weeks)

As Figure 2.4 shows, pre-season training can also be broken down into different periods:

- Base training
  - Base 1
  - Base 2
- Speed training
- Taper and peaking

Very simply, base training builds a foundation of fitness, and speed training helps you adjust to the demands of racing. Taper and peaking allow you to perform at your best on race day.

Base training (generally eight to twelve weeks)

Base training can last as long as six months, although it usually takes about two to three months. It really depends on how much time you have before the race or races you are aiming at, and how fit you are when you start base work. This phase of training consists mainly of high mileage/long duration workouts at a low intensity. These workouts are designed to improve your aerobic ability and muscular endurance.

As base training progresses you will find your tolerance to exercise improves – the so-called adaptation process. This enables you to recover from each training session more quickly. But, equally importantly, the base work will give you the endurance you need to cope with the increased intensity that comes later on in the programme.

Base training is divided into Base 1 and Base 2.

Base 1 – the preparation phase

The goal of this phase is quite simple: to get your body used to the type of exercise you are

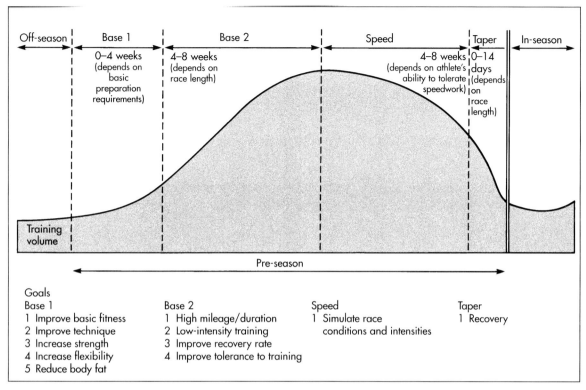

Goals

Base 1	Base 2	Speed	Taper
1 Improve basic fitness	1 High mileage/duration	1 Simulate race conditions and intensities	1 Recovery
2 Improve technique	2 Low-intensity training		
3 Increase strength	3 Improve recovery rate		
4 Increase flexibility	4 Improve tolerance to training		
5 Reduce body fat			

Figure 2.4 Pre-season training and periodisation

planning to compete in. For example, if you are a rower, you will become reacquainted with the boat and get back out on the water doing some easy technique work, if you haven't already been doing so during the off-season. Base 1 is also a good time to improve your strength and flexibility, refine technique and reduce body fat. The preparation phase is just that: a time that prepares you for the physical challenge that lies ahead.

Base 2 – the volume phase (mileage/duration)
During this phase, mileage is gradually increased. Training is still done mainly at a low intensity, although small amounts of speedwork can be done (particularly by experienced athletes). And *small* means *small* – you don't want to peak too early!

How much mileage should you do during this phase? That depends on how much you've done in the past. If you're new to the sport, then mileage will be less than for experienced athletes, and recovery from each workout will be slower. This means more time between workouts and fewer miles/km.

It is important to remember this when you are reading about a top athlete's training programme. It will have taken that athlete years of training to build up to that level. You copy them at your peril!

We all respond to training in different ways, and what works for one person may not work for another – that's what makes training such a personal adventure! Base training can be further broken down into sub-phases – easy,

11

hills, and sometimes up-tempo, which occurs more often at the start of speed. The first part of base is very easy training, followed by hill training during the middle to end of base. Finally, towards the end of base, up-tempo training is used to prepare your body for the speedwork in the speed phase (*see* chapter 4, 'Training Subphases'). Towards the end of Base 2 *some* up-tempo work (*slightly* faster than long slow distance) can be injected into the programme. This is to help the body begin to adjust to the real speedwork to follow. But remember this: base is *slow*! Training too fast during the base phase won't help you achieve race fitness more quickly and may even lead to injury, illness, peaking too early or over-training. So be patient. Rome wasn't built in a day, and nor is fitness.

Base training is designed to allow you to cope with the intense speed phase to come. The better you are able to do the speed phase, the better your race performance is likely to be. Therefore, base on its own does not improve performance greatly (unless you race ultra distances), but it is essential to your later training. Some athletes put too much effort into their base training and arrive at the start of speed training tired. They then end up performing below full potential despite all the hard work put in. You could say they got excited a little too early! Be patient during base and remember the speed phase is the 'critical zone' – be ready for it.

Speed training
(generally four to eight weeks)
After you have completed your base training it is time to add some speed to the programme. This will allow you to take advantage of the tremendous endurance you have built up in Base 1 and Base 2. The speed phase is the critical time. You need to be physiologically and psychologically prepared to put the 'hammer down' in the final four to eight weeks of training as this is where most

The racing mentality

When training, leave home without it – your racing mentality, that is. It's often tempting when training with friends (and would-be opponents!) to start racing them. Don't!

During the base phase it's vital you keep clocking up those miles/hours. You won't be able to do that if you train too fast, get tired and can't complete the next day's workout (a common mistake).

Some days, of course, long slow workouts are boring with a capital 'B'. On those days, and you will have them, it's okay to ease the boredom by doing two or three 'race-like' surges for a very short time. This applies mainly to training on the bike. To make sure these surges don't go on too long, decide where the surge will end before you begin it. If training with a group, make sure everyone regroups after the surge is finished; for example, sprint for a signpost and then regroup.

These surges should be limited to one workout a week. And remember, there will be plenty of opportunities for competing with your training partners during the speedwork phase. Indeed, simulating race conditions during that phase can be a great motivator and plenty of fun. But in the meantime, don't worry about winning the local club run or ride.

of your performance gains will be made. Speedwork usually lasts about four to eight weeks, depending on your training history and how you cope with faster work. During this phase, training volume decreases and training intensity *gradually* increases. Towards the middle or end of the phase, some workouts will closely match racing intensity. As speedwork progresses, the body will adapt to the new stress being placed upon it. This will eventually translate to a faster race pace.

Certain aspects of your speed, for example acceleration/power, top speed, speed endurance and maximum steady state pace, can also be worked on during this phase. This does not mean, however, that long slow workouts are neglected altogether. These still need to be done so that you retain your base conditioning.

Speedwork uses interval and sprint training, time trials and racing. It's very intensive (it often hurts like hell!) and therefore it must be managed carefully. Too little and you won't reach a peak; too much and overtraining can occur. The intensity of this phase also means there is more recovery time built into the programme. This time provides an excellent opportunity to refine technique. You must also contrast the intensities between speed training sessions and slow sessions. 'Creep' through your slow sessions as comfortably as possible so that you are able to 'hammer' the speed sessions.

Interestingly, some scientists suggest that for elite athletes a period of training overload ('superovercompensation', which would be overtraining if maintained for too long) should occur immediately before the taper, for example the third or second week before competition. This would only be done once or twice a year, however. Theoretically, a period of training overload enhances performance more than a traditional training programme in which overloading is not very severe. Why? Because the greater the training stress, the greater the body's adaptation to overcome it. This adaptation will, however, only occur if you follow the overload period with a long recovery period (the taper). Without this time to recover, overloading will become overtraining – the endurance athlete's 'death sentence'! (For more on superovercompensation *see* page 25.)

Taper and peaking (two to fourteen days)

A vital part of getting ready to race is freshening up. The tapering phase should happen before every race. The longer and/or more important the race, the longer the taper. Gradually easing back on the volume of training in the week or so before a race will bring you to a peak. The exact point at which you begin to reduce volume is determined largely by the event you're tapering for. For shorter events (around one hour's duration), two to four days is probably enough. For an Ironman triathlon, however, two weeks is probably best. A marathon taper is typically about ten days.

A common mistake in the tapering phase is to cut back on race intensity work too soon. Only in the final few days should race intensity training be stopped altogether. By maintaining training *intensity* right up until the last few days before a race, you retain a better 'feel' for the effort that will be required on race day. The volume of training, however, is reduced.

Tapering is a very personal part of training and what works for you may not work for someone else. It's up to you to experiment and find out what suits you best. Some athletes, for instance, feel that they 'lose their edge' if they ease back too much, although it's much more common for people to race tired because they don't ease back enough. Similarly, some athletes feel they need speedwork right up to the day of the race; others find speedwork 'flattens' them for quite a while and so they avoid it as race day approaches. Either way, tapering always involves reducing training volume. And if you are unsure just how much to taper, have a longer rather than a shorter taper.

Figure 2.4 (*see* page 11) shows the four preseason training phases described above.

In-season – competitive phase (generally eight to twelve weeks)

This is when the serious racing begins! The competition phase usually lasts about eight to twelve weeks, with performance sustained at 90 per cent plus with one or two 100 per cent or 'full peak' efforts (lasting one day to one week) during this time. Alternatively, a competition phase may involve several peaks requiring a cycle of peaking and recovering over a period of about four months. A good training programme will let you excel at either a single/double-peak season or a multiple-peak season and examples are given in figure 2.5.

Many athletes mistakenly believe they can hold a 'full' peak for three to six months. This is impossible. It can result in perfor-

mance dropping away, injury, illness or loss of motivation, or all four. For these reasons, training during the competition phase must be closely monitored. This means carefully manipulating training volume and speed-work.

It's best to focus on only one to six high-priority races per season, with lower-priority races in between used as 'training'. Most athletes can only achieve a 'full' peak (100 per cent performance for a single race) two to four times in a season. These peaks often coincide with provincial and national championships and training is organised accordingly. For elite athletes, the peaks may coincide with national trials and world champs. In cases where the peaks are well spread out, such as a national series (multiple races spread over ten weeks), it will be necessary to achieve

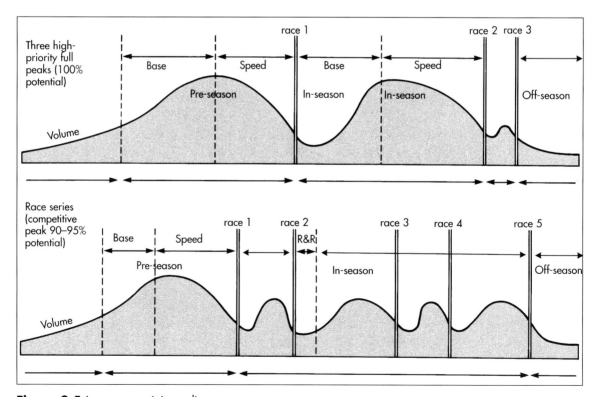

Figure 2.5 In-season training adjustments

'competitive' peaks throughout the season. These 'competitive' peaks require you to hold a high level of performance (95 per cent) over a series of races or a season. In this case, it is essential that fewer intensive training phases are inserted between races.

Speed training cycles and multiple peaks

These are normally used if you are in a race series. During the competitive phase you can set up peaks, or at least semi-peaks, from month to month. When trying to achieve multiple peaks it is essential that both the quantity (mileage) and quality (speedwork) are closely monitored from day to day and week to week. Too much of either will upset the programme and lower performance, or lead to injury.

These training cycles last about three to eight weeks. If the races are five or more weeks apart, a short period of base work with a small element of speed may be done immediately after races to allow for better recovery. Full speedwork can then be resumed. After racing, speedwork should not restart until recovery from the race is complete. And when you start speedwork again, keep the volume low initially. In the second week after a race, there is a gradual increase in mileage and speedwork toward the next race.

Multiple peak speedwork can be maintained over a competitive season that lasts two to three months. If the competitive season is any longer than this, a base training phase or an off-season becomes necessary again. And remember: too much speedwork can kill your season stone dead!

Off-season – active recovery or transition phase (generally four to sixteen weeks)

This phase usually lasts one to four months (four to eight weeks for elite athletes) and gives you a valuable chance to recharge the batteries (the 'recovery' bit) while still maintaining a reasonable level of fitness (the 'active' bit). Training during this phase is recreational (when you want, for example three times a week) and should be low intensity, low mileage. It's also a good time to work on technique or flexibility.

Off-season training doesn't need to be sport-specific either. Cyclists, for instance, could go mountain biking, swimming or running. As long as you are active it doesn't really matter what you do, although it is better if the activity continues to work your muscles and cardiovascular system in the same way your sport would. Elite athletes still need to spend a fair portion of their time doing their sport.

Overall, the key to the off-season is to make sure you begin the new season's base phase fresh, enthusiastic and ready to go, but also ready to build on last season's work and achieve a higher level of performance in the next season (*see* figure 2.6, page 16). It's a fine line between being rested and being 'wrecked', but one which will become easier to judge as you become more experienced. Don't worry about losing *some* fitness – it's all part of a planned, well-structured programme. Besides, you and your body have earned a break!

The key to performance lies largely in how you do your off-season. Too much training in the off-season results in tiredness and lack of enthusiasm for training. This will affect your following build-up. Too little training means loss of the hard-earned performance gains from last season. The result is less improvement in your following build-up. If you do a little training in your off-season you will maintain some of the gains in performance from your previous season resulting in greater improvements in the following year. Your off-season can help or hinder your performance improvement from year to year.

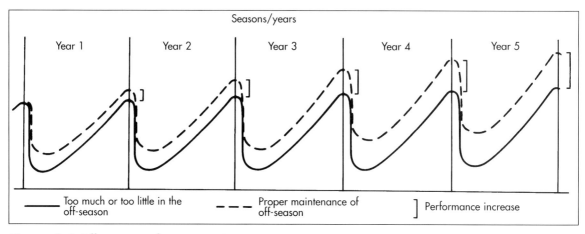

Figure 2.6 Off-season performance gains

♦ Training cycles ♦

Day to day: microcycles

A microcycle is used to maximise training on a day-to-day, workout-to-workout basis by balancing your training. The greater the recovery between workouts the more effective they become and the more progress you make. This can be achieved by using a hard/easy/hard/easy approach to training. As you get fitter, the harder sessions can, of course, become harder. Hard in base means more distance/duration; hard in speed means more speedwork. Intensity remains the same.

It is important that the hard sessions within a microcycle are not all of the same type of workout; that is, your hard sessions should rotate through long workouts, hill work, speedwork, and so on. If, however, you are training in a number of disciplines (running, cycling, swimming, kayaking), make sure similar workouts in the same discipline are kept apart. For example, long swims should not be done two sessions in a row. The key is to balance your training stress throughout the week. For a duathlete, a long run might be done in the middle of the week, so a long bike should be done at the end of the week. Similarly, a run speed session might be completed on Monday, and a bike speed session on Thursday.

Microcycles generally last 7, 14 or 21 days. For obvious reasons, the seven-day cycle is the most common (*see* examples on page 17–18).

The microcycle can be changed during the racing season with hard sessions mid-week and easy sessions towards the end of the week as part of the taper for Saturday/Sunday racing. You may require more rest before or after an intense workout (such as speedwork), and this then dictates whether the preceding and following workouts are in the morning or afternoon.

The following schedule, as an example, allows for longer rests after speed sessions.

Microcycle morning and afternoon adjustments

Mon	Tue	Wed	Thu	Fri	Sat	Sun
a.m.	a.m.	p.m.	a.m.	D/O	a.m.	p.m.
Easy	Speed	Hills	Easy		Speed	Long

Examples of microcycles for different sports

Cycling and mountain biking
Base phase

Mon	Tue	Wed	Thu	Fri	Sat	Sun
Easy	Hills	Easy	Hills	D/O	Long	Long
E	H	E	H	E	H	H

Speed phase

Mon	Tue	Wed	Thu	Fri	Sat	Sun
Easy (Hills)	Ints	Ints	Easy	D/O	Race	Long
E	H	H	E	E	H	H

Triathlon
Base and speed phases

Mon	Tue	Wed	Thu	Fri	Sat	Sun
Swim		Swim		D/O	Swim	
	Bike(Hills)		Bike(S)	D/O		Bike(Long)
Run(S)		Run(Long)		D/O	Run(Hills)	

Multisport
Base and speed phases

Mon	Tue	Wed	Thu	Fri	Sat	Sun
Run(Long)		Run(S)		D/O	Run(Hills)	
	Bike(Hills)		Bike(Long)	D/O	Bike(S)	
	Kayak(S)	Kayak(R)		D/O		Kayak(Long)

Running (10 km and marathon)
Base and speed phases

Mon	Tue	Wed	Thu	Fri	Sat	Sun
Easy	Med	Easy	Med	D/O	Med	Long
	(Ints)		(Long)		(Ints)	
E	H	E	H	E	H	H

Duathlon
Base and speed phases

Mon	Tue	Wed	Thu	Fri	Sat	Sun
					Run(Hills)	
	Bike(Hills)		Bike(S)	D/O	Bike(Long)	Bike(Long)
Run(S)		Run(Long)		D/O	Run(E)	Run(E)

Key: E = easy; H = hard; Ints = intervals; Tech = technique; D/O = day off; Med = medium; Land = land-based training; S = speed; R = resistance.

Examples of microcycles for different sports, continued

Rowing
Base phase

Mon	Tue	Wed	Thu	Fri	Sat	Sun
Tech	Med	Tech	Med	D/O	Long	Long
	Land		Land		Land	Land
E	H	E	H	E	H	H

Speed phase

Mon	Tue	Wed	Thu	Fri	Sat	Sun
Tech	Ints	Ints	Tech	D/O	Race	Long
E	H	H	E	E	H	H

Key: E = easy; H = hard; Ints = intervals; Tech = technique; D/O = day off; Med = medium; Land = land-based training; S = speed; R = resistance.

Week to week: mesocycles

A mesocycle is used to maximise training on a week-to-week basis and has a built-in recovery period to compensate for several weeks of long and/or intense training. This period usually lasts a week and is called a 'compensation week'. Mesocycles should occur regularly in the training programme, for example every second to fifth week, even during base training. These help you to steer clear of cumulative fatigue which, as the name suggests, can wear you down.

A mesocycle helps to keep you healthy and motivated: a great way to start the next period of hard training. It also allows for more improvement than a continuous build-up because of the adaptation to training that occurs when an easy period follows a hard period. Figure 2.7 gives examples of mesocycles to suit different types of athletes.

Most athletes have an easy week every third or fourth week, although some prefer alternating hard and easy weeks. Others, of course, can handle weeks and weeks of hard training without a break, but these athletes are few and far between and often perform at less than their potential because they never freshen up (*see* fig. 2.8, page 20).

Mesocycles are longer (five to six weeks) in early season base training due to the low training intensities, and shorter (three to four weeks) during the intense speedwork and competitive season.

Year to year: macrocycles

Macrocycles are used to plan the broad aspects of your training programme. This allows you to set out your training periods, training goals, and race priorities. As we have seen, this involves breaking down the year into three major seasons: off-season (active recovery), pre-season (base and speed training), and in-season (competition). These phases provide for seasonal/yearly recovery by including an easy period and a hard period in the training/competition cycle. Once you have established your macrocycles, you can slot in your mesocycles (week-to-week/month-to-month planning) and your microcycles (day-to-day planning).

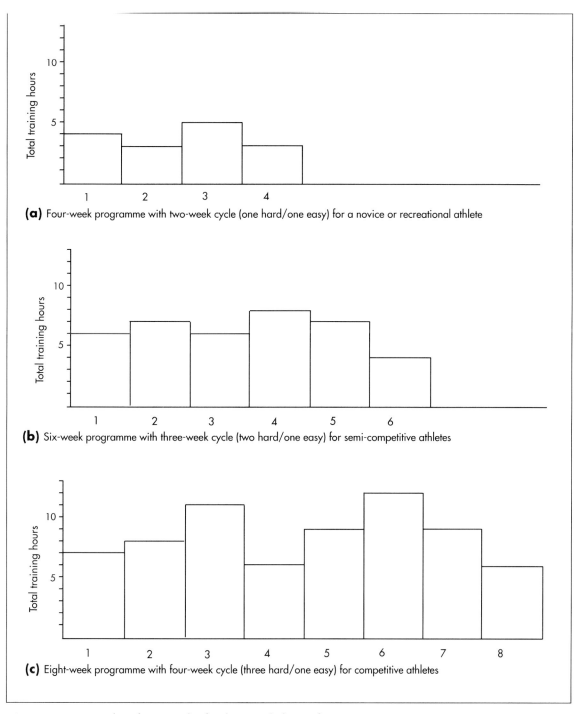

(a) Four-week programme with two-week cycle (one hard/one easy) for a novice or recreational athlete

(b) Six-week programme with three-week cycle (two hard/one easy) for semi-competitive athletes

(c) Eight-week programme with four-week cycle (three hard/one easy) for competitive athletes

Figure 2.7 Examples of mesocycles for the speed phase of training prior to competition

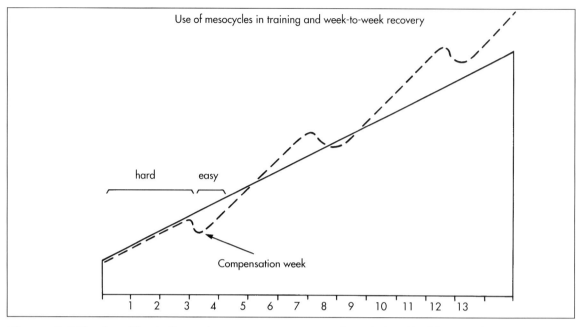

Use of mesocycles in training and week-to-week recovery

hard   easy

Compensation week

1 2 3 4 5 6 7 8 9 10 11 12 13

Figure 2.8 The dotted line indicates the variation in training volume (3 hard build-up weeks, 1 compensation week). The straight line indicates the continuous build-up method, which results in more chance of overtraining and generally results in less training being completed because of cumulative training fatigue.

Performance levels during competition build-up

Britain's great marathoner Ron Hill once said: 'A distance runner wakes up tired, and goes to bed tired.' Even with mesocycles this is, to some extent, both true and unavoidable for all endurance athletes.

In the build-up phase, 'cumulative fatigue' means you will always be training slightly tired – a natural side-effect of the body's adaptation to increasing training stress. This tiredness, however, needs to be carefully monitored.

This is the time when you must have faith in your training programme, because there seems to be a lot of hard work and little obvious reward. Once you start doing the lower mileages towards the end of the speed phase, you will feel less fatigue and your performance will tend to improve. Being slightly tired means you won't be breaking any world records in training. That's okay – they can wait until you start racing!

Alternative training cycle recovery strategies

In multisport and triathlon training, one effective strategy is to emphasise one discipline per week. The other disciplines are still done, but at a lower training volume. For example, in a three-sport discipline such as triathlon, swimming, cycling and running are emphasised on different weeks. This allows recovery from the mileage and intensity of each of the disciplines. Rotating the emphasis in this way may also be more convenient in terms of regular work, education or family commitments. For example, if your work takes you out of town and away from a pool for a few days every third week, this type of programme can easily accommodate this.

The schedule below shows how a 12-week triathlon programme may look with the emphasis alternating between the three disciplines.

Alternating the training emphasis in this way is an effective recovery strategy, similar in effect to a mesocycle. A mesocycle is probably best as it allows a complete recovery week, but this 'alternating strategy' may be useful for some athletes.

Week	1	2	3	4	5	6	7	8	9	10	11	12
Swim	H	E	M	E	H	E	M	E	H	E	M	E
Bike	M	H	E	E	M	H	E	E	M	H	E	E
Run	E	M	H	E	E	M	H	E	E	M	H	E

Key: H = hard; M = medium; E = easy.

Chapter 3

Recovery, Training Intensities and Heart Rates

♦ More isn't better ♦

When training for a major competition or a series of major races, it is important to understand the aims of training. Large amounts of very intense training or high mileage training on consecutive days can be detrimental to performance if the body doesn't recover between workouts. This, as has been mentioned, can lead to overtraining and injury. It is important, therefore, that the training is balanced with adequate rest and recovery.

Balanced training ensures the body recovers after each workout. Only then will the body be able to adapt to a gradually increasing workload. High training volumes are only worthwhile if you can cope. Of course, as you become fitter, recovery periods shorten. But these periods remain as critical as the workouts themselves. Why? Because training, alone, does not improve performance. Rather: Training PLUS adequate recovery improves performance! This principle should guide your training at all times.

Recovery – 'The forgotten edge'

Too many endurance athletes get 'hung up' on mileage. They think that the more you train, the stronger, faster, and fitter you get. It is not as simple as that. If it were, there would be no need for books on training principles. The winners would simply be those who trained the most. Fortunately, endurance training is a lot more interesting than that. This does not mean, of course, that you can get away with a couple of hours of training a week if you want to be successful. If you want to run a marathon, or complete an Ironman, or finish a cycle tour, then you will have to complete a certain minimum volume of training to do so. When the 'more is better' mentality takes over, the aspect of training most neglected is *rest*. Without rest and recovery you will not improve. This is hard for many endurance athletes to accept (even after repeated bouts of injury, illness and poor performance).

One 'problem', of course, is that endurance athletes tend to have a very, very strong work ethic. They also seem to get an 'attack of the guilts' if they think they are taking it easy. These 'guilts' may reflect a lack of knowledge concerning training, and/or a lack of confidence in their programme.

The key to improvement is not how much training you can do, but *how much training you can recover from*. That is what you should be thinking about when planning your training. A one-hour session that you don't fully recover from before the next workout will mean part of that next workout has been wasted. This is because insufficient recovery means the body has not been able to fully adapt. So, remember, *rest* is training too. Get into it!

Recovery strategies to boost performance

Your training is limited by two factors: how much you can do, and how quickly you can recover. These factors are obviously related and are very important in physically intense and endurance sports. Here are some ways to help recovery.

Warm-downs

These are particularly important after intense workouts such as strength and speed training. Warm-downs elevate heart rate slightly, increasing the blood flow to muscles. This helps to flush by-products such as lactic acid out of the muscles, providing a faster recovery than if you just stop training or competing 'cold'. The length of the warm-down is determined by the intensity of the workout. The more intense the workout, the longer the warm-down (15 to 30 minutes is appropriate most of the time). Of course, for low-intensity workouts (easy runs/easy bikes), the beginning and end stages of the session are used as a warm-up and warm-down respectively; that is, you start off easy and you ease down towards the end of the workout.

Warming down after a race will certainly help ease post-race soreness and aid recovery. Of course, the temptation after a race is to stop dead. A good way to overcome this is to warm down with friends or opponents. It's a great time to find out what happened up front or behind you, and share in the black humour that athletes seem to enjoy after racing hard. Just make sure the warm-down is very easy!

Fluid replacement

This is essential! Excess fluid loss during training will reduce the quality of the workout and slow recovery. Even mild dehydration will take 24 to 36 hours to reverse, and will impair the next day's workout. Clear urine indicates you have rehydrated. Note, though, that if you are on multivitamins, your urine may not be clear even when you are rehydrated. It is essential (that word again) that you consume water before, during and after training and racing, or better still, a sports drink containing glucose polymers to replace energy as well (*see* chapter 12).

Nutrition

If you're training hard, you need to eat a balanced diet. This means ensuring your energy output needs (training) are matched by your energy input requirements (diet).

Finding the right dietary mix of carbohydrate, protein and fat is vital. If you are unsure whether your diet is meeting your needs adequately, consult a sports dietician. Generally, your diet should be high in carbohydrate (complex sugars in foods like bread, pasta, potatoes), and low in fat. Eating high carbohydrate food immediately after training (within one to two hours) aids recovery significantly. For more on nutrition *see* chapter 12.

Sleep

Different people need different amounts of sleep. But for the athlete in training, eight hours a night is probably a good target to aim for. Perhaps more importantly, a constant sleep pattern is essential for recovery.

Before competition, it is the previous three to five nights' sleep that count, not the night before – which is just as well as nerves can sometimes make it difficult to sleep soundly the night before a race. This problem can be compounded if you are sleeping away from home.

Alternative activities as active recovery

Doing things other than the sport you compete in can be a great way to stay active, recover from competition and maintain your enthusiasm. Golf and walking seem to be particular favourites. For a runner or cyclist, easy swimming might do the trick.

Massage

Massage is one of the most underrated ways to look after muscles and prevent injuries. It also helps improve performance by promoting faster recovery from workouts – cyclists in the Tour de France use their end-of-the-day massage to hasten recovery from each day's racing.

Massage increases blood flow to the muscles, promoting the faster removal of by-products. This improves flexibility by reducing the 'tightening up' experienced after training and racing.

Knots of scar tissue are also broken up by massage. These knots are sites of potential injury as they adhere to the muscle, preventing smooth contraction.

For most athletes, a massage every week or two is sufficient to keep the muscles in good working order. Make sure you find a masseur who suits your needs and who is experienced in dealing with sportspeople (your fellow athletes will be able to recommend someone).

Relaxation baths, spas, saunas

If used properly, both spas and saunas seem to speed recovery by promoting relaxation and passive blood flow to the muscles and removing by-products. Just don't stay in them too long (especially the day before a race) as they can lead to dehydration and tiredness. Alternatively, ice baths are found to be beneficial for some athletes.

If you are in a 'leg sport', such as running or cycling, just putting your legs in a spa may be as effective as completely soaking the body, and less likely to induce fatigue. Hot water bottles on specific areas of the body can also be beneficial.

♦ Overcompensation ♦

Overcompensation is the physiological reaction of your body to training. It is, in a sense, an overreaction by the body to the stress placed upon it through training. This overreaction (adaptation) enables the body to cope with greater and greater training loads. This leads to improvements in performance (*see* fig. 3.1). This theory, that work and rest determine performance, is the basis for the use of training cycles (*see* page 16).

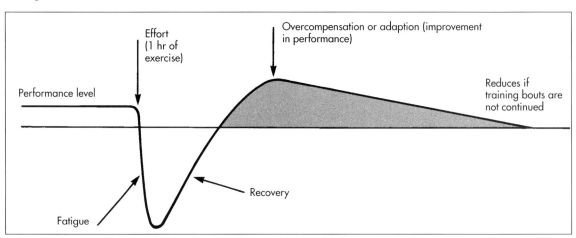

Figure 3.1 Cycle of compensation: regular alternation between exertion, fatigue, recuperation and overcompensation as the basis for training

Superovercompensation

Superovercompensation, apart from being the longest word in this book, is the same as over-compensation, only more so. Superover-compensation involves subjecting the athlete to greater training loads or stresses than is usual. This results in a 'superoverreaction' or 'overadaptation' to the training load. Super-overcompensation puts the athlete into a mildly overtrained state for a short time (a few days). As long as this period is only brief, adverse effects and overtraining can be avoided.

This technique seems to be most effective in sports where muscular stress is low, as in cycling and swimming. Runners need to be particularly careful when adopting super-overcompensation as a training technique because the risks of injury are high. Instead of running more, runners may choose to add cycling to their programme in order to create the superovercompensation effect.

Inexperienced athletes should not attempt superovercompensation as it is a physiologi-cally and psychologically severe form of training. Nor should superovercompensation be used more than once during a build-up. One bout of superovercompensation before tapering is most effective. Superover-compensation is most effective one to three weeks before a peak race. If done correctly it will produce a maximum peak above that of a traditional build-up (*see* fig 3.2).

Small bouts of overcompensation may work every third, fourth or fifth week immediately before an easy week. In terms of daily training this could look something like the following four-week schedule, which is illustrated in figure 3.2.

Weeks 1–3:

Mon	Tue	Wed	Thu	Fri	Sat	Sun
E	H	E	H	E	H	H

Week 4:

Mon	Tue	Wed	Thu	Fri	Sat	Sun
E	H	H	H	E	H	H

Then back to week 1 again. E = easy, H = hard.

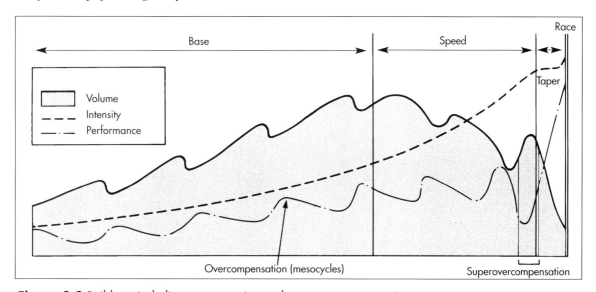

Figure 3.2 Build-up: including compensation and superovercompensation

◆ Training intensities ◆ and heart rates

When someone asks you, 'How much are you training?', they usually want to know how far or how often you train each week. Seldom does anyone ask, 'How hard are you training?' Yet understanding the 'hardness' or intensity of your training is the key to understanding how a progressive, balanced training programme is put together. While novice and elite athletes may be poles apart when it comes to how fast they train and race, the intensity (not speed) of the work each group does in each phase of their training is the same.

Training intensities have traditionally been categorised in many different ways. But they can easily be broken down into three basic types. Starting with the lowest intensity and moving up to the highest, these intensities are:

1 Low-intensity (which can include active recovery, long slow distance, and up-tempo training)

2 Submaximal intensity (anaerobic threshold training)
3 High-intensity (extensive and intensive sprints, and power training)

Low-intensity (LO) training is aerobic exercise (with oxygen) which can be performed for long periods of time. High-intensity (HI) training is anaerobic (without oxygen). High-intensity exercise (basically sprinting) can only be performed for brief periods before complete temporary fatigue occurs and you have to rest. Submaximal intensity (SM) training occurs at what some regard as the threshold or crossover between LO and HI training (*see* fig. 3.3).

Race pace (RP) training is a further intensity and fits into one of the three training types (LO, SM, HI), depending on the length of the race you are training for. This means RP will be slower (and less intense) if you are training for long races, such as a marathon, and faster (and more intense) if you are training for shorter races, for example a 10 km road run.

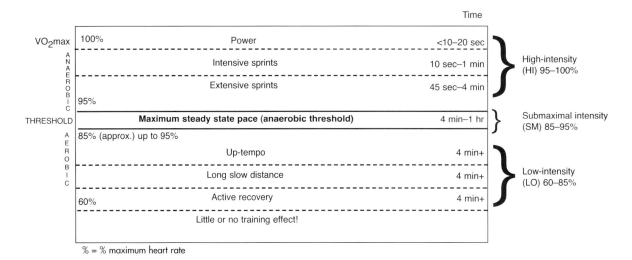

Figure 3.3 Training intensities

Before discussing training intensities in detail, we need to look at how training intensity and heart rate together form a powerful training tool.

Heart rate – the athlete's 'revs'

Heart rate gives you a constant indication of how hard you are working: the higher the rate, the harder the heart is working to supply enough oxygen to the working muscles. Indeed, your heart rate acts like a rev counter on a car, telling you at what rate your 'engine' is ticking over. From this you can decide whether to work harder (increase the revs) or ease off (decrease the revs). And just as rev counters have a 'red line' marking an excessively high rev level, you too can work out a 'red zone' that will guide your training and racing intensity. Many heart rate monitors have a function that allows you to set it to 'beep' at different rates. This means you don't have to keep looking at the monitor to see if you are in the right 'zone'.

Knowing your training heart rates is a simple yet sophisticated method of controlling training intensity so that you maximise your training time and effort. But before you can do this you need to know what you 'idle' at – your resting heart rate.

Calculating your resting heart rate

Endurance athletes tend not to take things lying down, but in the case of your resting heart rate, you can make an exception. By measuring your heart rate* each morning for a couple of weeks, you will be able to estab-

*Using a heart rate monitor is the best way to get your heart rate. However, it is possible to take your heart rate manually by placing your fingers (not thumb) on your wrist (palm side) at the base of the thumb. Count the number of pulses for fifteen seconds and then multiply by four. Alternatively, instead of using your wrist, you can place your fingers on your neck at the angle of your jaw.

lish your average resting heart rate. This is taken in bed, lying down, upon waking. If you wake up to an alarm, this can raise your heart rate slightly, so rest for two to three minutes before taking it. Make allowances if you have a busy day that day (anxiety), or if you need to urinate, as both may elevate heart rate slightly. The following is an example of resting heart rates during a week. The figures are the numbers of beats per minute (bpm).

Day	Mon	Tue	Wed	Thu	Fri	Sat	Sun
Heart rate	56	54	55	56	54	56	57

Total heart rates = 388, divided by seven days = 55.4. This gives you an average resting heart rate for the week of 55 bpm.

Calculating your maximum heart rate
Once you know your resting heart rate you will need to find out your maximum tested heart rate for each discipline you are training in: cycling, rowing, kayaking, running, swimming, and so on. These heart rates need to be worked out when you are not tired from training, so a couple of easy days before each test is necessary.

To find your maximum heart rate, warm up for ten to fifteen minutes. Once warmed up, work out as hard you can for four to eight minutes with the last one to two minutes at maximum effort until you 'blow'! (Sprinting up a hill is useful, but do not make it too steep or leg muscle fatigue may occur before you reach your maximum heart rate.) Do this for each discipline, but make sure you are fully recovered between tests (allow a few days), otherwise the tests won't be valid and you won't be able to calculate your correct training intensities. Your maximum heart rate is the highest reliable heart rate reached during testing. This is best worked out using a heart rate monitor, but you can work out your heart rate manually as long as you do it immediately after the test. A maximum heart rate test can be dangerous, so if you are in any doubt about whether you can physically cope with it, see your doctor.

The simplest way to work out maximum heart rate is to subtract your age from 220. Unfortunately, this not entirely accurate because of individual differences in heart size. Larger hearts beat fewer times per minute, so people with larger hearts will find it harder to reach their target heart rates using this calculation. This can result in overwork. Conversely, people with smaller hearts using the 220 minus age formula may find their target heart rates too easy to reach and therefore will not be working hard enough to meet their performance goals.

Karvonen heart rate calculation

By subtracting your resting heart rate from your maximum heart rate you can use the Karvonen formula to calculate your heart rates for various training intensities. These are usually expressed as a percentage.

For instance, submaximal (SM) intensity is considered to be an 85 to 95 per cent effort (0.85 to 0.95 for multiplication purposes). Thus, if your maximum heart rate (HR^{max}) is 196 and your resting heart rate (HR^{rest}) is 55, then your submaximal intensity range is worked out like this:

Karvonen Formula:

(HR^{max} - HR^{rest}) × % exercise intensity + HR^{rest}

HR^{max} 196 − HR^{rest} 55 = 141

141 × 0.85 (85%) = 120

120 + 55 (HR^{rest}) = 175

---

175 is therefore the low end of your submaximal range. Repeat the calculation using 95 per cent and you get 189. This gives you a submaximal heart rate intensity range of 175 to 189.

When you begin training at your submaximal intensity, you should start off at the lower end of the range, in this case 175 to 180. As training progresses and you get stronger, you will be able to train more often at the higher end of this range, e.g. 180 to 189.

Ideally, your HR^{max} and SM intensity pace (also known as anaerobic threshold or maximum steady state pace) should be worked out in a fitness testing laboratory. Mathematical estimates can be used, but these are not as accurate. Once you have got your HR^{max} and SM paces, you are then able to work out your heart rate ranges for the different training intensities, which are described in detail later in this chapter (*see* appendix 1). In essence, these ranges tell you how hard or easy to train in each phase of training. There is more on this in the sport-specific section later in this chapter.

Heart rates and what they mean

Heart rates at rest

1 A normal resting heart rate means you are fully rested and not fatigued.

2 An elevated heart rate, for example 10 per cent above normal, indicates fatigue and/or stress (e.g. 55+ for an athlete with a normal heart rate of 50). If it is only marginally elevated, continue to train and assess fatigue once training. Reduce training volume/intensity if required. If heart rate is only mildly elevated it is sometimes good to wait: you may be recovered and ready to train by the afternoon.

Unfortunately, resting heart rate is not foolproof when it comes to indicating your reaction to training stress. It can remain low even when you are tired (particularly in very over-trained athletes). Always subjectively monitor how you feel during training and when resting. If you feel tired, you probably are. Nevertheless, it is good to monitor heart rate during training. The orthostatic heart rate check (*see* appendix 5) may help.

Heart rates during training

Using a combination of resting heart rate, training heart rates and training speed you will be better able to check on your reaction to training.

1 Resting heart rate normal, training heart rate normal, training speed normal. This indicates training and recovery are well balanced.
Message: Everything's fine.

2 Resting heart rate normal, training heart rate elevated above predicted level, training speed above normal. This is particularly likely during base training and indicates you are training too hard.
Message: Slow down!

3 Resting heart rate normal, predicted training heart rate cannot be reached, training speed can't be reached. This indicates fatigue in major muscle groups, such as 'dead legs' in cycling; your legs are so tired that they are not able to take you to the speed/intensity that you are capable of in training when 'fresh'.
Message: Abandon programme for the day and have an easy day, e.g. 'spinning' in cycling, or go home and have a day off. This occurs more often when you are doing speed-work, like intervals or sprints.

4 Resting heart rate elevated, training heart rate elevated, training speed below normal. This indicates serious tiredness.
Message: Have a day off, you may be ill!

5 Resting heart rate normal, training heart rate goes from normal to elevated considerably above normal while training or racing, training speed constant or begins to drop.
Message: You may be dehydrated. Be very careful.

6 Resting heart rate normal, training heart rate above normal, training speed below normal.
Message: You are overtired.

7 Resting heart rate normal, training heart rate normal, training speed below normal.
Message: You are tired or you have 'dead legs'.

8 Resting heart rate above normal, training heart rate normal, training speed normal.
Message: You may be experiencing mild mental stress/anxiety. Be very careful.

9 Resting heart rate normal, training heart rate begins to drop and cannot be held in a long workout, training speed drops.
Message: You may have 'hit the wall', or 'bonked'.

10 Resting heart rate normal, training heart rate slow to drop after an effort (e.g. interval) or after a workout, training speed normal or marginally below normal.
Message: You are probably fatigued or over-trained.

Heart rates during racing

Heart rate monitors can be very good for working out or adjusting your race strategy. (Racing heart rates tend to be 5 to 10 bpm higher than in training, because of race hype.)

1 Heart rate drops significantly during the race. This indicates you:
• started too fast;
• had an inadequate taper (legs too tired to hold pace for duration of race);
• did not do enough base distance work (specific to race);

- were overtrained;
- 'hit the wall', 'bonked', legs 'blew up' in longer races.

2 Heart rate increases slightly during the race. This indicates you:
- started too slow;
- had an ineffective warm-up;
- did not do enough speedwork (specific to race).

3 Heart rate increases significantly during race. This indicates you:
- are dehydrated (drink lots of water and check for other signs of dehydration).

4 Heart rate starts and remains too high for the duration of the race. This indicates you:
- are too tired;
- are overtrained;
- are ill.

5 Heart rate 'jumps', or fluctuates greatly (150 to 220 bpm), in the space of a few beats:
- check transmitter, battery;
- wet your skin and the electrodes more;
- check signals aren't being affected by someone else's monitor or overhead power lines;
- accept it could be a heart abnormality. *Stop exercising and see a doctor as soon as possible.*

6 Heart rate remains constant at usual race pace level. This indicates you:
- had good race preparation and good race pace.

Things to know about heart rate monitors

Your heart rate monitor is a tool not a dictator.

1 You can't train at a specific heart rate constantly; it is almost impossible. Terrain, fatigue and heat affect heart rate significantly. Use the heart rate range as a guide. (Don't crawl up a hill just because your heart rate monitor tells you to.)

2 Heart rates take time to move into your training range (up to 5 minutes), particularly if training is quite intense.

3 Heart rates can drop significantly from the start of training as you become fitter. Reassess regularly.

4 Heart rates will differ between different sports – heart rates for running are higher than for cycling, and cycling is higher than swimming.

5 Heart rates are generally higher during racing. 'Race hype' artificially elevates the heart rate by 5 to 10 beats.

♦ Types of training intensities ♦

As described earlier, training intensities are divided into three types: low, submaximal and high. First let's take a look at the least intense of these, low-intensity.

Low-intensity (LO) training – aerobic (approximately 60 to 85 per cent training range)

LO training gives you basic aerobic and muscular conditioning and it will improve your ability to metabolise (use) fat as an energy source. LO training can also be used to aid recovery. LO training can be broken down into three types. These too have an order of intensity:

1 Active recovery
2 Long slow distance
3 Up-tempo

Active recovery occurs at the easy end of the LO training range, while up-tempo occurs just below submaximal intensity (SM) training. LO training is performed at approximately 60 to 85 per cent of your HR^{max}. The Karvonen method of calculating your LO training heart rate range therefore goes like this:

For 60%: 196 (HR^{max}) − 55 (HR^{rest}) × 60% (0.6)
  + 55 (HR^{rest}) = 140
For 85%: 196 − 55 × 85% (0.85) + 55 = 175

This gives you an LO training heart rate range of 140 to 175.

Most athletes will work at the middle to low end of this range (active recovery, long slow distance) most of the time until up-tempo training begins in preparation for speedwork. If you do not have access to a heart rate monitor or you don't wish to use heart rates as a guide to training intensity, LO pace can be described as an easy to medium effort (if you can't comfortably hold a conversation at this pace, i.e. you're gasping, then you're going too fast!).

Active recovery (up to approximately 60 per cent training range)

Active recovery (AR) is at the lowest end of the training heart rate range. It is only used in training to assist recovery, for example by removing by-products from the muscles, or when you feel tired. Light activity is generally better for recovery than no activity at all. AR should be used on those days when you feel too tired to do your intended workout. But if after 10 to 15 minutes of training you still feel tired, go home and rest! Further training on that day will do more harm than good. If you feel you need a day off altogether – take it (and forget about training until tomorrow).

Long slow distance (LSD) (approximately 60 to 75 per cent training range)

Most of your mileage work will consist of LSD, especially during base training. This is not a very specific intensity, just an easy conversation pace. The pace will improve as you get fitter. Most athletes need to remember the 'slow' part of long slow distance.

Up-tempo (UT) training (approximately 75 to 85 per cent training range)

This is an intermediate intensity that bridges the gap between LO and higher intensity training. It is used late in the base training phase to help get you ready for speedwork.

Up-tempo training can be performed continuously or in intervals. The intervals will progress from long and easy to short and fast as your fitness improves. It needs to be stressed that up-tempo intervals are much longer than the type used in submaximal/high-intensity training. An up-tempo interval can be 15 to 30 minutes long (with long rests) at the start of up-tempo training. This is because the intensity is relatively low. Two to three up-tempo intervals may be done in one workout towards the end of base training, or at the start of speedwork, depending on your race distance (shorter races have up-tempo at the end of base; longer races at the start of speedwork). The days on which you do up-tempo intervals should correspond to the days on which you intend to do your speedwork, once the speedwork phase is begun.

As you adjust to the small increase in pace that up-tempo training involves (compared to LSD), intervals will become shorter and more intense, particularly as you approach the end of base work. Once speedwork begins, up-tempo intervals are replaced by higher intensity intervals. The length of the intervals will then gradually be increased again. In many cases, particularly for races that are shorter than two to three hours, up-tempo training becomes redundant once speedwork begins (*see* page 60 for more information on interval training for speedwork).

The effects of low-intensity training

Base training improves basic aerobic and muscular conditioning (including muscular endurance), speeds recovery and increases your tolerance to training. These training adaptations enable you to cope with the speedwork to come (and they improve your hill climbing ability if you have trained on the hills – good for cycling and running, not so relevant for kayaking!). Low-intensity training also improves your ability to metabolise fat as a source of energy. This means you are better able to race over long distances with less likelihood of 'bonking' on the bike or 'hitting the wall' on the run. And that's got to be good for an endurance athlete!

Submaximal intensity (SM) training – maximum steady state/anaerobic threshold (approximately 85 to 95 per cent training range)

SM training raises your maximum steady state pace (often referred to as 'anaerobic threshold' pace) and increases overall endurance or fitness. SM training includes intervals, time trials and, in most endurance sports, low-key races. SM training forms a vital part of any training programme because it plays such a big part in improving your race pace.

These days, anaerobic threshold is a term frowned upon by some sports scientists. This is because there is no absolute threshold but rather a 'grey area' where your body moves from functioning at a mainly aerobic level (where most of your energy needs are being met by oxygen) to mainly functioning at an anaerobic level (you can't take in enough oxygen to sustain your current level of exercise intensity). Therefore, the term 'submaximal intensity' is used to describe

training that corresponds with that 'grey area'. SM training is usually about 85 to 95 per cent of HR^{max}, although these percentages vary a lot depending on your conditioning and the phase of training you are in. They can only be determined effectively through proper fitness testing (*see* page 89).

SM training should be performed at or slightly below the maximum steady state level; i.e. in the example calculated on page 28, this would be 175 to 189. If you have not been tested in an exercise laboratory, use the Karvonen formula and progressively increase intensity (and therefore heart rate) as you get fitter. That is, start at 85 per cent of HR^{max}, and using a five to ten beat range only, progress gradually to 95 per cent. In simple terms, SM training pace is medium to hard. You should find it difficult to converse at this pace.

The effects of submaximal intensity training

Various types of SM training will improve steady state racing speed and improve muscle endurance. Time trials and low-key races will help you prepare physiologically, mentally and technically for racing. The mental aspect is particularly important because you need to get used to coping with race intensity (and the nervous tension that often precedes it!).

As time trials are hard work, you should only do them over distances that are about 33 to 50 per cent of race distance (for sub-three hour races). For a 10 km race, for instance, 5 km time trials are sufficiently long for training purposes. For triathlons with a 40 km cycle, 20 km time trials are appropriate. Even then, they will be very tiring and may hinder training for the rest of the week (*see* page 63 for more information on time trials for speedwork).

Intervals are an alternative form of SM training (*see* page 60). These can be differentiated from high-intensity intervals by the fact that they are over four minutes in duration.

As you get fitter, the workload (number and length of efforts) will increase and the rests will get shorter until you are performing at a high steady state pace for a long time with little rest. At this point you are virtually doing a time trial.

For endurance sports, intervals should be longer than four minutes to ensure you are exercising at submaximal intensity – less than four minutes and there is a danger the exercise intensity will be too high (anaerobic). Submaximal training is particularly useful for cycling (time trial events and long break-aways), mountain biking, sprint and standard distance triathlon, running, duathlons, multi-sport and rowing racing. Submaximal intensity training is the cornerstone of your racing speed.

High-intensity (HI) training – anaerobic (approximately 95 to 100 per cent training range)

HI training bears some similarity to SM training, but it also improves your ability to cope with sprinting (acceleration, top speed and speed endurance), sprint recovery (oxygen debt), and high levels of exertion. High-intensity training can be broken down into sprinting (extensive and intensive) and power (acceleration). The Karvonen heart rate calculation for HI training goes like this:

$$196 \ (HR^{max}) - 55 \ (HR^{rest}) \times 0.95 \ (95\%) + 55$$
$$= 188 +$$

To exercise at 95 per cent plus of your HR^{max} means sprinting. It is the only time in training you should let all the brakes off and go for it. To some extent, it is hard to define and monitor exact heart rate levels at this intensity. If using a heart rate monitor, it is assumed that heart rates must be above 95 per cent HR^{max}

to have the desired effect. But it is better to use the duration of the sprint to control intensity. Why? Because in very short sprints your heart rate will not reach a constant, meaningful level. HI training pace can be described as hard to very hard. You should not be able to talk. Actually, even thinking should be difficult!

What makes up high-intensity (HI) training?

1 Extensive (EX) sprints (90 to 95 per cent effort/45 sec to 4 min duration): These are long sprints and are used to condition your body to extended sprinting (speed endurance). Extensive sprints are very good for cycle racing, any multisport races that involve some aspect of cycle racing in a bunch (peloton), mountain bike starts, distance running and rowing.

2 Intensive (IN) sprints (100 per cent effort/10 sec to 1 min duration): These are short sprints and are used to improve your top speed and speed endurance. This is effective for cycle racing, mountain bike starts and, to some extent, rowing. Intensive sprints are not as effective for the other endurance sports dealt with in this book, although both intensive and extensive sprints may, when done at the right phase of your training programme, improve leg speed.

3 Power (PW) sprints (100 per cent effort/less than 10 to 20 sec duration): This is used to develop explosive ability (efforts generally lasting less than 10 seconds) and is useful for cycling (to improve the 'jump' or acceleration). Power can also be effective for rowing. It is of little benefit to the other sports dealt with in this book.

High-intensity training improves your recovery from oxygen debt and your ability to sustain pace in oxygen debt (lactate tolerance). It is good for fast starts and finishes, it is also very good in cycling for pushing up and over hills, breakaways, sprint primes, sprint finishes and starts, and for bridging gaps between 'bunches'. Acceleration, top speed and speed endurance can be developed separately or in combination, generally progressing from EX to IN and finally to PW. Overspeed (an aspect of HI: lighter load and a muscle contraction slightly higher than race pace) can also be used for cycling. High-intensity training levels need to be manipulated precisely at the right time to improve racing ability. Too much speedwork over-trains; too little speedwork undertrains (*see* page 63 for more information on sprints for speedwork).

Race pace (RP) training

Race pace training simulates race conditions and intensities. It conditions the body physically and mentally to tolerate race pace. Which training intensity it fits into depends on general race pace. RP training is determined by your racing distance. The longer the race, the lower your RP. It is also determined by your fitness and ability. For this reason, it is difficult to calculate RP accurately. Nevertheless, it can be defined simply as this: race pace is the pace you feel you can maintain for the entire race.

RP can best be gauged by using a heart rate monitor with memory to record racing heart rates. This gives a clear indication of this training intensity. But note, it must be checked within four to six weeks of a major race. Although RP training should be done at this established level, pushing too hard (intensity too high) in this type of training will not improve racing ability. The transition from submaximal training to race pace training is made during the speedwork period. A combination of SM training and RP training should be used only in the last few weeks before

peaking. In preparing for longer races (over three hours), a slightly different approach is used as SM training is used relatively less than RP training. RP training is also initiated before SM training.

♦ Sport-specific heart ♦ rate monitor use

Time trial

The best way to race any form of time trial distance event is to maintain an even pace or effort. This enables you to use your energy resource in the most 'economic' way possible. Changes of pace or effort are expensive and drain your 'energy bank account' quickly. The even pace, of course, should be the fastest pace you can sustain for the entire race or time trial. This pace, for example, may be for a race of one hour at your submaximal (SM) or anaerobic threshold pace.

As described previously, your submaximal pace will have a corresponding heart rate (85 to 95 per cent of HR^{max}). Once you know this heart rate you can use it to help keep your effort strong and steady for an entire race or time trial. This is particularly useful when racing over hills or in windy conditions, as both situations contribute to heart rate fluctuations. It is worth remembering also that different disciplines produce different heart rates at similar intensities.

To find your target racing heart rates (as opposed to your SM training heart rates) for each discipline, you should do a time trial at a pace you think you could sustain for the race distance. Time trials are 33 to 50 per cent of race distance for sub-three-hour races, and 50 to 75 per cent for races over three hours. For example, time trials should be 2 to 3 hours for a 4 hour plus race; 45 to 60 minutes for a 1.5 to 2.0 hour race; and 15 to 30 minutes for a 30 minute to 1 hour race. If possible, try to do the time trial over a course similar to the one you will be racing over.

These time trials should be done every two to four weeks during speedwork, and they are substituted for another speed session (they're not an extra one!). Because of the lack of race hype, your heart rate in these time trials may be 5 to 10 beats lower than actual race pace intensity. If this is the case, the only way to obtain racing heart rates will be by racing.

If you are racing a lot, use the races as time trials. These time trials will give you a starting heart rate, for example 160 to 165. If you found this too comfortable, then next time out increase it by 5 beats. Keep increasing the heart rate until you can't hold it for the entire time trial. When this happens, drop back to the previous heart rate and retest. This will probably be your current racing heart rate. This method is especially good for working out the heart rate for long races. For shorter races, low-key races can be used instead of time trials. Be careful, though, that other training factors, such as tiredness or speed-work, are not affecting time trial results (*see* page 63 for details on time trials and speed training).

Cycling – heart rate/cadence link
When on the bike it is useful to link heart rate to cadence (how fast you're pedalling). This allows you to optimise gear changes as well as pace. Optimal time trial cadences are around 85 to 95 revs per minute (rpm).

Example of the heart rate/cadence link
Optimal race pace heart rate (tested) = 170 to 175
Optimal cadence = 85 to 95

Heart rate	Cadence	Analysis
172	87	Excellent. Hold effort.
180	89	Heart rate too high; you are going too hard. Change to easier gear.
140	92	Heart rate too low; too easy. Change to a harder gear.

Note: You will need to watch heart rate and cadence constantly as both change as the course changes and you become fatigued.

Using a heart rate to monitor effort on the bike is particularly useful for inexperienced cyclists, though notable improvements in performance have also been achieved by experienced riders. Inexperienced cyclists often push too big a gear, causing severe leg fatigue. End result? They end up 'legless' late in the race. This is because the lower the cadence (big gears), the more muscular the effort is. The higher the cadence (small gears), the more cardiovascular the effort is.

The optimal cadence, of course, lies some-where in the middle; for example 90 to 110 rpm for a road race, 85 to 95 rpm for a time trial. It is important for triathletes and duath-letes to understand this because not only will monitoring heart rate on the bike help your bike time, but the less leg fatigue you can incur on the bike the better you will go in the run.

Heart rate can also be used to check whether you have warmed up properly, and on the bike it can measure bike/rider effi-ciency, aero position, biomechanical variables, bike set-up, and the like, although each test should be done in identical conditions and at race pace. Heart rate can also be productively used in combination with new cycle comput-ers that measure not only speed but also work (watts).

Cycling – road race

Aside from being used to maintain your SM pace (and an even effort), heart rate monitoring can be used to find out where in the bunch (peloton) you travel most easily. Heart rate can also be used to help you decide when to chase (heart rate low beforehand) and when not to chase (heart rate high beforehand). A low heart rate while in the bunch indicates you are fresh and strong and ready to attack. If heart rate has been high for some time, it is best to relax in the bunch until you recover. Finally, don't become a slave to heart rate, especially towards the end of races. Sometimes you've just got to go for it.

Cycling – stage race

In addition to the guidelines outlined above for road races, heart rates can also be used to monitor energy levels from day to day. For instance, if rest and exercise heart rate is as predicted or below on a particular day, the stage suits your strengths, and your legs feel fine, this might be the day to attack. If, on the other hand, your heart rate is high, then it would probably pay to sit in the bunch and wait for another day. Resting heart rates can also be taken each morning to see how well you've recovered from the day before (*see* previous time trial and cycling sections).

Multisport

The important consideration here is that each discipline will have a different racing heart rate, with a significant difference between upper and lower body exercises (*see* time trial section above).

Mountain biking

Mountain biking is like cycle time trials, so a constant heart rate and intensity is desirable once the start is over and your position is established (*see* time trial section above). As it is difficult to look at your monitor when mountain biking, make sure you get one that can be set to beep at different levels.

Running

Maintaining a constant pace is crucial when running. A heart rate monitor provides constant feedback on effort, as opposed to 'splits' which are often too infrequent to help with pace judgement.

Rowing

The best way to use a heart rate monitor in rowing is to strap it to the stroke in successive races. You can only use one monitor in the boat at a time as they transmit on the same frequency. The stroke is the best person to wear it as he/she determines pace. Use the memory mode to collect a number of time trial/racing heart rates two to three weeks before the major race, then assess what the race pace heart rates are for each 500 metres and work out the crew's race pace.

Generally in rowing, pace is constant, although the first and last 500 metres are marginally faster. Once race pace is known, the coxswain can indicate to the stroke whether to work harder or 'back off' to achieve optimal pace. However, it shouldn't be forgotten that you are racing and sometimes race strategy will override heart rate considerations.

Each rower's heart rate can also be assessed before the start of speedwork so that appropriate training intensities can be worked out (each rower will probably have a different racing heart rate). Heart rates could also be used to check rowing efficiency, for example inboard versus outboard ratio on oar, racing stroke rate. The aim, of course, is to achieve the fastest boat speed at the lowest heart rate.

Chapter 4

Training Subphases

♦ The training phases ♦

As discussed previously, training for endurance sports can essentially be broken down into two phases – the base and speed phases. But that doesn't just mean slow and fast! Indeed, there are a number of training factors that must be addressed under the headings of base and speed. But before we look at what these factors are, and how they form the 'subphases' of training, let's briefly revisit the base and speed phases.

Base – endurance/technique (Base 1)
  – strength endurance (Base 2)
Speed – speed

The base phase

The base phase is primarily designed to build basic sport-specific 'fitness'. It does this by increasing your tolerance *to* training, and by promoting faster recovery *from* training.

Base 1

Base training initially focuses on technique and endurance. This first period of the base phase is called Base 1. Base 1 is designed to get you conditioned to training. It provides basic fitness and gives you time to address any weaknesses, physical and technical, you may have. Examples of Base 1 training are:

- Cycling – pedalling easily for a long ride
- Rowing – rowing with half/three-quarter pressure on the blades
- Running – easy long runs

Essentially, Base 1 allows you to complete the race distance (or, for longer races, get close to completing).

Base 2

After Base 1 comes Base 2 – strength endurance training. This period of base training gives you the ability to apply more 'grunt' (strength, power, force) as you complete the race distance. Examples of Base 2 training are:

- Cycling – riding in a bigger gear (low cadence; on hills and flat ground)
- Rowing – rowing with some form of drag (e.g. bungy, rope tow)
- Running – long strides uphill, uphill bounding and stride outs

Strength endurance training involves the application of more and more muscular effort to training, through to the point where speed begins to gradually increase in speedwork.

Overall, the main purpose of the base phase is to allow you to do effective speedwork or, more accurately, race-specific conditioning, later on.

The speed phase

The human body responds to training stress by *adapting specifically* to that training stress. In order to prepare for the stress of racing, therefore, speedwork needs to more and more closely resemble racing intensities and conditions. Consequently, speed training generally follows this order:

- Up-tempo training (occurs at the end of base or start of speed training depending on the race length)
- Anaerobic threshold/maximum steady state training
- Long sprints (if required)
- Short sprints, power, and overspeed (in that order if these types of training are required)

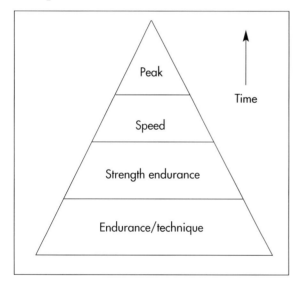

Figure 4.1 Training progression

To summarise: during the base and speed phases, training moves from endurance/technique to strength endurance to speed to peak (*see* fig. 4.1).

Now, let's look at the 'subphases' of training.

♦ The training subphases ♦

The nine training subphases are shown in Figure 4.2 below. Note that there is a progression from endurance/technique training, through to sport-specific strength endurance training, through to speed training. In other words, your training moves from less race-specific training to more race-specific training as your goal race approaches.

Subphase		Period/Phase
1	Preparation (easy)	Endurance/technique (Base 1)
2	Load	Strength endurance (Base 2)
3	High Load	
4	Load/Speed	
5	Low speed	Speed
6	High speed	
7	Sprints (if required)	
8	Power (if required)	
9	Overspeed (if required)	

Figure 4.2 Training subphases in relation to the main training phases of base (Base 1 and Base 2) and speed

We can then apply these subphase requirements to specific sports and training programmes. Figure 4.3 (opposite) illustrates the subphases for individual sports and events and how they relate to the two main phases, base and speed, of an endurance training programme.

Each of the nine subphases will now be described based on the graph illustrated in figure 4.3. The descriptions include sport-specific guidelines and examples of training weeks. The workout themes used in the training weeks are: (H) = hills; (S) = speed; (L) = long; (ML) = medium long; (S/H) = speed or hills; E = easy.

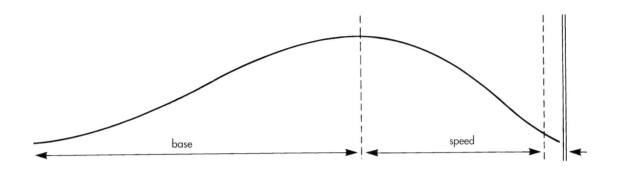

Subphase	1 easy	2 load	3 high load	4 load/speed	5 low speed	6 high speed	7 sprints	8 power	9 over- speed
Triathlon	easy	hills/ pull buoy	hills, big gear hills, long stride paddles/band	flat, big gear stride outs (bound) pull buoys	up-tempo	anaerobic threshold			
Duathlon	easy	hills	hills, big gear hills, long stride	flat, big gear stride outs (bound)	up-tempo	anerobic threshold			
Multisport	easy	hills/ bungy	hills, big gear hills, long stride bungy/rope tow	flat, big gear stride outs (bound) bungy	up-tempo	anerobic threshold			
Running	easy	hills	hills, long stride	stride outs (bound)	up-tempo	anaerobic threshold	extensive sprints		
Mountain biking	easy	hills	hills, big gear	flat, big gear	up-tempo	anaerobic threshold	extensive sprints		
Rowing	easy	bungy	bungy/ rope tow	bungy	up-tempo	anaerobic threshold	sprints	power	
Road cycling	easy	hills	hills, big gear	flat, big gear	up-tempo	anaerobic threshold	sprints	power	over- speed

Note: The subphases for triathlon, duathlon and multisport include the requirements for cycling, running, swimming and kayaking as applicable. The low speed subphase (5) and up-tempo training may occur at the end of base or at the start of speed training, depending on the race length (*see* pages 51–52).

Figure 4.3 Explanation of subphases

BASE PHASE

All heart rates in the base phase are at long slow distance rates (60 to 75 per cent HR^{max}) unless otherwise specified.

Period: Endurance/technique (Base 1)

Subphase 1: Preparation (Easy)

Preparation involves easy conditioning and occurs as you start back into a more structured training programme after your off-season. Preparation gets the body ready for what lies ahead. The preparation subphase is also a good time to look at problems (e.g. flexibility, strength imbalances, etc.) and continue work on rehabilitation if needed. Depending on your background and the amount of training done in the off-season you might be able to skip the preparation subphase. Alternatively, it could take many weeks if problems need to be resolved. In particular, technique should be emphasised at this time, especially for running, cycling, swimming, rowing, and kayaking. Preparation occurs at the start of Base 1 and can last zero to eight weeks (generally two to four).

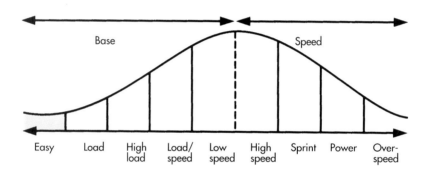

Specifics: Light/easy conditioning in all sports

Effort: Easy conversation pace (50–60% effort)

Sports
Swim: Easy/technique
Bike: Easy/small gears. Cadence 85–95 rpm if time trial or Tri/Du/mountain biking; 95–105 rpm for road cycling
Run: Easy
Kayak: Easy
Row: Easy (½ pressure, low stroke rate: 18–22 strokes per minute)

Training weeks

Triathlon/duathlon/multisport

M	T	W	T	F	S	S
S/K (H)		S/K (S)		DAY OFF	S/K (L)	
	B (S)		B (H)			B (L)
R (H)		R (L)			R (S)	

Cycling/mountain biking/running/rowing

M	T	W	T	F	S	S
E	S/H	E	ML	DAY OFF	S/H	L

For **bold** workouts, use the form of training specified for each sport.

Period: Strength endurance (Base 2)

Subphase 2: Load

Load represents the beginning of strength endurance, or what a lot of endurance athletes call 'strength training'. After the preparation phase you should be conditioned enough to benefit from an increase in training effort. This increase in effort can be undertaken with a reduced risk of injury thanks to the conditioning work already done.

Running and cycling
In running and cycling, hill training is used to build strength (more accurately, strength endurance). Hill training progresses from more moderate, shorter climbs, to longer, steeper, multiple climbs.

Swimming
Pull buoys are used for periods in the pool (200–2000 m) and then progresses to paddles (200–500 m).

Kayaking and rowing
Bungy cords attached to the hull are used to create drag. This progresses from longer periods of low drag, to shorter periods of high drag. This occurs over 1–6 reps of 10–40 minutes.

Load would progressively occur in training from one to two times per week in early Base 2. The load subphase could last from two to eight weeks (generally four).

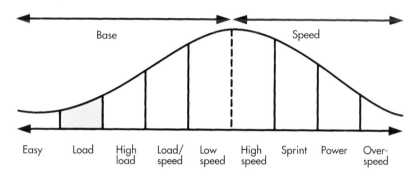

Easy	Load	High load	Load/ speed	Low speed	High speed	Sprint	Power	Over- speed

Base ⟷ Speed

Specifics: Strength endurance training

Effort: Generally easy conversation pace (60–70% effort); slightly higher under load (75–85%, but no higher)

Sports
  Swim: Pull buoy to paddles
  Bike: Hills (easy gears); small to big hills
  Run: Hills; small to big hills
  Kayak/Row: Bungy drag

The **bold** workouts are the training sessions where load would be applied. The 1 and 2 show where load would be emphasised first and second.

Training weeks						
Triathlon/duathlon/multisport						
M	T	W	T	F	S	S
S/K1 (H)		**S/K2** (S)		DAY OFF	S/K (L)	
	B2 (S)		**B1** (H)			B (L)
R1 (H)		R (L)			**R2** (S)	
Cycling/mountain biking/running/rowing						
M	T	W	T	F	S	S
E	**S/H1**	E	ML	DAY OFF	**S/H2**	L

Period: Strength/endurance (Base 2)

Subphase 3: High load

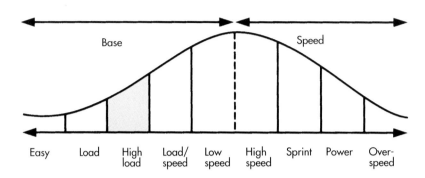

| Easy | Load | High load | Load/speed | Low speed | High speed | Sprint | Power | Over-speed |

High load is a further extension of strength endurance training. As you become conditioned to load training, the load is then increased further.

Cycling

Big gear hill training involves training on hills in gears 1–5 cogs higher (approximation based on conditioning/training history) than you would normally climb in. Pedal cadence is low (30–50 rpm). The aim is not to work too hard but to 'turn over' a large gear – the focus is on the legs not the lungs. If you have never done this before, be very careful, as it is easy to injure your knees. You should warm up at the start of your ride and do a further warm-up on some hills before progressing into the big gear training. In cold conditions keep your knees warm and stop if your knees are even slightly irritated. Move from 1–2 cogs above normal to higher loads. Between hills, normal gears are used to recover. Do from 1–12 reps on the hills.

'Pure strength' training may also be used to improve acceleration for cycle racing. From a stationary start at the bottom of a hill in the biggest gear you have, cycle 15–30 pedal revo- lutions up a hill until you almost stall. Then turn and roll back down the hill. This can be performed 2–6 times, but be very careful as this exercise can injure your knees. To recover between reps, ride around in easy gears for 5–10 minutes. Athletes under 16 years of age should not attempt high load or load/speed training (subphase 4) as this could cause long-term injury. If your back or knees are predis-posed to injury do not do high load or load/speed training, or at least do them care-fully. If your back or knees become irritated, stop training and see your doctor.

Running

Running training includes extended strides up hills to further develop strength. Use a long stride length and low stride rate to avoid making it too aerobic (keep the focus on the legs not the lungs). Do 1–12 reps of 200–400 m on the hills. Bounding uphill may also be used for shorter events (<10 km).

Swimming

Move from paddles (200–500 m) to band (100–400 m), depending on your training background.

Kayaking/Rowing

There is now an emphasis on greater drag using bungies or other forms of drag (e.g. rowers in a coxed four may do pair rowing while the other two rowers don't row; or rope tow for a single sculler). Bungy/pair rowing, 1–6 reps for 10–40 minutes; rope tow, 1–6 reps of 5 minutes.

High load training would occur one to two times per week over two to eight weeks (generally four).

Specifics: High strength endurance

Effort: Easy conversation pace (60–75% effort; during high load efforts, 75–85% effort)

Sports
  Swim: Paddles to band. Paddles 200–500 m; band 100–400 m
  Bike: Hills, big gears (1–5 cogs higher than usual; 30–50 rpm, 80% seated and 20% standing)
  Run: Long strides uphill (low stride rate) Bounding uphill, short races
  Kayak/Row: Low drag to high drag (bungy/rope tow) Bungy 1–6 × 10–40 min; rope tow 1–6 × 5 min

---

Training weeks						
Triathlon/duathlon/multisport						
M	T	W	T	F	S	S
S/K1 (H)		**S/K2** (S)		DAY OFF	S/K (L)	
	B2 (S)		**B1** (H)			B (L)
R1 (H)		R (L)			**R2** (S)	
Cycling/mountain biking/running/rowing						
M	T	W	T	F	S	S
E	**S/H1**	E	ML	DAY OFF	**S/H2**	L

The **bold** workouts are the training sessions where high load training would be applied. The 1 and 2 show where high load is emphasised first and second.

Period: Strength/endurance (Base 2)

Subphase 4: Load/speed

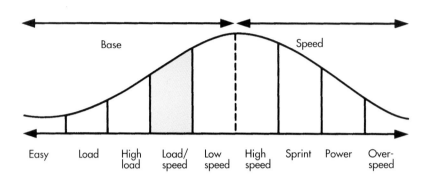

Load/speed is a transitional type of training. It ties strength endurance training to speed training. So far you have conditioned yourself through endurance/technique training, strength endurance training, load and high load. But you can't just go from high load–low speed to high speed. So load/speed is used to begin speedwork while maintaining an aspect of strength. This allows a gradual introduction to speed (your body hates sudden changes!). It also allows strength to be applied to speed.

Cycling
Load/speed in cycling is similar to high load except that training is carried out on the flat in a big gear. Long intervals of 10–20 km (up to 100 km in a week) are often used. The focus should still be on the legs not the lungs. Therefore, cadence is generally lower than for racing (50–70 rpm). Once again, watch your knees.

Running
Previous training is maintained but stride outs are now incorporated (long strides over 200–300 m on the flat).

Swimming
Swimming would move back to pull buoys with slightly more speed.

Kayaking/Rowing
The drag (bungy) is reduced and speed continues to be increased.

Load/speed training would occur one to two times per week over two to eight weeks (generally three to four). Load/speed is emphasised at the end of Base 2.

Specifics: Strength endurance moving to speed endurance

Effort: Easy conversation pace (60–75% effort)

Sports
  Swim: Band to pull buoy (as for the previous subphase)
  Bike: On flat, big gear (big chain ring, e.g. 52 × 16), 50–70 rpm
  Run: Stride outs
  Kayak/Row: Drag is reduced and speed is increased (as before)

Training weeks						
Triathlon/duathlon/multisport						
M	**T**	**W**	**T**	**F**	**S**	**S**
S/K (H)		S/K (S)		DAY OFF	S/K (L)	
	B (S)		B (H)			B (L)
R (H)		R (L)			R (S)	
Cycling/mountain biking/running/rowing						
M	**T**	**W**	**T**	**F**	**S**	**S**
E	**S/H**	E	ML	DAY OFF	**S/H**	L

The bold workouts are the training sessions where load/speed training would be applied.

SPEED PHASE

Once base training is completed, you are ready for the speed phase. Now the real work starts. You can begin to increase the tempo of your training. Everything up until now has been important, but the final weeks of the speed phase 'make or break' your chances of a top performance.

The following subphases are progressively combined into one to three speed sessions per week (1 = novice, 3 = elite) over the last four to eight weeks of the speed phase.

Sometimes racing over shorter distances is a better (more specific) form of speed training and can be substituted for a speed session. But remember: a race does not act as an extra speed session. Speedwork is very intense and demanding. Too much speedwork can quickly overfatigue you and destroy your build-up. Therefore, be careful. There is a fine line between too much and too little speedwork. As a rule of thumb, 10 per cent of your training in your biggest speedwork week can be at anaerobic threshold intensity or higher (or 20 per cent up-tempo or higher, and 80 per cent long slow distance).

Each of the following subphases is introduced progressively each week during the speed phase.

Period: Speed

Subphase 5: Low speed

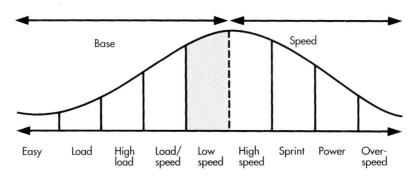

Base — Speed

Easy | Load | High load | Load/ speed | Low speed | High speed | Sprint | Power | Over- speed

Cycling, running

For cycling and running, up-tempo work marks the beginning of the conditioning work for speed. This form of training is faster than easy conversation pace but not as high as 10–60 minute race pace. When cycling, for example, you should be riding fast (70 to 75 per cent effort) and feeling strong (i.e. Ironman/marathon race pace), but not 'hammering'. Because low speed training is only moderately intense, the interval periods can be quite long (10–20 minutes). This would occur one to two times per week and would be gradually phased in over a period of one to four weeks (generally two).

Specifics: Long intervals at up-tempo pace (Ironman race pace). You should feel fast and strong.

Effort: Moderately difficult to converse (70–75% effort)

Sports
   Swim: 600–1000 m intervals
   Bike: 10–20 min intervals
   Run: 10–15 min intervals
   Kayak: 10–20 min intervals
   Row: 10–20 min intervals

Training heart rate: Up-tempo rate (75–85% HR^{max}) for intervals; long slow distance rate (60–75% HR^{max}) between intervals.

Training weeks

Triathlon/duathlon/multisport

M	T	W	T	F	S	S
S/K (H)		S/K (S)		DAY OFF	S/K (L)	
	B (S)		B (H)			B (L)
R (H)		R (L)			R (S)	

Cycling/mountain biking/running/rowing

M	T	W	T	F	S	S
E	**S/H2** E		ML	DAY OFF	**S/H1**	L

The **bold** workouts are the training sessions where low speed training would be applied. The 1 and 2 show where low speed training should be emphasised first and second.

Period: Speed

Subphase 6: High speed

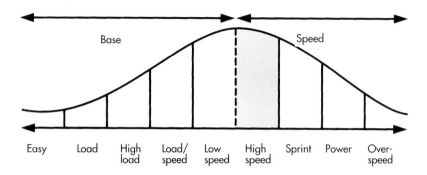

| Easy | Load | High load | Load/ speed | Low speed | High speed | Sprint | Power | Over- speed |

Base — Speed

Anaerobic threshold is defined as the highest intensity that an athlete can maintain for approximately one hour. This equates to about a 40 km time trial pace on your bike or 16 km run pace. Anaerobic threshold training can be conducted as time trials or as less psychologically demanding intervals (e.g. 5–10 minutes). It improves your anaerobic threshold pace, thereby improving your race pace or your high steady state race pace. This subphase would occur one to two times per week and would last two to eight weeks (generally four).

Specifics: Short intervals (16 km run or 40 km bike time trial pace). You should feel like you are 'hammering'.

Effort: Difficult to converse (75–85% effort)

Sports
   Swim: 250–500 m intervals
   Bike: 5–8 min intervals
   Run: 5 min intervals
   Kayak: 5–8 min intervals
   Row: 5–8 min intervals

Training heart rate: Anaerobic threshold rate (85–95% HR^{max}) for intervals; long slow distance rate (60–75% HR^{max}) between intervals.

Training weeks						
Triathlon/duathlon/multisport						
M	**T**	**W**	**T**	**F**	**S**	**S**
S/K (H)		S/K (S)		DAY OFF	S/K (L)	
	B (S)		B (H)	DAY OFF		B (L)
R (H)		R (L)		DAY OFF	**R** (S)	
Cycling/mountain biking/running/rowing						
M	**T**	**W**	**T**	**F**	**S**	**S**
E	**S/H2**	E	ML	DAY OFF	**S/H1**	L

The **bold** workouts are the training sessions where high speed training would be applied. The 1 and 2 show where high speed should be emphasised first and second.

Subphases 7–9:
Sprints, Power, Overspeed

The subphases of sprints, power and overspeed are not always applicable to most endurance sports, but are some exceptions. The exceptions are:

- Mountain biking, distance running (particularly 10–21 km events) and some multi-sports require extensive sprints;
- Rowing uses sprints and power, and road cycling uses sprints, power and overspeed.

Subphase 7: Sprints (extensive/intensive)
The sprints subphase involves different forms of anaerobic or sprint training. Extensive sprints (45 seconds to 4 minutes) are used to improve sustained sprint speed at the start or end of a race, to bridge gaps, to break away from the peleton (pack) close to the finish, and to initiate breakaways. Intensive sprints (usually 10 seconds to 1 minute) are used to improve top sprinting speed. Intensive sprints can be broken down to uphill (50 m), crest (20–30 m uphill/20–30 m over the top) and flat (200–400 m) for running and cycling.

(Incidentally, uphill sprints occur during the load and high load subphases, crest sprints occur in the load/speed subphase, and flat sprints occur in the speed phase.) Extensive and intensive sprint training occurs one to two times per week over one to four weeks (generally one to two)

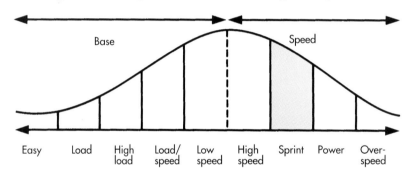

	Base					Speed		
Easy	Load	High load	Load/ speed	Low speed	High speed	Sprint	Power	Over-speed

Specifics: Extensive sprints (long sprints) are 45 sec to 4 min sprints. Intensive sprints (short sprints) are 10 sec to 1 min sprints.

Effort: Very difficult to talk (90–100% effort)

Sports
  Swim: 100–400 m sprints
  Bike: 200–4000 m sprints
  Run: 100–1000 m sprints
  Kayak: 100–500 m sprints
  Row: 100–700 m sprints

Training heart rate: Not applicable

The **bold** workouts are the training sessions where sprint training would be applied. The 1 and 2 show where sprint training should be emphasised first and second.

Training weeks

Multisport

M	T	W	T	F	S	S
K (H)		K (S)		DAY OFF	K (L)	
	B (S)		B (H)			B (L)
R (H)		R (L)			R (S)	

Cycling/mountain biking/running/rowing

M	T	W	T	F	S	S
E	S/H2	E	ML	DAY OFF	S/H1	L

Subphase 8: Power (acceleration)

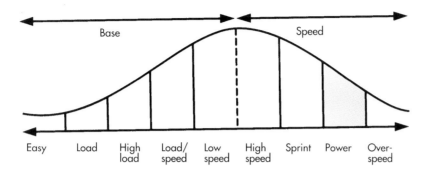

In cycling, power training is used to improve your ability to attack or 'jump' a rider, or the peleton. Power training can be conducted using plyometrics, by big gear wind-outs, or by using a dip in the road to gain speed down a hill in a big gear, and then sprinting in the same gear up a short climb on the other side of the dip, stopping when you are not 'on top of the gear'. Power training for rowing usually involves weight training but may also involve power training in the boat.

You should feel strong during power training (i.e. you should not struggle to turn a gear over). The power subphase can occur one to two times per week over one to four weeks (generally one to two).

Specifics: Explosive acceleration

Effort: 100% effort

Training heart rate: Not applicable

Training week						
Cycling/rowing						
M	**T**	**W**	**T**	**F**	**S**	**S**
E	**S/H2**	E	ML	DAY OFF	**S/H1**	L

The **bold** workouts are the training sessions where power training would be applied. The 1 and 2 show where power training should be emphasised first and second.

Subphase 9: Overspeed

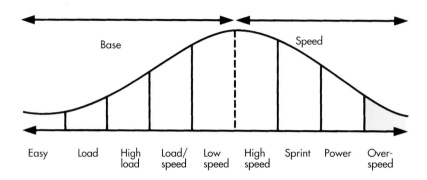

| Easy | Load | High load | Load/ speed | Low speed | High speed | Sprint | Power | Over- speed |

Overspeed training involves increasing muscular contraction speed. It is the final aspect of speedwork. In cycling, downhill spinning sprints (sprinting downhill in a small gear at a high cadence) and motor pacing (high cadence drafting behind a vehicle to decrease the effects of wind resistance) are useful forms of overspeed.

> *Specifics:* Short downhill sprint intervals or motor pacing (drafting behind a motor vehicle) at above race pace speed to enhance muscle contraction speed.
>
> *Effort:* Moderate/low load and high speed
>
> *Reps:* 100–200 m downhill, 120–200 rpm
>
> *Continuous effort:* 5–100 km drafting behind a motor vehicle

Training week						
Cycling						
M	T	W	T	F	S	S
E	**S/H2** E	ML	DAY OFF	**S/H1**	L	

The **bold** workouts are the training sessions where overspeed training would be applied. The 1 and 2 show where overspeed should be emphasised first and second.

Intensities and subphases – a piece of cake

In most cases, once you start to use a training intensity you continue to use it (to varying degrees) right up until race day. Each training intensity is slowly introduced and progressively increased over one to four weeks prior to the time when you begin to focus on the specific training subphase. Once a subphase reaches its peak emphasis, it is then maintained as other training subphases are initiated. Training subphases 1–5 (preparation, load, high load, load/speed, low speed) are introduced, focused on, and then maintained in progressively smaller amounts throughout the build-up (*see* appendix 12 for an example for cycling). Sport-specific strength training must not be underrated. This must be maintained all the way through the programme.

So, there it is. Those are all the ingredients needed for a good training recipe. But remember, training is a bit like baking a cake – it's not the ingredients that make a good cake, it's the way the chef puts them together.

To help you do this, an experienced athlete or coach could be called upon to advise you. They can use their experience to take the guesswork out of your training – this will save you learning the hard way!

Timing of subphases

When determining the timing of training subphases, you or your coach need to assess the racing intensity/pace for the competition you are aiming at. For example, if you are doing a long or ultra distance event (e.g. Ironman, marathon), race pace will be at approximately up-tempo training intensity.

For these events, up-tempo training occurs in the low speed subphase, i.e. at the start of speedwork, when race pace training always begins (*see* fig. 4.4). However, if you are doing a standard distance triathlon or 10 km run, the race pace will be closer to anaerobic threshold training intensity. This race pace intensity occurs in the high speed subphase, so this subphase would occur at the start of speedwork. This would push the low speed subphase back into base training (*see* fig. 4.5). Finally, be specific about what you require in training for your event. You might not need to use every subphase because:

- you might not have enough time;
- you might not require some of the intensities;
- you might want to spend more time on a specific subphase if you have a particular weakness.

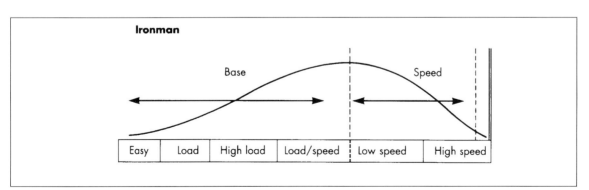

Figure 4.4 Subphase timing for a long distance event

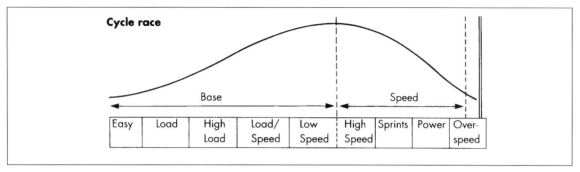

Figure 4.5 Subphase timing for a shorter event

How to use subphases

In the programmes in chapter 14, the bold subscript numerals denote the subphase that is appropriate to the workout. For instance, in the cycling programme on page 223, Tuesday's workout in the week beginning 6 January is '33.8$_2$'. This tells the cyclist to ride 33.8 km in load, i.e. with the main emphasis of the ride being hill training. Each subphase involves a different aspect of training; the subscript numerals tell you how to perform the training within a workout.

♦ How to structure a ♦ training session

1 *Try to keep similar types of training well apart.* For example, keep endurance sessions away from strength endurance, and strength endurance away from speed. This harks back to the principle of microcyclic training (*see* chapter 2, 'Day to day: microcycles'), where 'like' modes of training are kept as far apart from each other within the training week as possible. This helps recovery and therefore the absorption of training (very important!).

There are, of course, some situations where you might deliberately combine similar training modes (e.g. for triathlon: strength endurance hills on the bike followed by speed on the run to get used to running tired) but these situations are infrequent.

2 *If doing more than one type of training in the same workout, use the following order* (cycling example):

Training type	Time
Warm-up	10 min
Technique	20 min
Speed	sprints 2 x 1 min (10 min rest between reps)
Speed	up-tempo and anaerobic threshold 3 x 5 min (5 min rest between reps)
Strength endurance	20 min, flat, big gear
Endurance	60 min endurance
Warm-down	10 min
Total time:	172 min

Note: These forms of training would not normally be combined in one session!

The reason for training in this order is that you must be 'freshest' in order to do technique work correctly and train at the higher intensities. This order not only applies in a workout but also in terms of prioritising recovery between workouts – speed and technique training require the longest recovery time, whereas endurance training requires the least. Here are two examples (wrong and right) of day-to-day scheduling that includes a speed training session:

Wrong

	Mon	Tues	Wed
a.m.	—	speed	endurance
p.m.	endurance	—	—

Training Monday night and Tuesday morning leaves too little recovery time before the speed session.

Right

	Mon	Tues	Wed
a.m.	endurance	—	endurance
p.m.	—	speed	—

By training Monday morning and leaving the speed session until Tuesday night, adequate recovery time is scheduled. Once again, there are exceptions to the rule (e.g. learning to do speedwork when tired) but in most cases this is the best format.

Chapter 5

Manipulation of Training Principles

Now that you understand the training principles for endurance events, it is time to start looking at how those principles can be manipulated to get different training effects. It is also time to look at how you can customise your programme to suit your racing and training commitments.

◆ Length of seasons ◆

In-season (generally eight to twelve weeks)

The timing and length of the competitive season varies according to how competition is structured and what your goals are. Some sports have a single peak in a year, for example national or world champs, where it is vital you peak on race day. In such cases, the in-season lasts only the day of the race (talk about pressure!). Other sports have a series of races, such as national series, best athlete over a series. In this case, the in-season can last several months.

The in-season generally lasts eight to twelve weeks with the athlete holding a 90 per cent plus performance level during that time. A 100 per cent performance level can only be maintained for approximately two to fourteen days; this can occur one to three times during the in-season for most athletes. When an in-season lasts longer than ten weeks, the athlete will need to repeat some aspects of pre-season training.

Pre-season (generally twelve to sixteen weeks)

The length of the pre-season depends somewhat on how long the race is. A long pre-season is required for long races (Ironman), while short races (10 km, cycle criterium) require a shorter pre-season. Training for a race series is highly variable and depends on your training history, the length of the series and the length of each race. Why does the pre-season vary in length? Simply because it will take you longer to reach the peak training mileages necessary for longer races, (marathon, Half-Ironman), than for a shorter race (10 km, sprint triathlon). Remember that pre-season is made up of a base (two to six months) and a speed phase (four to eight weeks).

Off-season (generally four to sixteen weeks)

There is no problem with having a long off-season (although longer than six months is not advisable), as long as you maintain an active recovery programme, i.e. light, low-intensity activity. Four to twelve weeks is reasonable, less than four weeks is not advised. Elite athletes may have four to eight weeks whereas novices will have eight to sixteen. Too short an off-season can tempt disaster because you may not recover completely before you begin your next base phase. This may lead to . . . you guessed it, overtraining!

Single versus double periodisation

If an athlete's peak races fall in the same season they will only need a single training periodisation (*see* fig. 5.1). However, international athletes often have a different seasonal make-up to their year with multiple seasons, for example competitions in both the northern and southern hemispheres, or in the case of a runner, a marathon in spring and autumn. This may result in a year looking like this:

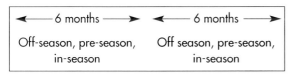

This type of double periodisation is illustrated in figure 5.2. In such cases, training periods are compressed, including off-seasons, though this needs to be carefully monitored as short off-seasons may increase the risk of burn-out. Note, though, that the more races you aim to peak for, the less chance you have of getting it right each time. International athletes with four or more peaks a season have to work very hard and very intelligently to peak precisely at the right time every time.

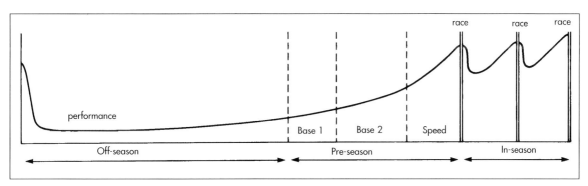

Figure 5.1 Athlete racing peak races in the same season (in one year) – single periodisation

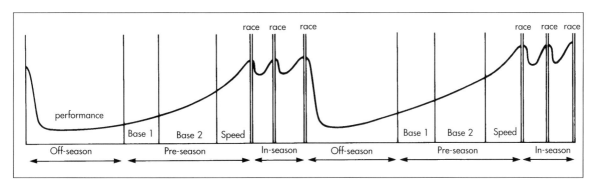

Figure 5.2 Athlete racing in two major events in one year – double periodisation

◆ Length of training ◆ periods

Training periodisation (Base 1, Base 2, speed, taper) varies according to a number of variables. These are:

- Experience (how long you have been competing in the sport, your training history)
- Your ability and training tolerance
- Your age
- The length of the race you are training for

Experience has a big effect on training. If you have been involved in your sport for years, you can train harder and longer than if you are new to it. Tied up with this is age – up to a point, older athletes tend to be able to tolerate higher training volumes (one of the few advantages of getting older!)

Ability also affects training. Some people are better suited to some sports than others; we have all seen those 'naturals' who perform well with relatively little preparation. These 'thoroughbreds' tend to be able to get away with less training than the rest of us. Of course, the history of sport is littered with examples of hard workers beating 'naturals'. Moral: it's hard to beat a good intelligent work ethic! Some athletes may also be able to naturally cope with greater training volumes and workloads than others.

The length of the race also determines the length of the training periods. As mentioned previously, longer races require higher mileages in training, and it takes time to build up to high mileages.

Let's look at the lengths of each of the training periods in turn.

Base 1
Base 1 can last between zero and eight weeks, depending on the number of problems that require work. If you have no real problems, Base 1 can be eliminated. But if there is a lot of work to be done, then Base 1 will probably last eight weeks. If you have a major injury problem to overcome, Base 1 can last for months.

Base 2
The length of Base 2 (eight to sixteen weeks) is primarily determined by the length of the race: the longer the race, the longer this phase needs to be to reach the required training mileages. To a lesser extent, Base 2 length is also determined by experience, age and ability. The younger or less experienced the athlete, the shorter the phases (Base 1, Base 2, speed) they can cope with.

Speed
This phase (four to eight weeks) is also determined by your experience, age and ability. Once again, younger and less experienced athletes will have a shorter phase (four weeks). More experienced athletes will cope with a longer speed phase (eight weeks). The length of the race (for sports dealt with in this book) has only a marginal effect on the length of the speedwork phase. This is because endurance events, unlike shorter races and sprint-oriented sports, don't require as great an emphasis on speed. Endurance events aren't called endurance events for nothing!

Taper
The length of the taper (two to fourteen days) is again determined by the length of the race. The longer the race, the greater the training volume required, the greater the cumulative fatigue, and therefore the longer the taper. Taper is also affected by your recovery rate: the better you recover, the shorter the taper.

Variations in build-up time

What happens if you have more time than you need in build-up? Or not enough? In such situations (not uncommon, especially the latter), a programme may require major surgery.

Too much time

Having too much time is the better of the two problems to have. Generally, this means you can relax a little and start your build-up very gradually. You will also be able to concentrate on any small problems (flexibility, strength imbalances, niggling injuries) that may affect performance. Technique can also be emphasised for a while. Don't get sucked into building your training up too soon. The key is to build up *gradually*. With a long, gradual build-up, intermediate races should be done to help you maintain your enthusiasm, as well as help condition you for the major race or races ahead.

In cases where there is plenty of time, base training can be lengthened and one to two mini peaks can be scheduled into the programme. If you have more than six months until the start of your peak race build-up, you may want to focus on some similar events to help build your proficiency in the sport. For instance, if a build-up for Ironman takes about four months, and you have seven months, it would be useful to do a marathon or a long bike race in the three months before you begin your full Ironman build-up (*see* fig. 5.3). This will all add to your experience and performance.

If you have between three and six months until your peak race build-up begins, the 'more than six months' formula applies, except you would have only one mini peak involving a similar event. If you have less time than this, concentrate on slowly building up training and addressing specific problems.

Not enough time

If the time left until the race you want to aim at is too short for a complete build up, your programme will need to be compressed. This is a difficult and undesirable situation that long-term planning usually gets around. However, injuries, illness and the importance of an event (for example, an Olympic Games), sometimes mean you have to make the best of a bad situation. Nevertheless, if you have missed more than one-third to a half of your build-up, you should probably look at another event.

If you have lost less than one-third to a half of your build-up, the compression of your programme depends on the type of race you are facing and your previous background and experience. If it is a long race, the speed phase should be compressed or eliminated. If it is a

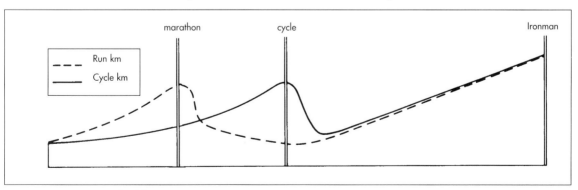

Figure 5.3 Ironman build-up

short race, you will need to compress the base phase mainly, or compress slightly both the base and speed phases. Remember, though, that you need to do enough base work so you don't become overtrained or injured by speedwork.

◆ How to manage training ◆ during the 'in-season'

Generally, you have two choices in peaking for races:

1 Spacing – peaks are spaced approximately six to eight weeks apart
2 Clumping – peaks are clumped together over two to three weeks

The following outlines what to do for peak races at various periods.

Peak races two weeks apart:
• less than two hour race – two weeks speed
• two to four hour race – two weeks speed
• longer than four hour race – two weeks speed

Four weeks apart:
• less than two hour race – one week base/some speed; three weeks speed
• two to four hour race – two weeks base/some speed; two weeks speed
• longer than four hour race – three weeks base/some speed; one week speed

Six weeks apart:
• less than one hour race – two weeks base/some speed; four weeks speed
• two to four hour race – three weeks base/some speed; three weeks speed
• longer than four hour race – four weeks base/some speed; two weeks speed

Ten weeks apart:
• less than one hour race – four weeks base/two weeks some speed; four weeks speed
• two to four hour race – four weeks base/two weeks some speed; four weeks speed
• longer than four hour race – six weeks base/one week some speed; three weeks speed

Fifteen weeks apart:
Do another pre-season build-up, possibly with a small off-season.

◆ Mileage determination ◆ and peak mileage

'How many miles are you doing?' When one athlete wants to find out how much or how 'hard' another athlete is training, this is usually the question they ask. The question implies that more is better – which it very rarely is. Training is a dynamic process of which weekly mileage is just one ever-changing part, and often the least important part. Nevertheless, there is one week when you do need to count the miles in order to establish what your training volume will be in build-up. 'Peak-mileage week' is the highest training volume week in a training build-up.

Peak-mileage week placement in a build-up depends on the length of the race and, therefore, on whether distance or speed is the main training requirement. For a long race, peak mileages will occur closer to the race as mileage or distance is the main requirement (doing too much speedwork will stop you doing the mileage you need to do). For a cycle road race or tour, Ironman or marathon, the peak-mileage week will occur approximately three to five weeks before the event. For a short race, peak mileage is done further away from the race as speed receives a greater emphasis (too much mileage close to the race won't let you do the speedwork you need to do). For shorter races (standard distance triathlon or duathlon, rowing, most mountain bike races), peak mileage will be done six to ten weeks before the event.

Mileage increase

A common mistake is to increase your training mileage too quickly. In the first four to six weeks, a 5 to 10 per cent increase per week is sufficient, for example from 50 km to 55 km, or six hours to six hours 36 minutes. This doesn't seem like much, but it soon adds up over the weeks and months. After this, 10 per cent increases are okay while mileage is still fairly low. Finally, as you get close to peak mileage, 5 to 10 per cent increases are again acceptable.

First, though, you need to work out when you want your peak-mileage week to occur. You can then work out the weekly mileages for your build-up, working back from the peak-mileage week. The way to do this is explained, step-by-step, in chapter 7.

Peak-mileage workouts (that is, the longest workout you will do in training for a particular event) vary depending on the length of the race and the sport you are training in. In general, for longer races, athletes tend not to train up to the full race distance (as this can be too taxing, unless they are training in a low-impact/stress sport), whereas shorter races often involve overdistance training (workouts longer than the race distance). High-impact/stress sports, such as running, are less likely to involve training up to full race distance for longer races than low-impact/stress sports such as cycling. The following table includes some examples of peak-mileage workouts.

Peak-mileage workouts for long races

Sport	Race length	Approx. longest workout
Running		
Marathon	42 km	30–36 km
Half-marathon	21 km	21–26 km
10 km	10 km	16–21 km
Triathlon sprint		
Swim	700 m	700–2000 m
Bike	20 km	20–80 km
Run	5 km	5–16 km
Olympic		
Swim	1.5 km	1.5–3 km
Bike	40 km	40–120 km
Run	10 km	10–21 km
Half-Ironman		
Swim	2 km	2–3.5 km
Bike	90 km	90–140 km
Run	21 km	21–26 km
Ironman		
Swim	3.8 km	3.8–4.5 km
Bike	180 km	160–200 km
Run	42 km	26–36 km
Mountain biking		
Standard race	2–3 hr	3.5–4.5 hr
Cycling		
40 km	40 km	80–120 km
80 km	80 km	80–140 km
160 km	160 km	160–200 km
Tour	700–1100 km	160–200 km
Rowing		
Standard race	2000 m	15 000–25 000 m
Duathlon		
Short		
Run	5 km × 2	16–21 km
Bike	40 km	40–120 km
Long		
Run	10 km × 2	20–26 km
Bike	60 km	60–120 km
Multisport – depends on race		
Run: up to duration or add 40–60% to race length for sub-3-hour races		
Bike and kayak: up to race distance or add 40–60% to race length for sub-3-hour races		

♦ Types of speedwork ♦

Speed training is required to some degree for most racing situations. It increases your competitive capabilities by simulating race conditions and intensities, and this helps you adapt physically and psychologically to the demands of racing. Speedwork can be performed at various intensities, but it needs to be specific to your racing needs – going flat out may feel good, but it won't help your performance if you don't need to race flat out!

Speedwork during training will generally move from short distances with long rests at the start of speedwork, to longer distances with shorter rests at the end. This allows you to develop your tolerance to speedwork gradually. Without this gradual approach you are likely to become overtired and you will not achieve the desired training response. Submaximal work improves your steady state speed.

Sprint or anaerobic speedwork generally follows a slightly different format. Progression here is from longer sprints (for speed endurance development) to shorter sprints (for top speed, power and acceleration development). Rest periods between sprint intervals vary from very short (to improve sprint recovery or recovery from oxygen debt) to long (between maximal sprint efforts). Variations in sprint training depend on the sport or on the requirements of particular races – you can emphasise speed endurance, top speed or acceleration/power as you need to. Common forms of speedwork for endurance athletes are racing, intervals, time trials and sprints.

Basic progression of speedwork

Intervals →	Time trials, intervals →	Time trials, intervals
	(if no specific races)	Sprints (if needed)
	Races	Races

The tables on pages 61–2 summarise the types of submaximal and high-intensity training for speedwork as discussed in chapters 3 and 4. Details on types of low-intensity training are also included.

Intervals (aerobic/anaerobic threshold)

Intervals are designed to increase gradually the amount of race pace stress on your body. Initially, you need to start your intervals off with short periods of work and large periods of rest. You will progress gradually to large periods of work and short periods of rest as you adapt to the increasing volume and the interval intensity. Eventually, you will train at race intensity for most, if not all, of the distance you are aiming to race over.

Heart rate monitors can be used to achieve not only the correct interval intensity, but also the correct rest periods between intervals. Correct interval intensity, as indicated by a heart rate monitor, is generally determined by laboratory testing. This can also be determined, although less accurately, by indirect calculations (*see* appendix 1).

Most aerobic/anaerobic threshold intervals for endurance sports are performed at or near maximum steady state pace. Recovery between intervals can be set to a pre-selected time or the time it takes for your heart rate to drop to a specified level (e.g. 40 to 50 beats below interval exercise heart rate). The less fit you are the longer the recovery period because your heart rate will take longer to return to the specified level. Figure 5.4 (*see* page 61) gives an example of interval sessions used by a runner during a four-week training period.

Very short intervals with long rests should be used in your taper week before races. This will help you maintain race pace form, but avoid fatigue as race day approaches.

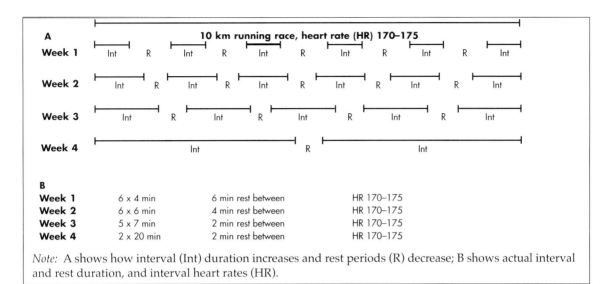

Figure 5.4 Speedwork preparation for a 10 km running race

Types of speedwork and their use in each sport

Training type	Effort (approx.)	Duration (approx.)	Tri/multi	Run	Cycle	Mountain bike	Row
Power	100%	<10–20 sec	—	—	Jumps	—	Stroke
Intensive sprints	100%	10 sec–1 min	—	—	Jumps, bridge gaps, final sprints	Accel	first, and last 500 m
Extensive sprints	95–100%	45 sec–4 min	—	Leg speed, some starts	Bridge gaps, final sprints	Accel	first and last 500 m
Submaximal intervals	85–95%	>4 min	Approx. race pace	Approx. race pace	Peloton, riding, TTs, breaks	Approx. race pace	Approx. race pace

Key: Accel = acceleration; TTs = time trials; — = intensity not used.

Note: Low-intensity training (up-tempo, LSD and active recovery) are not classed as speedwork.

Training intensities and their effort

Training type	Duration (approx.)	Effort (approx.)	Subjective pace	Training effect	Interval example
Power	<10–20sec	100%	V. intense V. short	Improves initial accel.	V. short 10–15 sec then rest to recovery; plyometrics
Intensive sprints	10 sec–1 min	100%	V. intense, unable to converse	Improves max. explosive sprint	short 30 sec–1 min then rest to recovery (in most cases)
Extensive sprints	45 sec–4 min	95–100%	Intense, very difficult to converse	Improves max. sustained sprint pace	Moderate 1–3 min; variable recovery
Submaximal intervals	>4 min	85–95%	Moderately intense, moderate to difficult to converse	Improves max. steady state pace	Long Ints usually 4–20 min, or TTs; dec recovery
Up-tempo	>4 min	75–85%	Moderately easy to converse	Progressive intensity, inc bridge btwn LSD and speedwork	V. long Ints, progressive intensity inc and duration dec; rest to recovery
Long slow distance	>4 min	60–75%	Easy to converse	Inc training tolerance and inc ability to cope with dist; basic conditioning	Continuous
Active	>4 min	<60%	V. easy to converse	Assists recovery, no real training effect	Continuous

Key: Int = intervals; inc = increase; dec = decrease; dist = distance; LSD = long slow distance; accel = acceleration; TTs = time trials.

Time trials

Time trials involve long periods of continuous exertion close to race pace. They usually last 30 to 60 minutes for most sub-three-hour races. The only exception to that in this book is rowing. Rowing time trials last approximately three to seven minutes, because rowing races are over a relatively short distance (2000 m). In essence, time trials are mini race simulations. They should start at very short distances and progress to longer distances. They can be very tiring and preferably should only be done late in the speedwork phase after intervals have already been done.

If there are no effective warm-up races available, then time trials are the next best thing. But remember that races and time trials are similar workouts and so both should not be done in the same week. Neither should time trials be done the week before or the week after a race. No more than one time trial should be done each week, and it is best only to do them every two to four weeks (elite, every one to two weeks; intermediate, every two to four weeks; novice, no time trials, just intervals). *See* page 131 for more details on time trials and training.

Racing

Races are very much like time trials, but with the added bonus of competition. Races should preferably only be done towards the middle and latter stages of the speedwork phase after a period on intervals. Do not race every week unless it is necessary (e.g. a race series), or unless it has been built into your programme. Avoid speedwork two to four days before and after a race (*see* 'Tapering for races', page 72).

Sprints and sprint intervals (anaerobic)

Sprints are a type of high-intensity interval. They are used to develop your ability to cope with oxygen debt and to develop maximum pace. The difference between sprints and aerobic/anaerobic threshold intervals is that sprints are shorter and do not always require a reduction in the rest period.

Some sprints will have reduced rest periods, while others will have rests that allow full recovery as the sprint is designed to improve short distance speed and not sustained top speed.

The only so-called endurance sports that use sprint training are cycling (road and mountain biking) and rowing, although very short sprints or 'stride outs' may be used to develop leg speed for running. A speedwork session may look like this: 6×1 min at 100 per cent effort with a 2 min rest between efforts.

Other forms of speedwork

Another form of speedwork is 'fartlek' (a Swedish term meaning speedplay). Your interval/sprint lengths are varied in both duration/intensity and recovery time, based on how you feel.

Overspeed is used by cyclists and short distance runners to increase muscular contraction speed. This involves exercising at a slightly faster biomechanical pace than race pace.

'Dead leg' speedwork can also be used to get your body used to exercising on tired legs. This may involve hill training immediately followed by speedwork.

In general, doing speedwork in the afternoon is best. Your body seems to perform better then.

◆ Use of speedwork ◆

Determination of training intensities

When looking at your training requirements for a specific race, think about what training period you are in, and the intensity of the training you will need to do. In the base period, low-intensity training is required. During the speed phase, though, you will need to do some training at race pace and practise aspects of racing such as accelerating, extensive and intensive sprints, and hill climbing. This all helps to simulate race conditions. The questions you need ask yourself, therefore, are *which* training intensities, *when* and *how much*? Let's start with *which*.

If the race is going to involve some long or extended sprints, then you will need to do some high-intensity (HI) training incorporating extensive sprinting. This is the rule of specificity! You need to work out what intensities you should train at and when (*see* chapter 14 specific sample programmes for help). If you are doing speed phase training for a 40 km cycle criterium, for instance, mileage is not as important as speedwork. You would need to concentrate on high steady state speed (SM), sprinting/acceleration (HI; extensive, intensive and power), and cornering, as criteriums are generally on short, fast, tight courses.

If, on the other pedal, you were training for a 1400 km cycle tour over nine days, most of your training would consist of high mileage at low intensity (LO). After all, there is no point in being fast if you can't complete the tour. LO training would still be done in the speed phase to maintain base, but at low volume. Different sports also have different demands in terms of training intensities. Rowing, for example, requires greater volumes of high-intensity training than mountain biking. Ironman triathletes require greater training volumes at lower intensities than short-course triathletes. Now for the *when* part.

Different races and different courses in the same sport require slightly different approaches in terms of training intensities. Deciding which training intensities you will need to emphasise is only half the challenge. You have to decide *when* during the training period the different intensities need to occur. For example, SM starts in the speedwork phase, HI towards the middle to end of speedwork. Realise that your body has a good memory for duration/distance training (i.e. base). This means you can drop your training volumes to 50 to 70 per cent of peak volumes and your body will remember the long work you did for some time. On the other hand, your body has a lousy memory for speedwork. If you eliminate speedwork from your programme, you start to slow down virtually immediately (approximately four to fourteen days). So speedwork needs to be maintained until a few days before the race. Now, *how much*? Or to put it less succinctly, what proportion of the training is done at each intensity?

To work this out, you will also need to work out how much each intensity contributes to a race and then allocate training accordingly *during the speedwork phase*. For example, for elite marathoners, since a marathon is 99 per cent submaximal and below, no high-intensity training is necessary! If a race is short and hilly with a lot of sprinting, such as a cycle race, the main training requirement will be SM, with some HI work for the sprints, and LO work to maintain base. A lot of hill training would also be carried out. The hill training and the low-intensity work would occur mainly in the base phase, with submaximal and high-intensity work (including hill intervals and sprinting) happening in the speed phase. You can even assign percentages to each intensity. SM, extensive and intensive sprints, and power will only account for a maximum of 10 to 15 per cent of total mileage in the speed phase. The rest will be up-tempo, long slow distance (LSD) and active recovery.

In general, match your training intensities to those of the race. But remember that training generally progresses from long and slow to short and fast, relative to the race pace you are trying to achieve. And don't forget that if you need to do some high-intensity training during the speed phase, do some submaximal training first. The body does not like to jump from slow to fast in one leap.

Here's an example. The final two to three weeks of base before speedwork starts might look like this:

Mon	Tue	Wed	Thur	Fri	Sat	Sun
LO	UT	LO	UT	D/O	LO	LO (Long)

Key: LO = low-intensity; UT = up-tempo (intermediate intensity); D/O = day off.

Up-tempo days slowly progress from very slow training in the final weeks of the base period to speed training during the speed phase. This should be a careful progression. No sudden changes in training tempo should occur from week to week. Not only would a sudden tempo change increase the likelihood of injury, it might lead to you peaking too early, or training overload in the last few weeks of the base phase. Up-tempo workouts should be done on the same days of the week you will later do your speedwork on. All other days are maintained at LO.

The tables below and on page 66 are an example of how base and speed phases might be set out for a road cyclist. They show that speed is introduced into the programme very gradually.

Road cyclist: base and speedwork phases

BASE Week	Mesocycle	Mon	Tue	Wed	Thur	Fri	Sat	Sun	HR
1	H	28 kph Cont	LO	28 kph Cont	LO	D/O	LO	LO	135–140
2	H	28 kph Cont	LO	28 kph Cont	LO	D/O	LO	LO	135–140
3	E	28 kph Cont	LO	28 kph Cont	LO	D/O	LO	LO	135–140
4	H	28 kph Cont	LO	28 kph Cont	LO	D/O	LO	LO	135–140
5	H	28 kph Cont	LO	28 kph Cont	LO	D/O	LO	LO	135–140
6	E	28 kph Cont	LO	28 kph Cont	LO	D/O	LO	LO	135–140
7	H	32 kph Cont(UT)	LO	30 kph Cont(UT)	LO	D/O	LO	LO	145–150/ 140–145
8	H	34 kph Cont(UT)	LO	32 kph Cont(UT)	LO	D/O	LO	LO	150–155/ 145–150

SPEED									
Week	Mesocycle	Mon	Tue	Wed	Thur	Fri	Sat	Sun	HR
1	E	LO	50% Ints* 38 kph	LO	LO	D/O	50% Ints* 38 kph	LO	165–170
2	H	LO	Ints* 39 kph	LO	LO	D/O	Ints* 39 kph	LO	170–175
3	H	LO	Ints* 40 kph	LO	LO	D/O	Ints* 40 kph	LO	175–180
4	E	LO	50% Ints* 40 kph	LO	LO	D/O	50% Ints* 40 kph	LO	175–180
5	H	LO	Ints* 41 kph	LO	LO	D/O	Ints* 41 kph	LO	180–185
6	E	Taper							

Key: HR = Heart rates; H = hard week; E = easy week; kph = kilometres per hour; Cont = continuous; LO = low-intensity; UT = up-tempo; D/O = day off; Ints = intervals; 50% Ints = 50% number of usual intervals; * = submaximal intensity.

Note: Speeds and heart rates are given as examples only to show increases in speed; these will vary from person to person; all low-intensity workouts are done at a heart rate of 135–140; 5–10 k on/10–15 k off; 5–10 k on/10–15 k off = up-tempo interval in the final two weeks (weeks 7 and 8) of base.

Mesocycles and speedwork

During the easy weeks of a mesocycle, training volume is reduced. The volume of speedwork is also reduced. The training intensity, however, is not reduced!

Here's an example of how this works in the speedwork phase.

Week	Mesocycle	Interval
1	Hard	2 × 5 min with 4 min rest between
2	Hard	4 × 5 min with 3 min rest between
3	Easy	3 × 5 min with 4 min rest between
4	Hard	5 × 5 min with 2 min rest between
5	Hard	6 × 5 min with 1 min rest between
6	Easy	Taper

Note: The work period is reduced and the rest period is increased during the easy week.

Maximum number of speed days per week

In most single-discipline sports, for example rowing or running, speedwork can only be performed as a complete session a couple of times per week during the speed phase. All other workouts are done at a low intensity (tired athletes please note!) to maintain base. One exception is swimming, as it is less taxing on the body because the bodyweight is being supported. Indeed, some speedwork can be done every session in swimming. Generally, low-impact, high-fluidity sports allow more speedwork sessions per week, for example swimmers and cyclists can tolerate more speedwork than runners. In multidiscipline training, one speed session can occur in each discipline each week. However, more speed sessions can usually be done overall as the sessions are spread across a number of disciplines.

The amount of time you have been in the sport and your recovery rate also determine how many speedwork sessions you can handle during the speedwork phase. Here are some recommendations:

Category	Speed sessions per week
Novice	0–1 speed sessions per week (speed phase only)
Semi-competitive	1–2 speed sessions per week (speed phase only)
Elite	2–3 speed sessions per week (mainly in the speed phase, but small amounts should also be done in the base phase, particularly towards the end of base)

For swimming, the number of speed sessions may be doubled. Triathletes and multisport athletes may have one run and one bike speed session per week (plus swimming or kayaking), or one run, one bike and one swim/bike/run combined speed session.

Where practical, do your speedwork using the same equipment that you will use during your peak race. This helps to simulate race conditions. It is sometimes good, however, to save one piece of previously race-used equipment or gear just for major races, for example special shorts, shoes or wheels. When you use this equipment, or put on that piece of gear, you know it's time to *ruuummmble*!

Contrasting intensity of training sessions during speedwork

Most athletes do not have enough of a contrast between their slow sessions and their speed sessions during the speed phase. In other words, they tend to do their slow workouts too fast, which results in them being too tired to do their speedwork fast. They do not, therefore, get the maximum benefit from their speedwork (*see* figs 5.5 and 5.6) Ideally, you should train very slow in your easy sessions during the speedwork phase so that you can 'hammer' your speed sessions. Generally, the better your speed sessions, the greater your performance gains.

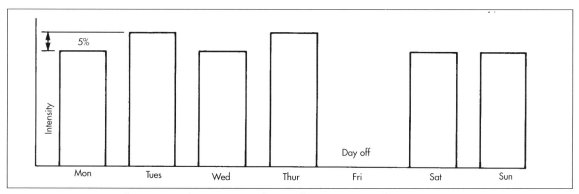

Figure 5.5 Incorrectly contrasted training (too fast on lower-intensity days, too tired to do speedwork on Tuesday and Thursday)

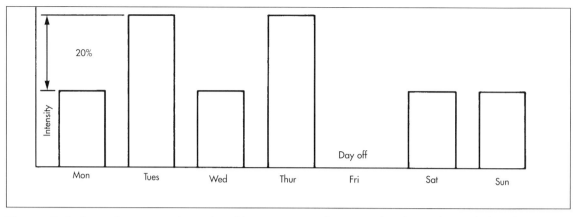

Figure 5.6 Correctly contrasted speed and lower-intensity days (speedwork Tuesday and Thursday)

♦ Racing during training ♦ periods and racing a race series

Choose your races

Do not race all the time. Racing should be used for peak performances or to set up a peak performance. Racing all season will reduce your base (you won't be able to maintain mileage), flatten you physically, and will throw water on your 'competitive fires', making it very difficult to get psyched up for a race. It may also lead to burn-out. Besides all that, racing is supposed to be fun and special. It will be neither if you race every weekend.

Race priority

Prioritise your race goals. Pick the main race or races you want to peak for and make them top priority. Over a year you may have between one and six 'high-priority' races (usually one to four) where peak performance is vital, for example national champs, club champs and race series. These races should be evenly spaced (every six to eight weeks) to allow recovery and to build towards race peak (*see* fig. 5.7, page 69), or they can be grouped close together (every two to three weeks) –'clumping' – with recovery after this sustained peak. Prioritising races in this way enables you to build low-priority races into the speed phase. These will help you to race yourself into shape. Low-priority races should come before the major peak in the speed phase.

'Super-priority' events such as major international or national races override all other races during the year. There is generally only one 'super-priority' race a year, although some athletes may choose to have only one super-priority race (or race series) every four years to coincide with the Olympics.

Number of high-priority races to focus on per year

Level	Race priority		
	Super	High	Low
Novice	1	—	2–6
Intermediate	1	1–2	2–8
Elite	1	1–3	2–10

Number of races to peak for per year

1–3 hour race

Level	100% peak	90–95% peak
Novice	1	2–3
Intermediate	1–2	3–4
Elite	1–2	4–6

4 hour+ race

Level	100% peak	90–95% peak
Novice	1	1–2
Intermediate	1	1–2
Elite	1–2	2–4

Racing during training periods

The correct placing of races during training periods (base, speed) is vital to ensure that peaking is achieved and broader training objectives are not compromised. During the base period, racing should be kept to a minimum. Too much racing at this time may see you peaking too soon or overtraining and burning out. Nevertheless, one or two races during base are good for motivation and break up the routine a bit – a change is as good as a rest, as they say. Any racing during base training should be done towards the middle or end of base to lessen the chance of injury. But don't expect great results. You haven't done speedwork yet! If you do not want to race during base, it will not harm your build-up.

During the speed phase, warm-up races are important as they prepare you for the high-priority races you have planned. A warm-up race or two before your priority races is a good way of adjusting to the racing environment. If your highest priority race is a 10 km, then some 5 to 10 km races at race pace (or close to it) will help you get used to a combination of race pace and distance. Running a 21 km event in preparation for a 10 km race is not effective, however. When choosing races to use as speedwork, be race specific. For long races, such as half-marathons, choose warm-up races that are long enough to simulate race pace. For a half-marathon, 15 km or 10 miles is a good distance to test yourself over.

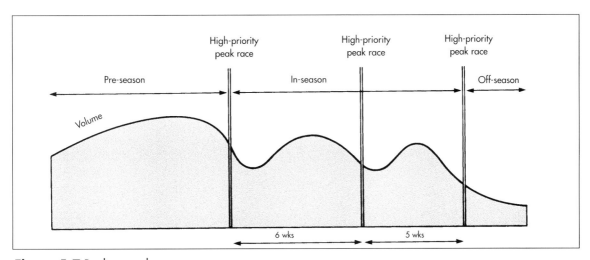

Figure 5.7 Peak race placement

When should you race? Racing too long before your peak race can mean your form is good too early. Racing too near your peak race may mean you don't recover in time for the big day. The optimal racing period starts six to eight weeks out from your high-priority race. How many races you have in this period depends on the distance of your peak race. But generally, two or three races are enough, with the last one likely to be between two and four weeks before the peak race.

Try to space your races during speedwork so as not to get too tired: race every two weeks if you are an intermediate/elite competitor; every three weeks if you are a novice. A good example of spacing low-priority races would be to race the second, fourth and sixth weeks out from a peak race (*see* fig. 5.8).

Some people find racing the week before a peak race very effective, though it depends a great deal on race distances. The longer the race, the longer the gap between your last warm-up race and your peak race. Here's a guide to how soon before your peak race you should have your last warm-up race.

- Ironman: At least 3–6 weeks (for a Half-Ironman it should be less)
- Standard triathlon/duathlon: At least 2–3 weeks (a standard or sprint race is fine)
- Rowing: 5 days to 2 weeks
- Cycle (road race): 2–3 weeks (depending on race length)
- Cycle (tour): 2–3 weeks
- Mountain biking: 2–3 weeks (depending on race distance)
- Multisport: 2–4 weeks depending on race distance (half distance or less for races over 6 hours)
- 10 km run: 2–4 weeks (remember, running is more damaging to the legs)
- Marathon: 4–6 weeks (for a half-marathon it should be less)

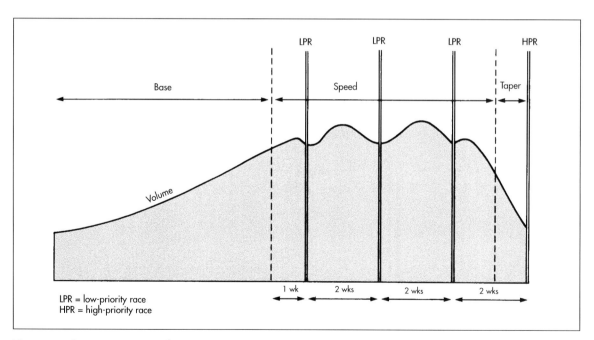

LPR = low-priority race
HPR = high-priority race

Figure 5.8 Warm-up race placement

For long races, warm-up races should be limited to a few, and these should be shorter than race distance. Each successive warm-up race should be closer to the race distance, for example when preparing for an Ironman, do a standard distance triathlon first, then a Half-Ironman. For shorter races (races under two hours for most of the sports dealt with in this book), limit your racing to a maximum of once every two weeks at the most.

It is important to remember that warm-up races are being used to bring you to a racing peak. Therefore, do not thrash yourself into the ground during these races (but still go for it). Just let your body gradually adapt to the stress of racing. Don't expect peak performances in these warm-up races and make sure you recover properly after each one.

During a race series, it is often vital to peak at the end of the series (when more points are often up for grabs). Again, try not to peak too early in the series (*see* 'Racing in a race series' below).

Finally, *never race* during taper or during the off-season!

Racing in a race series

When training for a race series, the idea is to hold a consistently high level of performance over a period of time. This means holding a *competitive peak* rather than a full peak. A full or absolute peak (100 per cent potential) cannot be held for longer than a week or two, so a slightly lower, more sustainable 'competitive' peak (95 per cent potential) is needed for a race series lasting longer than this. What you are trying to do is hold performance at the top of the performance arc (*see* fig. 5.9), although it is really a series of mini

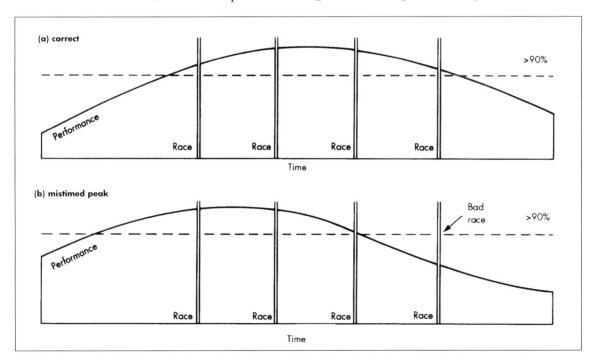

Figure 5.9 Timing peak performances over a series of races

peaks and troughs in performance. The arc equates to you coming into top form, holding it, and then losing form. Remember: you cannot hold a peak indefinitely. Therefore, don't peak too early or you will reach the top of the performance arc too soon. This means holding off on speedwork longer than you would if you were aiming at a full peak.

If you have a very long race series (more than eight to ten weeks) and you don't feel you can hold a high performance for that long, you may need to ease off in the middle of the racing season and build up again. This would give you a performance arc with twin peaks. This approach is particularly useful if during a series only a certain number of races count. You can then have your higher peaks coinciding with selected races and a rest in the middle (*see* fig. 5.10.)

◆ Tapering for races ◆

Tapering involves a gradual reduction in training volume (duration/distance) in the lead-up to a race. Intensity, however, is generally maintained virtually until race day because, as mentioned earlier, your body has a bad memory for speed – it quickly forgets how to go fast! Recovery during tapering can either be partial or full, depending on the priority of the race. Only when fully rested (for a high-priority race) are you able to fulfil your racing potential.

Most tapers involve a 40 to 60 per cent reduction in peak training volumes in the final week before competition. The last week, especially, involves low volumes and little speedwork. The intensity of that speedwork,

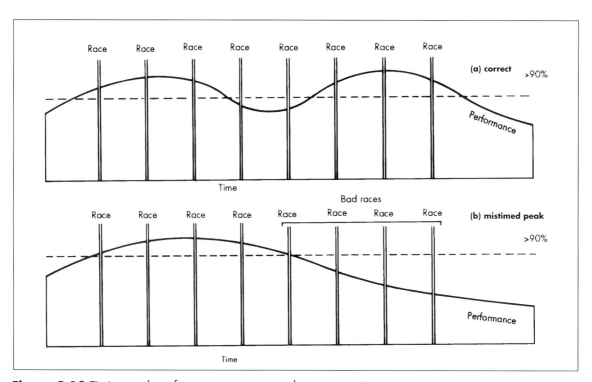

Figure 5.10 Timing peak performances over a very long race series

however, is maintained. In the last two to four days, there is little or no training, and any training is low-intensity. This is the time to rest (that four-letter word so many athletes hate!). The final week before a race can be a good time to work on technique; for example a triathlete may focus on transitions.

The general rule with tapering is the longer the race, the longer the taper. Rowing, standard distance triathlons and duathlons, half-marathons or shorter runs, and many mountain bike races, require a four- to seven-day taper. Marathons require ten days. In the case of ultra distance, single-day races, and multiple-day races, the taper will start ten to fourteen days before competition. Tapers for these events require a large reduction in training volume.

The length of the taper is also determined by how much stress the training puts on your body (particularly muscular stress). In terms of training stress, running is highest, followed by rowing and cycling, followed by kayaking and swimming. Taper length should reflect this.

You also have to allow for individual differences in recovery rate. Different tapers suit different athletes. As a rule, less experienced competitors need longer tapers than 'seasoned' athletes. In a nutshell, a good taper will get you and your body to the startline fresh and ready for action.

Basic taper examples (days)

Race duration	Elite	Intermediate	Novice
5 hr+ race	8–10	10–12	12–14
3–6 hr race	6–8	7–9	8–10
2–3 hr race	4–5	5–6	6–7
6 min–1 hr race	4–5	5–6	6–7

Specific examples of taper lengths

Here are some basic guidelines on how long (days) to taper for various races. The rule of thumb is that the more experienced you are the shorter your taper (within the range indicated).

Run	
10 km	4–7
Half–marathon	5–8
Marathon	8–12

Triathlon	
Sprint	4–5
Olympic	5–7
Half–Ironman	7–10
Ironman	10–14

Multisport	
< 3 hrs	4–5
3–5 hrs	5–8
5–7 hrs	8–10
7 hrs+	10–14

Rowing	
2000 m	4–5

Mountain biking	
< 3 hrs	4–5
3–5 hrs	5–8
5 hrs+	8–10

Cycling	
40 km	4–5
80 km	5–8
160 km	8–10
Tour	10–14

Duathlon	
Run 10 km / Bike 60 km / Run 10 km	5–8
Run 5 km / Bike 40 km / Run 5 km	4–5

Taper in, taper out

Now that you have an understanding of the whys and hows of tapering before an event (tapering in), let's look at an idea few athletes seem to have grasped – the importance of tapering after an event to recover (tapering out).

Tapering out of an event means progressively increasing training in the period following a race. As with tapering in, the longer the race, the longer the tapering out should be. In addition, the higher the priority of the race, the longer the taper.

Some examples of tapering out (post-race recovery)

Sport	Low priority	High priority
Standard triathlon or duathlon	2–4 days	2 weeks plus
Ironman triathlon		4–8 weeks plus
Cycle road race (80–160 km)	4–7 days	2–4 weeks plus
Cycle tour	4–7 days	2–4 weeks plus
Mountain bike race	2–4 days	2 weeks plus
Multisport (short)	2–4 days	2 weeks plus
Multisport (long)		4–8 weeks
Rowing	2–4 days	2 weeks plus
Marathon	1–3 weeks	4–8 weeks plus
Half–marathon	1–2 weeks	2–4 weeks
10 km run	7–10 days	2–4 weeks plus

♦ Peaking ♦

Correct training + correct timing = peaking

The key to top performance is being able to peak effectively. Most athletes, particularly inexperienced ones, tend to reach very good racing form, but do not peak fully. And there is a big difference between good form and peak form. (At a world champs that difference may mean finishing tenth instead of first!)

Base and speed phases, and warm-up races, are all deliberately set around a high-priority race or races so that you reach peak and perform at your best on the day or days that matter. Peaking encompasses all facets of training. Important points for peaking:

- Correct structure of programme
- Specificity of programme
- Applicability to athlete
- Elimination of training errors (too much, too little, too fast, too slow)
- Timing of the programme (too early, too late)
- Correct programme balance (work/rest, sport vs sport, workout requirement vs workout requirement, training frequency)
- Understand your training
- Analysis of training

If you take all these key points into account, you will achieve a peak performance on the right day. And as you get more experienced, your ability to peak will improve as you learn to refine your training.

Peak too early or too late, and you will race slow. Remember, a true peak brings all facets of training together at precisely one time. Most athletes manage to bring most facets together and some athletes none. By manipulating the principles above, you will be able to bring all facets of training together and maximise performance whenever you need to. Remember, peaking is rather like walking a tightrope – a matter of balance.

◆ The big mistakes ◆

Big Mistake Number One: Too much, too early

Training is not only about hard work, it is also about timing. Doing too much too early can have an adverse effect on performance. Many endurance athletes start doing their high-volume work way too early in their build-up. It's often a confidence problem – 'Can I go the distance?' They then try and hold those volumes for too long. This leads to cumulative fatigue and a slow deterioration in performance (sound familiar?). Try and hold the high-volume work back as long as practically possible. Otherwise you will peak too early and by the time race day rolls around you will probably be as 'flat' as the proverbial pancake.

Big Mistake Number Two: Too fast, too early

A whole smorgasbord of mistakes could be listed here. Some of them are:

- Way too fast, too early – within a short period of time (days to weeks) you will most likely be ill or injured.
- Too fast, too early – within a moderately short time (several weeks to months) you will probably be overtrained, ill or injured.
- A little too fast, too early – you will peak too early (probably by a few weeks).

Big Mistake Number Three: Too much speedwork

For endurance athletes, speedwork makes up only a very small percentage of the total training volume. Endurance athletes not only can't do speedwork every day (it's too tiring), they don't need to. During the speed phase, speedwork should only be done one to three times per week, depending on your experience (novices, one; advanced, two; elite, three). Speedwork may only account for 5 to 15 per cent of training volume (novices, 5 per cent; advanced, 10 per cent; elite, 15 per cent). Too much speedwork can destroy a good build-up. You end up exhausted.

Big Mistake Number Four: Too much racing, too long an in-season

Racing week after week for long periods of time will not, generally, improve performance. Instead, you end up tired. Set up your racing schedule so that 'peak' races and 'lead-up' races are clearly defined. Use the lead-up races as an opportunity to get in shape for the 'big one'. Spending more than eight to twelve weeks (novices, eight; advanced, ten; elite, twelve) racing at one time can also harm performance as it is difficult to sustain both a physical and psychological peak for that long. Some people can naturally cope with more than others. You can be an elite athlete and still be a 'one peak wonder' (one peak per season).

Big Mistake Number Five: Too much effort in base before speedwork

Base is used to increase recovery rate and tolerance to training to prepare you for speedwork. Base doesn't actually make you go fast. You need speedwork for that. Base will make you fit enough to complete the race. A lot of athletes either don't do speedwork, which means a fit but slow athlete in competition, or they train so hard that they are too mentally and physically fatigued to endure the rigours of speedwork. The result is poor quality speedwork, and since speedwork is what makes you fast you end up with performances below peak potential. It's also a waste of a lot of hard work in base. Don't 'hammer' yourself in base, and do good quality speedwork (*see* fig. 5.11).

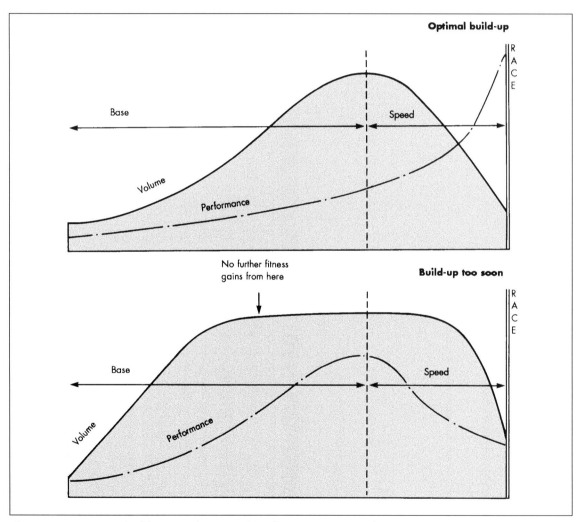

Figure 5.11 Timing build-up to achieve peak performance on race day

Big Mistake Number Six:
No speedwork in taper

Tapering is all about recovery. You must taper off your training volumes just before racing to be fully recovered and race at your best. Most athletes get the tapering of training volumes right but also stop doing speedwork. Your body has a great memory for training volumes, but a bad memory for speed. If you stop doing speedwork your body will quickly lose the speed you worked so hard to improve. Therefore, even in your taper, training volumes gradually reduce but you must still do some small quantity of speedwork to retain your speed. No speedwork in your taper will usually result in a small loss of speed on race day.

Chapter 6

Fundamentals that Aid Training and Performance

Warming up and warming down are an extremely important part of each workout. The format for warming up/warming down should look like this:

warm- → stretch→ workout → warm- → stretch
up   down

Warm-up

Warm-ups are aimed at gradually bringing the body up to the exercise pace/intensity level at which you will be training. For instance, a warm-up for intervals will involve a longer warm-up, gradually building to interval intensity, than a warm-up for a long slow distance workout. Warm-ups prepare you for exercise, reduce the chance of injury and increase the effectiveness of the workout (particularly for higher intensity workouts). The main goals of the warm-up are to increase muscle temperature, metabolic rate, blood flow and lubrication of joints, and to improve muscle contractile capacity. Here are some of the benefits of a good warm-up.

1 Muscle temperature increases, resulting in:

- the muscle contracting more forcefully;
- the muscle relaxing more quickly;
- speed and strength enhancement.

2 The blood temperature increases as blood flows through the warmed-up muscle. This also makes more oxygen available to the muscle.

3 Hormonal changes occur, resulting in:

- a greater production of hormones responsible for regulating energy production;
- more carbohydrate and fatty acids being made available for energy production.

4 The metabolic rate increases, which improves the body's ability to process energy.

The higher the training intensity of a workout, the longer the warm-up should be, for instance 15 to 20 minutes for intervals, 20 to 30 minutes for races. Breaking out in a sweat means that your warm-up is satisfactory as it indicates that you have raised your body's internal temperature. Stretching should follow the warm-up (*see* below).

Warm-ups and tiredness
If you have difficulty during the warm-up and workout in reaching your normal steady state heart rate, or you feel very heavy legged, this could indicate tiredness; for example, you may experience leg fatigue in your intervals if you are a runner or cyclist. If you can't reach your heart rate in the warm-up you should either go home and rest or continue with a short, active recovery (very low-intensity) workout.

Warm-up stretches

Stretches during warm-up increase your range of movement, thereby allowing you to work out optimally. Stretching can also help prevent injury. Stretches should be specific to the workout. Lack of flexibility can result in inefficient movement, causing loss of speed and poor technique.

Each stretch should be performed in a slow, controlled manner. Move slowly into the stretch until the *first sensation* of a stretch is felt – any more tension in the stretch can cause muscle overstretching which results in muscle tightening rather than loosening. You should not bounce during the stretch, and no sudden, jerky movements are advised as both can cause injury. Hold each stretch for ten to fifteen seconds (less is not really beneficial) and try to fully relax the muscle being stretched, and the surrounding muscles.

Be sensitive to tension in the muscle as this will determine how many repetitions you should perform. This also acts as a guide to improvements in your stretching and prevents overstretching. Be aware of any flexibility imbalances between left and right limbs. Emphasise the less flexible side until balance is achieved. And note that more stretching and a longer warm-up will be required in the morning as you will generally be less flexible at this time of the day.

Warm-down

A warm-down is a drop in exercise intensity designed to promote recovery. It will help prevent blood pooling at your extremities, which can make you feel light-headed (common after speedwork). In a cyclist, for example, blood pools in the blood vessels in the legs and not enough returns to the heart. As a consequence, the heart beats faster in an attempt to increase blood flow. The result? You feel dizzy.

During a workout exercise-induced by-products are accumulated in the body and these affect performance in the following workouts. If you stop exercise cold, by-products remain in the body and removal will take much longer as your metabolic rate (the basic speed at which your body functions) drops to resting. Ideally, you should lower your training intensity to a light activity which does not stress the body, that is, does not produce further by-products. At low training intensities, exercise by-products are removed at a much faster rate as your metabolic rate is still higher than at rest. This will improve the rate of recovery, allowing for 'fresher' and more effective exercise in following workouts. The higher the training intensity used in the workout the longer the warm-down: for example 20 to 30 minutes for intervals and races.

Warming down after a race can take a lot of discipline – you'd often much rather have a drink, eat and talk – but get that warm-down done first!

Warm-down stretches

This is the best time to develop and improve your flexibility. Warm-down stretching should be targeted at the specific muscles used in the exercise just performed; for example, after a running workout stretch your running muscles. Most flexibility gains are made following exercise. Warm-down stretching is aimed more at improving performance than preventing injury. For example, hamstring (back of thigh) stretches could improve stride length for running which in some cases may improve speed.

For lazy stretchers

Some athletes do not like stretching. If you are one of those athletes, at least try and stretch up to three times per week rather than not at all (it might help to think about which you hate more: stretching or injuries!). It's best in this case to stretch before and after your shorter workouts, when you have more time and are less tired. Stretching is always more important in the warm-down than in the warm-up. If you decide to stretch only during warm-down, do a longer exercise warm-up before starting your workout.

'Carbo-up'

If you take in carbohydrates within 60 to 120 minutes of completing exercise, the body will recover much faster than if you didn't (and it'll love you for it!). In the first hour after exercise the body is in an energy-depleted state and if provided with carbohydrates it will 'supercompensate' for the loss of energy due to the workout. This means more energy can be taken in the first one to two hours after exercise than in following hours. This extra energy boosts recovery rate and therefore increases the effectiveness of the next workout. *See* chapter 12 for more on this.

◆ Racing tips ◆

Race warm-ups

Warming up for races involves 20 to 30 minutes of exercise in the sport you are about to race in. If you are racing in a multi-sport/triathlon type of race where two or more different sports are performed during the same race, warm up in each of them. This will not only allow you to warm up all race-specific muscle groups, but it will also allow you to check your equipment.

Always work backwards from the last sport to the first sport: for example, a triathlon warm-up should look like this: run, cycle,

swim. This is because you need to do the most thorough warm-up for the first event as in the following events you will already be warmed up extensively by each of the preceding disciplines (*see* fig. 6.1). If you start the first event cold it will take between 5 and 20 minutes of racing to warm up, which obviously affects your race performance – and you won't feel good either.

Race warm-ups should begin 20 to 30 minutes before the race start. Long races such as Ironman triathlons, where race intensity is moderately low and energy demand high, may not require a significant warm-up, especially when it's hot.

Start with about five minutes of light activity specific to the race, followed by about five minutes of easy specific stretches. Continue your warm-up after stretching with light activity, building gradually over five to ten minutes to race pace. You should spend up to five minutes at race pace to be fully warmed up. The intensity is then dropped back to light activity (for another five to ten minutes) to keep warm. This should continue until the race starts. Allow sufficient time for full recovery before the race begins.

Do not warm up too early as you will have to spend too long staying warm before the race starts. In fact, the closer the warm-up is to start time, with adequate recovery, the better. Spending 30 minutes warming up with several minutes at race pace will not harm your performance. If you are well conditioned, this should enhance your performance significantly. If you are doing a multisport/triathlon race, warm up with light activity in each discipline except for the sport you are to race in first. In that discipline, warm up to race pace and use it to stay warm before race start.

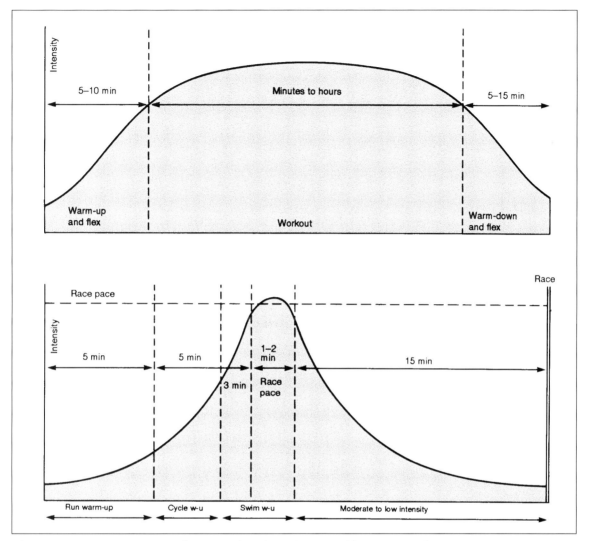

Figure 6.1 Warm-ups, warm-downs, and workouts (top); triathlon warm-up (bottom)

Psych-ups and psych-outs

If warming up near where the race starts, with all the pre-race hype, gets you psyched up to race, always arrive early and warm up in the race atmosphere. However, if this psychs you out, or makes you nervous, arrive early at the race site and obtain all the race information you need, then go off and warm up away from the race hype and come back just before the gun.

If you don't know the course, try to get a car and check out the whole course before you warm up. This will help you see what is required in terms of equipment, and it will also help with tactics and pace judgement.

81

Knowledge of the course is particularly crucial if you are planning to be in or near the front! It is obviously better to train over the course if you can, but this isn't always possible.

The week following the race

Most athletes try to continue their standard workouts in the week following a race. This is a big mistake. A race stresses the body considerably and the following week should be a recovery week (at least in part), with less mileage and low-intensity training.

A day off or one of very light activity is best the day after a race, with a gradual build-up back to your normal training regime over the next one to five days, depending on your conditioning and race distance/intensity. Longer races, such as an Ironman or marathon, may need to be followed by two or three weeks of light activity.

If you have raced for over 20 minutes there should be no speedwork in the week following a race, or at least not until late in the week. Don't forget that a race is speedwork. More experienced athletes will recover faster and therefore will be able to start doing their speedwork earlier than less experienced athletes.

If you have muscle soreness following a race, exercise lightly, at a very low intensity, with no muscle stress on the sore muscles. Exercise in a low-impact and fluid form of exercise, for instance, if you have just done a triathlon, don't run with muscle soreness – swim or cycle gently for a short period.

♦ Missing workouts ♦

In almost every build-up you will miss workouts and training days due to overtiredness or lack of time. This is normal and an expected part of training. An athlete generally misses up to four days/workouts per month, over and above prescribed days off. This varies depending on the individual, but missing workouts is a fact of training life and nothing to get concerned about. If you miss a day unexpectedly, never try to catch up the missed mileage the following day, or do extra on your day off. If a workout is missed, it is gone! It is better to look at a missed day in a positive way – it is both a physical and mental day off. It is a day where your body rests, recovers and improves. Trying to catch up mileage destroys the balance (exercise versus recovery) of the programme and may lead to excessive fatigue and extended negative effects on your training programme.

Listen to your body. If you feel tired, adjust your training to take this into account. Trying to do prescribed mileage in a fatigued state is of no benefit whatsoever. Put another way, resting for a day because of fatigue may mean only one day of training is affected. However, trying to do the workout despite fatigue may affect several days or even weeks of training, with far greater potential for overtraining. Think about it: what would you rather have? One day off or one week off? Now, that's a no-brainer!

If you miss three or four days in a row through tiredness or lack of enthusiasm for training, then it is likely that total mileage or speedwork is too excessive. If not quickly reduced or adjusted, overtraining may occur.

Monitoring your fatigue levels is always the most important guide to training. Listen to your body first, then listen to your coach or follow your programme.

♦ Flexibility and ♦ stretching

The accepted reason for stretching is primarily injury prevention through greater flexibility. However, a more important reason for stretching is to improve performance through an increased range of motion and a reduction in fatigue (loose muscles don't fight against each other). Loose muscles contract/relax faster and technique work can be performed more accurately with no limitations due to inflexibility. Flexible muscles also recover more quickly as they suffer less exercise trauma and damage, and have a better blood flow.

Good flexibility is thus an important factor in sports performance. Of course, flexibility varies widely between individuals, but most athletes can benefit from being more flexible than they are. And there's nothing worse than failing to finish an event because of muscle tightness, such as a sore back in rowing, cycling or kayaking.

Muscle imbalances, for example, where the left hamstring is tighter than the right, can also harm performance and may lead to injury if not dealt with.

Either assess your own flexibility while doing your stretching – you may feel tight in a specific area or one limb/side – or get your flexibility checked by a fitness testing lab.

Types of stretching

Static
- Slow, held stretching. The joint is taken to a certain point and held. This form of stretching is particularly recommended.
- PNF (proprioceptive neuromuscular facilitation) stretching is static stretching, but the joint is taken to a point where a mild stretch is felt and then you contract the muscle against the direction of the stretch. The

contraction is held for five to ten seconds. The muscle will then be able to be moved through a greater range of motion. This technique is continued until no further movement gains are made for the stretch. PNF is particularly useful for inflexible athletes.

Dynamic
Through forceful movement, the joint/ muscle is taken through a greater range of motion than it can normally achieve, for example a high, straight leg kick to stretch the hamstring.

How to stretch

1 Always do a warm-up and warm-down. Don't try and hurry your stretching.

2 You don't have to stretch every muscle every time you stretch (good news if you don't enjoy stretching). Do the stretches that are most specific to the workout. If you need to do a lot of stretches for a particular area, do these in the warm-up and warm-down, with the key area getting the most attention in the warm-down. Split the other stretches between the warm-up and warm-down.

3 Make time to stretch! Many athletes use lack of time as an excuse not to stretch. You're better off cutting your workout by five minutes at each end and stretching, than risking injury/poor training performance because you're tight.

4 When stretching, concentrate on technique. Understand where you feel the stretch and aim to reproduce it over and over. As you become more experienced with your stretching you will find that simply assuming a stretching position may not be enough to add to your flexibility. You will then need to look carefully at technique and at fully relaxing the stretched muscle.

5 Move into all stretches slowly and be sensitive to the tension being placed on the stretched muscle. You should slowly move into the stretch until you feel the first sign of comfortable mild tension in the muscle. Hold this for 10 to 15 seconds.

6 Stretching will be enhanced if you are relaxed. Relax not only the muscle groups you are stretching, but your entire body. Stay loose! Stretching is also enhanced if you visualise the muscle being slowly stretched. Imagine you can look inside your leg or arm and see the muscle slowly being stretched out. You may even want to imagine it as a piece of chewing gum or putty. See and feel the muscle slowly and gently being stretched. It's a great feeling!

7 Your muscles are protected by a 'stretch reflex'. This means that if you overstretch a muscle by bouncing or pushing the muscle past its natural elastic capabilities the muscle's reflex response is to contract (tighten). This contraction stops you from stretching to the point where serious damage could be done.

If you are already very tight in an area, be particularly careful, as overstretching this area will see the muscle contract and get very tight. This may lead to pain and/or injury through microscopic tears in the muscle fibres. These tears can form scar tissue on the muscle and may decrease muscle elasticity. This also occurs if you begin vigorous activity without first warming up. Overstretching actually increases the tightness of the muscle you are trying to loosen!

8 The limb you are stretching should not be shaking due to excessive muscle tension. Don't 'bounce' – controlled movements only.

9 Never try a new stretch before a race! Stick to those you have been doing regularly. A new stretch at this late stage only invites injury or soreness.

10 Be careful stretching during exercise. Generally, your perception of pain drops during exercise so there is a danger you may overstretch without realising you're doing so.

11 Finally, when it comes to stretching, the 'No Pain, No Gain' philosophy *does not apply*. Stretching can improve performance, prevent injury and make your movements more fluid. But only if it is done slowly and gently. A more flexible, supple body is worth working for, but remember that overstretching can be as ineffective as understretching. Bottom line: if you don't relax when you stretch, your flexibility will not improve.

See appendix 11 for stretching exercises.

♦ Strength and strength ♦ training

Strength is defined as the ability of a muscle group to exert maximal contractile force against a resistance. It is widely regarded as the foundation of speed and endurance. Strength tests on elite endurance athletes appear to indicate that standard gymnasium strength training may not significantly improve performance. Nevertheless, there are many athletes (novice to elite) who will claim that strength training has helped their performance.

Despite this, strength training does appear better suited to short distance, 'explosive' sports, such as rowing, track riding and sprinting, than to endurance oriented sports like marathons, tour cycling, and Ironman. The best answer is to try strength training for yourself and see if it benefits you. Young athletes should approach strength training with care as it can be harmful, although lighter sport-specific strength training during a workout or use of light weights at high reps is possible.

If you do use strength training, make sure you do it correctly. An important aspect is timing – it should be done early in the build-up, preferably in Base 1 or even in the off-season. This is because strength training will severely fatigue the strength-trained muscles and this in turn will have a major effect on your ability to complete training mileages. In Base 2, as training becomes more sport-specific, strength training is generally discontinued or greatly reduced, for example once or twice a week instead of three or four times, or it may be restricted to a particular body area; a cyclist may continue to work on upper body in Base 2, for example.

As a rule, the shorter and more explosive the race distance, the more strength and bulk training required. Athletes competing in short races will do anywhere from 1 to 12 reps depending on what they are trying to achieve; those competing in longer races, if doing strength training, will do about 12 to 20 reps in order to increase strength endurance without significantly increasing body weight.

Correctly done, strength training should strengthen the muscles that you will use in your sport *in the same way they will be used in the sport*. This is a key consideration for it appears that strength and power training must simulate not only the movement and specific range of motion, but also the speed of movement if it is to enhance performance. For example, leg extensions are not nearly as effective as the leg press as a form of strength training for cyclists and rowers. If strength training is to be successful, it must be very specific.

The main problem with weight training is that it is difficult to mimic sport-specific movements precisely. For that reason, and because it is better suited to short, explosive events, strength training is of limited value for triathlon, duathlon, multisport, distance running and mountain biking. Rowers and track cyclists will get some value from strength training, however. If you decide to include strength training in your programme, do it in addition to your sport-specific sessions, not instead of one.

Of course, strength training doesn't have to be done in a gym or with weight equipment. Strength, or more accurately, high level muscle endurance (strength endurance), can be improved in a sport-specific manner by increasing the resistance or workload while doing the sport. For example:

Swimming
- Isokinetic swim bench
- Pull buoy (arms only)
- Kick sets (legs only with kick board)
- Paddles
- One arm only
- Swim tether

Time trial cycling for triathletes, multisporters, mountain bikers, cyclists
- Hills, low-intensity
- Riding into a headwind
- Stationary bike, high load
- Riding flats in big gears
- Riding hills in big gears

Cyclists and multisporters who do bike races (racing in a bunch)
- Hill sprints, intervals, power sprints
- Plyometrics (flat and incline bounding, no bike!)
- Riding hills/flats in big gears

Running
- Hills, low-intensity
- Hill intervals
- Running in soft sand
- Running in water (wading)

Rowing
- Pair oar rowing
- Slow stroke rate (18 to 22) full pressure
- One-armed rowing
- Rope tow
- Bungy attached around hull for drag

Kayaking
- Slow paddle rate at full pressure
- Bungy attached around hull for drag

Resistance training using cables attached to weights and the use of bungy cords can also be very effective as they allow you to mimic your sport's specific movement more closely than standard weightlifting equipment. To avoid injury, it is necessary to adapt gradually to these types of high-resistance training. It is also important to train as specifically as possible.

As with your overall training programme, strength training should be built around periodisation. There are specific phases in strength training that will lead to peak competitive performance.

Strength training programmes should change at least every eight weeks to restimulate neural activity in the trained muscle. After eight weeks on the same programme improvement gains are greatly reduced as a result of your body's adaptation to the type of strength training you have been doing. A plateau in improvement will tend to occur at this point. It is therefore necessary to change the programme in order to stress your trained muscles in slightly different ways. But do not waste your time on extra exercises that are of no practical benefit; if they're not specific enough to aid your performance, don't do them! Many strength training programmes have a lot of impractical exercises in them. These waste time and energy, both precious commodities for an endurance athlete. Remember that you do not need to be at a gym for two hours to benefit. Twenty minutes on several specific exercises may be as effective as or more effective than spending hours on exercises that are not specific to your sport.

Split routine programmes (strength programmes broken into several parts which are done on different days) are not as effective for endurance athletes as single routine programmes. Split routines, favoured by bodybuilders, would require between four and six workouts a week. This is an inefficient use of time and energy for an endurance athlete since specific training also needs to be done during the week.

Here is a basic guide to strength training repetitions, sets and recovery periods:

Training loading required	% 1RM outcome	Rep range	No. of sets	Rest between sets
Very light power	30–60	15–25	3	To recovery
Light muscular endurance (short, intermediate and long)	<70	12–20+ (up to 200)	2–3	20–30 sec
Moderate hypertrophy (muscle bulking)	70–80	8–12	8–12	30–90 sec
Heavy strength (very little bulking)	80–100	1–8	3–5+	2–5 min

Key: 1RM = one repetition maximum – the heaviest weight that the athlete can lift only once for an exercise.

Unless you require strength training for a specific reason (for example, if you are a track cyclist), use the light schedule in the off-season and early pre-season only. If you are doing 'true' strength training (moderate to heavy) for a particular reason, maximal strength gains will only be established if you pay close attention to technique. Always warm up well for strength training and watch the order of your exercises, as pre-exhaustion exercises can be very useful. Avoid any hard aerobic workouts following 'true' strength workouts as this causes too much muscle fibre damage (micro tears in the muscle fibres as a result of strength training need time to repair). The rest period should be greatest between the strength workout and the following aerobic workout. For example, your programme early in Base 1 could be:

Mon	Tue	Wed	Thu	Fri	Sat	Sun
p.m.	p.m.	D/O	a.m.	a.m.	p.m.	a.m.
SP	ST		SP	ST	SP	ST

Key: SP = sport; ST = strength.

This programme allows long rests after strength training and before sport-specific training, when recovery is very important, and shorter rests after sport training. Contrasting workouts are also alternated in a microcycle to maximise recovery. A mesocycle format is also used.

The next decision to make involves the type of equipment to be used. Free weights or machines? Again, the so-called experts can't seem to agree. A combination of the two is probably best. Don't forget to use sport-specific exercises during workouts and use bungees (elastic or stretch cords) or pulleys. A recommended order of strength training for rowers and track cyclists is:

1 Light/machines: basic conditioning, 2–4 weeks
2 Moderate/machines: strength, 4 weeks
3 Heavy/free weights/machines: strength, 4–8 weeks
4 Light: muscle endurance; and heavy: strength maintenance, 4 weeks
5 Very light: power, 4–6 weeks

There is a great deal written on strength training and it is beyond the scope of this book to summarise it all. Follow the guidelines outlined above and if you feel the need to investigate further, buy a good book (*see* Bibliography) or see a reputable coach or strength training consultant.

♦ Fitness testing ♦

While fitness testing cannot measure performance itself – only racing can do that! – it can measure certain variables related to performance. Indeed, thorough fitness testing allows an athlete to pinpoint accurately any weaknesses (for example low aerobic capacity, poor flexibility) that may exist, without having to go through the drama of racing or the frustration of injury. In other words, fitness testing allows you to fine tune your training and race preparation by ensuring all factors contributing to performance have been addressed in a systematic and specific way.

Physiological exercise testing

1 VO_2max

In order to exercise, your body needs a supply of energy. This energy comes from the breakdown of the body's carbohydrate (glycogen) and fat stores. If exercising for more than two to three minutes continuously, that energy will be supplied aerobically, or with oxygen. Of course, the more oxygen you can consume (and supply to the working muscles), the greater your energy supply, the longer you can keep exercising, and, theoretically, the fitter you are.

But what is VO₂max?

As you exercise more intensely (harder, faster), the body's need for energy increases. Initially you will be able to meet this increasing need by simply consuming more oxygen (breathing harder or more deeply). Eventually, though, as the exercise intensity keeps rising, and the minutes tick by, you will reach a point where you are consuming as much oxygen as you can. And no matter how hard you try (or how hard you breathe), you are unable to get more oxygen into your lungs. At this point you have reached your VO_2max. In other words, VO_2max provides a measure of the maximum (max) volume (V) of oxygen (O_2) you can consume during physical activity.

Generally, the higher your VO_2max, the higher your aerobic fitness and the greater your endurance potential. (Incidentally, your VO_2max potential is largely, though not wholly, inherited. So you can blame or thank your parents, as the case may be.)

By expressing VO_2max as a function of weight it is possible to make comparisons between athletes as to their aerobic potential, remembering that larger athletes generally will be able to consume, in absolute terms, more oxygen than their smaller colleagues.

How do you calculate VO₂ max?

To get a VO_2max score that can be compared to another you divide the maximum volume of oxygen that the athlete can consume in millilitres per minute (ml/min) by body weight in kilograms (kg). For example: A 70 kg athlete may consume 4500 ml O_2/min. By dividing 4500 by 70 you get a VO_2max score of 64 ml O_2/kg/min. By comparison, an 80 kg athlete with the same oxygen consumption (4500 ml O_2/min) would rate a much

lower VO_2max score of 56. This is because the larger athlete must distribute the same volume of oxygen around a larger body mass. As a result, the larger athlete potentially has less aerobic power.

Top male athletes generally have VO_2max scores of around 70–85; top female athletes 60–75. Women average slightly lower VO_2max scores than men because of their naturally higher body fat percentage, smaller muscle mass, lower oxygen binding capacity in the blood, and less powerful muscles.

Despite the strong hereditary influence on VO_2max, it can be increased through training, but only to a limited degree: about 20 to 30 per cent. The good news is that VO_2max is not the only indicator of performance. Indeed, world class athletes with almost identical VO_2max scores show a surprisingly wide range of times.

Initial physiological testing can determine your fitness level and your athletic potential or endurance ability. With a series of tests spread out over months and years, fitness levels (via VO_2max) can be reassessed frequently, giving an indication of the effectiveness of training. VO_2max can be tested directly (by gas analysis) or indirectly (using heart rate). Direct measurements, which are reputed to be more accurate, involve a progressive increase in load until you reach temporary exhaustion (maximal exercise). Indirect VO_2max testing is submaximal (you do not exercise to exhaustion). VO_2max is sometimes expressed as a final workload (in watts) reached during testing. In all forms of VO_2max testing a far more accurate score is recorded if the exercise closely mimics your sport; cyclists, for example, should be tested on a bike ergometer or preferably on their own bike, and runners on a treadmill. VO_2max scores and, therefore, aerobic ability, vary from sport to sport, so if you have more than one discipline in your sport it is best to be tested in each discipline.

While VO_2max gives a measure of maximum oxygen uptake, it doesn't tell you how efficiently you are using that oxygen. To use a motoring analogy, a VO_2max score tells you how big your petrol tank is, but it doesn't tell you how many miles per gallon you get. How economical are you to run? Exercise or oxygen economy (efficiency of oxygen used at a given speed) is now being used more and more as an indicator of elite athletes' performance abilities. Clearly, an endurance athlete who uses oxygen very efficiently will have an advantage over someone who does not.

Oxygen economy, which can be improved slightly through training, is tested by gas analysis or by heart rate, and can be expressed as a level of oxygen consumption or heart rate at a particular pace. It is represented by a 'flattening' on a graph of heart rate versus time/load. Obviously, exercise economy can also be affected by equipment, weather, physical readiness, and so on. In cycling, drafting, rolling resistance, fluidity of moving parts (hub, bottom bracket, pedal, axle), equipment set-up, hull shape, weight of equipment, and aerodynamics will affect exercise economy and, therefore, performance.

See appendix 2 for a basic VO_2max test.

2 *Maximum heart rate*
Maximum heart rate is the highest heart rate you can achieve. This occurs during maximum effort. True maximum heart rate usually occurs at around VO_2max, although during VO_2max testing, leg fatigue accumulated during the test can result in a slightly underestimated maximum heart rate; approximately five to ten beats below true maximum (*see* page 27 for a way to determine maximum heart rate without lab testing).

Maximum heart rate can be used to predict anaerobic threshold heart rate and other intensities. However, it is more accurate to obtain anaerobic threshold (AT) heart rate through testing (*see* below). AT heart rate can change over a matter of weeks. Using calculations based on maximum heart rate (such as 220 minus age) to predict AT pace may not be entirely accurate.

3 *'Anaerobic threshold' intensity and corresponding heart rate*
Firstly, it needs to be said that the term 'anaerobic threshold' is not wholly accepted by sport scientists. Instead, they use the terms 'ventilatory threshold', 'lactate threshold', and 'onset of blood lactate accumulation'. All are basically ways of determining maximum steady state pace, which, incidentally, can vary considerably depending on a number of factors. The reason for the sport scientists' dislike of the term 'anaerobic threshold' is that there is no absolute threshold between aerobic and anaerobic exercise. There is simply a zone where the body moves from predominantly using the aerobic energy system to predominantly using the anaerobic energy system.

Nevertheless, for practical purposes, anaerobic threshold (AT) is still a useful concept for discussing maximum steady state training and racing. AT is still the most recognisable and widely used term and it adequately describes the transition zone from aerobic exercise (with oxygen supplying the energy to continue for a long time) to anaerobic exercise (without oxygen, e.g. sprinting), where the pace cannot be sustained for very long at all. AT is basically the maximum pace you can sustain for around one hour.

AT can be tested both in the laboratory and in the field, using direct gas analysis testing, indirect heart rate tests (Conconi test) or through lactate testing. The last involves taking blood samples and testing for lactic acid concentrations. All of these tests involve a gradual increase in test workload and exercise intensity. Each test will show a marked change when the athlete reaches a predominantly anaerobic state: loss of controlled breathing, heart rate plateaus (causing a deflection on a graph), or a very sudden lactate accumulation (concentration of lactic acid in the blood). Some exercise labs now express AT as a workload, e.g. 200 watts, as athletes seem to relate well to this measure.

At AT pace there is, of course, a corresponding heart rate (monitored throughout testing). This identifies the specific intensity that is very close to the maximum aerobic pace an athlete can race at and train at to improve. This is where it gets exciting! Having identified AT and the corresponding heart rate, you can now use a heart rate monitor to accurately gauge and control the highest sustainable pace for particular races. No more slow starts; no more fast starts; no more wasteful surging. Instead, a way to maintain a steady sustainable pace for the entire race or time trial. This is particularly good for time trial-type races in running, triathlons, mountain biking, cycling, and to some extent rowing. It is also good for AT training in the speedwork phase, enabling you to simulate race intensities accurately.

Sound simple? It is. But you should still talk to an exercise physiologist about the most appropriate way of determining your training and racing heart rates. Quite often this is best determined by looking at recent racing heart rates, including the proportion of time spent in each intensity zone, and the average heart rate for the entire race.

Once you have worked out your AT heart rate, resting heart rate and maximum heart rate, all other training intensities can be determined (*see* appendix 1). It should also be noted that AT can be raised and lowered by speedwork. The more speedwork you do, the higher your AT is likely to be as long as the speedwork is not too anaerobic. Therefore, your AT will vary according to the type of training you are doing. AT can be increased through training by approximately 40 per cent.

When assessed concurrently with VO_2max, AT can also be expressed as a percentage of VO_2max, i.e. AT can be described as a percentage of the maximum workrate at which you can perform (*see* fig. 6.2). Thus, AT (maximum steady state pace) might be described as 75 per cent of VO_2max. Expressing AT as a

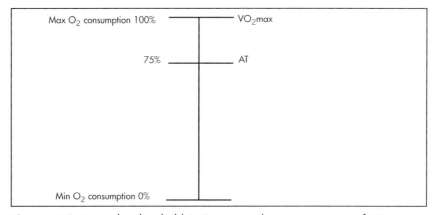

Figure 6.2 Anaerobic threshold (AT) expressed as a percentage of VO_2max

percentage of VO$_2$max is a good diagnostic tool for determining how much low-intensity distance work or AT speedwork needs to be done in training.

Aerobic threshold can also be predicted through testing. This is a transitional phase between slow and medium intensity training. Aerobic threshold occurs at 35 to 70 per cent of VO$_2$max.

VO$_2$max and AT figures vary from sport to sport. So your bike figures may be different from your swim figures depending on the training you have done in each sport. If you are a multisport athlete, you need to get tested for VO$_2$max and AT figures in each discipline.

Figure 6.3 indicates that in both time trials and variable tempo races, the athlete with the higher AT will have a faster race pace and he/she will spend less time in oxygen debt (shaded area) with each successive sprint or surge. This means the athlete is less likely to be dropped and should be 'fresher' later in the race.

See appendix 3 for basic anaerobic threshold tests.

Flexibility testing

Flexibility testing should be done on the major muscle groups used in the sport you compete in. If possible, the flexibility test should be as specific as possible to the sport, that is, muscle groups should be stretched as they would be in the sport. The results will not be absolute, but they will provide some useful information. Inflexibility in key areas and imbalances between limbs (sometimes due to past injuries that have not fully recovered) can affect performance and lead to injury. It is important, therefore, that a physiotherapist or exercise consultant assesses static flexibility.

A flexomeasure or tape measure can be used to obtain linear measures of range of motion. Otherwise a goniometer or flexometer can be used to obtain angular measures of range of motion.

The following lists the major muscle groups and muscle action used in the sports covered by this book.

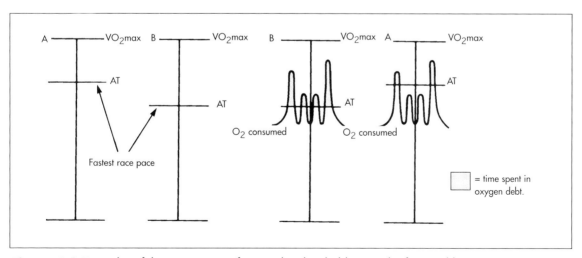

Figure 6.3 Examples of the importance of anaerobic threshold: 'A' is the faster athlete

Areas to be flexibility tested

Cyclists, runners, duathletes, mountain bikers: back, calves/Achilles, quads, hamstrings, hip flexors, hip extensors, hip rotation, adductors.

Triathletes, multisporters, rowers: back, calves/Achilles, quads, hamstrings, spinal rotation, pectorals, hip flexors, hip extensors, adductors, hip rotation, shoulder rotation.

Fat levels – body composition testing

Body fat is usually expressed as a percentage, and is commonly measured using up to seven site skinfold tests. Excessive fat, and therefore weight, will hinder performance, particularly in weight-bearing sports. There is no point, for instance, in having an ultra-light bike if you are carrying extra kilograms! If necessary, fat levels should be reduced gradually (no more than 1 kg per week). But remember that too little body fat can predispose you to illness.

The recommended lowest levels of body fat for athletes are: elite male 5 to 10 per cent; elite female 12 to 15 per cent; semi-competitive male 10 to 16 per cent; semi-competitive female 15 to 21 per cent. When it comes to body fat, women are genetically cursed; like it or not, they tend to carry more fat than men. Women also need to be careful about dropping body fat too much as this can lead to a range of health problems including amenorrhoea (ceasation of periods) and osteoporosis. When it comes to body fat, women athletes should not try to compete with their male counterparts!

There is currently a movement away from using percentage fat measures. Instead, skinfold (in mm) measures are being promoted. Body composition (adiposity) ratings for body fat can also be used.

Speed and power testing

For sports that require speed and power, tests can be done on these performance variables. Power testing involves assessing how much work can be done by the athlete over a short period of time. In the context of the sports addressed in this book, this type of testing applies mainly to cyclists and rowers. The other sports are not explosive enough to warrant power testing. Cycle racers should use a windgate test carried out on a bicycle ergometer where cumulative power, peak power, time to peak power (usually between one and three seconds) and current power are measured.

A fatigue index over a set period of time can be used to measure speed endurance. This can be an effective diagnosis of the cyclist's ability to 'jump' and hold an extended sprint. It also gives an indication of top speed. A timed sprint on the road between a series of set points, for example 50, 100, 200, 500 and 1000 metre marks, can also be used. There is also a rowing ergometer designed to test power via maximal load over 5 to 20 strokes.

Power and short-distance speed are predominantly genetic, whereas speed endurance is far more trainable. In other words, sprinters are born fast, the rest of us have to work at it!

Strength testing

Strength can be tested in the major muscle groups but it should be done using the same action/speed/resistance needed for your sport (without risking injury), that is, strength should be tested in a form that replicates the movement and speed of your sport. This, unfortunately, is a lot easier said than done when it comes to endurance sports. If the testing isn't sport-specific, then the results will be adversely affected. Nevertheless, it is possible to gain basic information that may help pinpoint weak areas or strength imbalances between limbs or opposing muscles. Weaknesses or imbalances can limit performance and lead to injury. Strength imbalances, for example, may see one limb favoured over the other, with the resulting increase in workload leading to breakdown of the 'strong' limb or overtraining of the weak limb.

Strength testing can be carried out on weight-training equipment, but it is preferable to use sophisticated strength testing machines, such as Cybex, where testing is controlled. Young athletes should use strength tests with care and only under the supervision of an qualified coach.

The following is a basic guide to strength testing for the sports covered in this book.

Mountain bike/cycling
- Leg press
- Leg curl

Rowing
- Leg press
- Leg curl
- Rowing machine
- Bench press (for safety, no cleans)

Triathlon/multisport
- Leg press
- Hamstring machine (straight leg)
- Pectorals
- Lat pullover
- Triceps

Running/duathlon
- Leg press
- Hamstring machine (straight leg)

Unless you are very experienced with free weights, always test on machines. And only test at the beginning and end of base training (never test close to competition). It is most effective to strength test on high reps, not only to avoid injury, but because weight resistance levels are more specific; 10 reps minimum, 15 to 20+ preferred. Remember, gym strength testing on weight machines is far from accurate and provides very basic information only.

When to be fitness tested?

Testing generally occurs at the beginning and end of the base phase (beginning of speed). It is often useful to be tested immediately after recovery from peak to assess the effectiveness of the training programme and to see how well you peaked. Ideally, testing should occur every six to eight weeks (*see* fig. 6.4).

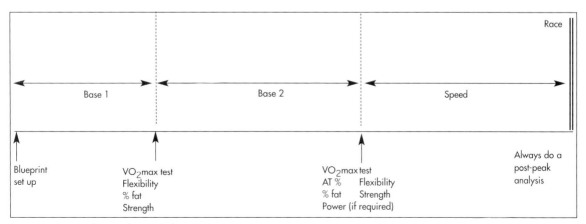

Figure 6.4 When to be tested

Testing in relation to mesocycles

Only get tested at the end of an easy week in a mesocycle. If you are in a high mileage phase, have one or two easy days before testing to help overcome the cumulative fatigue of training. Otherwise, have a day or two off before testing. That way you are fresh and the results will be meaningful. Remember, though, only a full taper would allow you to be fully fresh.

If you don't want to miss a workout on the day of testing, train in the morning (low intensity) on the day before testing, and get tested at lunchtime the next day. You can go out again and train afterwards. Try to get tested at the time of day you usually race and stick to that time for future tests. You need to have the same tests in the same order, using the same equipment with the same pre-test taper (*see* fig. 6.5).

Adaptation vs overload

Adaptation – your body's ability to adjust to exercise stress placed on it and then improve – is a far better training strategy than overload. In overload, the body cannot tolerate the exercise stress being placed upon it and this leads to fatigue (exercise and general), loss of performance and training burn-out. All that adds up to one thing: *overtraining*. Overtraining is a state of prolonged fatigue and is caused by excessive training; it is characterised by decrements or plateaus in performance despite continued training (*see* fig. 6.6).

In chronically overtrained athletes a decline of as much as 5 to 15 per cent in performance is not uncommon. One study showed a drop of 11 to 15 per cent in training pace and a 43 to 71 per cent drop in training distance. So, write this down now: training too much, too hard, or too quickly will not lead to long-term

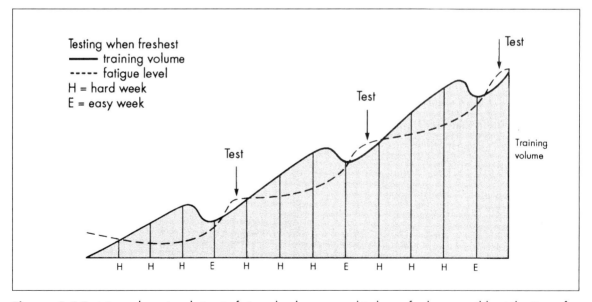

Figure 6.5 Training volume in relation to fatigue levels: you need to be as fresh as possible at the time of testing, so it's a good idea to be tested at the end of a compensation week

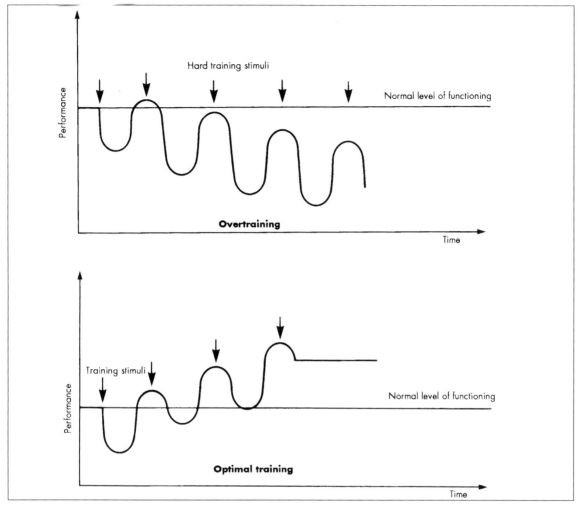

Figure 6.6 The effects of overtraining, and optimal training, on performance

performance gains. But it will lead to injury, fatigue, illness and staleness.

In a study of elite runners, it was found that 60 per cent overtrained at some point in their career. Too many athletes are lost to sport, especially young athletes, because they train too hard too soon, break down, and lose interest, or they are unable to train at the levels they once did because of continuing health problems.

Adaptation via a slow controlled increase in training volume and intensity is the aim of any good training programme. If given the chance, the body has an amazing ability to adapt and improve its performance through training.

While overtraining is a common problem in endurance athletes, particularly athletes training for ultra-distance races and those who race often, it also occurs in athletes who try to fit training in around work and social obligations and leave little time for recovery (physical and mental). Overtraining can occur through heavy training mileages towards the end of base training, during intensive speed training or after a series of races within a short period of time.

The main causes of overtraining

1 Inadequate recovery between training sessions
2 Excessive amounts of high-intensity (and sometimes high-volume) training
3 Sudden changes in training load (distance, duration or intensity)

Other training factors that contribute to overtraining

1 Intense strength training
2 Frequent competition and travel
3 Monotony in training programme
4 No off-season

Non-training factors that contribute to overtraining

1 Inadequate nutrition
2 Insufficient sleep and rest
3 Anxiety about life events, e.g. new job
4 Occupational stress
5 Mental conflict
6 Changes and irregularities in lifestyle
7 Successive failure to achieve goals

Overtraining needs to be differentiated from the short-term tiredness that occurs whenever training load increases. Overtrained athletes may be doing no more training than their peers, but due to outside pressures, medical problems or even their personal tolerance to training, may be feeling fatigued. Remember, to achieve performance improvement, the body must be allowed to adapt gradually to increased training mileages and intensities. But it is not absolute mileages and intensities that matter, but rather the amount of mileage and speed-work you personally can recover from – no recovery, no improvement!

Your ability to recover, of course, depends largely on your training history. The more years you have been in the sport, the bigger your base, the more training you can do and recover from. Elite athletes are particularly susceptible to overtraining as double seasons (winter and summer) can mean an inadequate off-season with too little time for recovery. Young athletes and inexperienced athletes are also susceptible to overtraining because of their lower tolerance to training. Common training errors that lead to overtraining are too long a season, high levels of competitive stress, frequent racing, intense training over an extended period of time, lack of effective recovery and lack of positive results / enjoyment.

Symptoms of overtraining

Emotional and behavioural changes
- Lethargy and excessive fatigue, especially at rest
- Loss of purpose, energy and competitive drive; poor attitude, confusion, loss of enthusiasm to train
- Feelings of helplessness and being trapped in routine
- Feeling emotionally unstable and excessive emotional display
- Loss of libido (loss of interest in sex)
- Increased anxiety and depressive feelings
- Increased irritability and anger (mood changes)
- Sleep problems (difficulty getting to sleep, nightmares, waking often during the night)

- Decreased self-confidence
- Poor concentration, inability to relax

Physical changes
- Weight loss, weight fluctuations and loss of appetite
- Heavy painful muscles, 'weak-feeling' muscles
- Excessive sweating
- Increased susceptibility to infections and illness (colds, rashes, fever)
- Increased number of persistent injuries
- Reduced performance in training and racing
- Inability to reach target heart rate while training
- Above expected heart rate at rest, during and after exercise
- Drop in blood pressure on standing, elevated resting and post-exercise blood pressure
- Swelling of lymph glands (sore throats)
- Gastrointestinal disturbances (diarrhoea and nausea)
- Hyperactivity
- Inability to maintain training load
- Chronic fatigue
- Hormonal changes, e.g. testosterone/cortisol levels in males
- Low serum ferritin levels
- Slower heart rate recovery
- Headaches
- Deterioration of sports skills
- Menstrual irregularities

Although there is no single physiological or psychological measure or symptom to identify overtraining, the symptoms when considered together give a strong indication that you are overtrained or approaching that state. These symptoms will vary across athletes and sports. The difficulty is that overtraining comes on gradually, so you and your coach must be vigilant at all times. Using a log book to record thoughts, feelings, mood, heart rates, medical tests, performances and so on can be a great help in picking up overtraining indicators before it is too late. If you exhibit several of these symptoms (you don't have to have all of them) over a period of more than two weeks, you are probably overtrained and you should consult a specialist doctor. If overtraining is not picked up early, it can wipe out an entire year's training! So watch for the signs.

The chronic fatigue experienced by overtrained athletes seems to be caused by too much stress being placed on the central nervous system. There appear to be two stages in the 'Chronic Overtraining Syndrome'. In the first stage, the athlete's body goes into a kind of overdrive, enabling it to cope with the excess load being placed upon it. During overdrive, the body seems to draw on the physical, emotional and mental reserves normally kept for emergencies. If overtraining is caught in this overdrive stage, damage can be kept to a minimum and recovery can be swift. However, if you carry on into the second stage of Chronic Overtraining Syndrome, the 'depletion' stage, then you are heading for big trouble and a long, slow recovery.

Indicators of central nervous system 'overdrive'
- Reduced performance (training and racing)
- Higher than expected heart rate at rest and during exercise
- Sleep problems
- Emotional instability
- Elevated blood pressure
- Delayed recovery of heart rate after exercise

Indicators of central nervous system 'depletion'
- Reduced performance (racing and training)
- Lower than expected heart rate at rest and during exercise
- Excessive sleeping
- Unstable behaviour, depressive feelings

- Low blood sugar response to exercise
- Low blood pressure
- Rapid recovery of heart rate after exercise

Medical considerations

It is important, of course, that overtraining is distinguished from normal fatigue and medical problems. Medical factors that may affect the body and contribute to overtraining symptoms include:

1 Illness – colds, glandular fever, post-viral infections: Be very careful when training after an illness as a relapse is normally far worse than the original problem. Recurrent illness should be checked. *Do not train through an illness*. Not only is it better to rest for two days now rather than ten days later, but you could do yourself long-term or permanent harm.

2 Inadequate nutrition: Prolonged inadequate carbohydrate intake (chronic glycogen depletion) can cause continuing fatigue. Lack of adequate protein, lack of some minerals and trace elements, and low fluid intake can all affect performance. This is particularly so in hot climates. Persistent or recurring infections (remember, intensive training weakens the immune system) and frequent training injuries suggest it's time to look at your nutritional intake or see a dietician.

3 Anaemia – iron deficiency

4 Exercise-induced asthma

5 Physical changes due to ageing (you can't do what you used to); not coping because present fitness level is not as high as previously

6 Psychological factors
- Non-physical stressors that can affect performance
- Education (all levels)
- Working environment
- Living conditions

- Training facilities
- Financial situation
- Social environment – sport administration

7 Travel problems – disruption of circadian rhythms (e.g. jetlag)

During the off-season, basic medical screening can be done to establish baseline levels and to ensure there are no underlying medical problems that may affect health and performance, or endanger your life.

Prevention of overtraining

The best way to avoid overtraining is to *listen to your body*! Athletes spend time listening to coaches, listening to their peers and keeping the numbers straight in their training log, but too little time listening to what their body is saying. And very often it is screaming, 'Give me a day off!', or 'Take it easy today, okay?' If you hear your body telling you this, follow its advice – it knows what it's talking about! Otherwise, yep, you'll be overtrained before you can say, 'I don't feel like training today.' The main areas that should be monitored to prevent overtraining are:

- careful planning of training schedules and seasons (particularly during the competitive season)
- optimal training strategies and effective recovery techniques; effective nutrition
- attention to and control of study, work and relationships

Clinical testing for overtraining is ineffective; prevention is a far better option. Recent research indicates that a downturn in psychological states is a good indicator of overtraining (*see* earlier section on 'Symptoms of overtraining'). If you notice your motivation, confidence and general satisfaction are low for days on end, and performances are poor, then it is time to reassess your training. By reacting quickly and correctly to these signals (this usually means lowering training stress) you can prevent a disaster, or at least control the damage. Training stress should not be increased again until all the symptoms have gone.

It should be mentioned, however, that it seems that mild overtraining just before your taper or in the second and/or third week out from competition, followed by a taper, can produce a higher performance than that obtained through standard training schedules (for more on this *see* 'Superovercompensation', page 25).

Of course, overtraining can easily be avoided by undertraining. But this is not an option if you want to be a competitive endurance athlete striving to fulfil your potential. Besides, undertraining wouldn't be nearly as much fun as 'giving it heaps' now and again, would it? Just don't overdo it!

Minimising the risk of overtraining

1 Avoid sudden increases in training load, both mileage/duration and speedwork (which needs to be gradually phased in). This is especially important at the beginning of build-up.

2 Avoid too much speedwork and frequent competition. The more stress, intensity and time involved in training, the less speedwork and racing that can be done.

3 Avoid monotonous training, particularly during the high mileage phase. If you can, train at a variety of venues.

4 Be aware of all the other physical and psychological stressors which may affect your training. If possible, try and arrange a stress-free life away from your sport! If this can't be done, then at least be aware of your stress levels and train accordingly. Do not push on regardless.

5 Do not get caught up in the 'train harder' response to a performance plateau or drop. Training longer and harder will not get you out of a slump. On the contrary, you will just dig a bigger hole for yourself.

In most cases, a performance plateau or drop (if you haven't increased training and aren't ill) is due to excessive fatigue or a natural performance drop following a peak. This means a recovery period is required. Once recovery is complete, training loads can increase again. Remember, rest is as important as exercise – *no recovery, no improvement*!

Use of heart rate monitors to avoid overtraining
Heart rate in an overtrained athlete will tend to be higher at rest (but not always) and during exercise, and it will drop more slowly following exercise. Remember, though, that heart rates can be elevated if you are ill, under stress, in high temperatures, when you are dehydrated, after recent exercise or if you have eaten recently.

Tests to monitor overtraining
Easy tests of overtraining are:
• Morning heart rate
• Training heart rate/speed
• Orthostatic heart rate test (*see* appendix 5)
• Exercise economy tests (*see* appendix 4)
• Time trials (*see* appendix 5)
• Perceived level of fatigue

Other tests include:
• Blood tests
• Physiological lab tests

Management of training if already overtrained

Okay, so you made a mistake, and you pushed on one week longer than you should have. Or you just tried to squeeze in one more week of high mileage when you shouldn't have. Result? You're overtrained (not tired, overtrained!). What do you do now? Well, first check for medical problems as mentioned above. If no medical factors are involved then you have two options:

1 *Rest*

Take three to five weeks off! Have a good time. Forget about training completely (but try not to put too much weight on). After this time, start training lightly again. Keep the number of sessions and mileage low, and do no speedwork! Over the next two to four months slowly increase your training, but don't race. It is absolutely essential that you take this conservative approach, because if you relapse it will take even longer to recover. Do it once, do it right! And remember, sport is supposed to be fun, and the first part of health and fitness is health.

2 *Use a gentle similar non-competitive exercise*

Exercise at low intensity (LO), but only when you want to and only for as long as you want. Forget about the pressures of how far and how fast. If you're an overtrained competitive cyclist, ride your mountain bike in the forest once a week, and do no other cycling! This type of training obviously won't increase performance, but that doesn't matter at all. All you are trying to do at this stage is aid recovery and maintain a little fitness. Using a variety of regenerative techniques may also help. These include massage, physiotherapy, hydrotherapy (spas, flotation tanks), stress management techniques (relaxation exercises).

Length of recovery

Recovery from overtraining can take from three weeks to three months, depending on how severely overtrained you have been. Don't forget, recovery consists of two types: physical recovery (cumulative fatigue has vanished) and psychological recovery (you are enthusiastic about training again). You need to be careful, though, that once you start to feel good again (often around three months into recovery) you don't pile on the training too fast. It is a good idea, therefore, in cases of chronic overtraining, to have four months of controlled reduced training with no speedwork and little, if any, competition. Only after that should a full training programme be recommended.

♦ Moving back into training ♦ following injury or illness

Moving back into full training after injury or illness is a delicate operation for endurance athletes – too soon and you risk becoming sick or injured again; too late and you waste good training time (particularly close to competition). If you are in any doubt about when to start full training again, consult qualified people (coach, doctor, physiotherapist), listen to your body, and err on the side of caution.

Illness

Never train through illness – it can be very dangerous. The best guides to whether you are over your illness are: how much energy you have, your motivation, your doctor, and blood tests. Once fully recovered, move back into training gradually.

If you have been sick for a few days

Reduce mileage/duration and intensity based on the amount of time you have been sick. As a basic guide, if you have been sick for a few days start back gradually for the first one to three days with low mileage/duration and low-intensity workouts. Only go back to a normal schedule the following week.

Of course, it really depends on what your body is telling you. If it is tired, make the next session easy. If it is very tired, have a day off. If, however, you're feeling good, continue to build up through the next workout. Pay attention to your body both during and for the first few hours after the workout. If you have a general tiredness a few hours after your workout, you are probably not fully recovered from your illness. So back off a little.

If you have been sick for more than a week

Reduce training back to what you were doing two to three weeks before the illness. Again, build back into training gradually over one week. But only up to the level you were at two to three weeks prior to the illness. If you have been ill for two weeks or more, consult your doctor and coach before resuming training, and listen to what they say! Common sense dictates that the longer you have been ill, the slower and more gradual the comeback needs to be.

Injury

If you are injured, that is, feel persistent pain during a workout and/or at rest, seek medical advice, preferably from a reputable sports doctor, or physiotherapist (if in doubt, check with your local sports medicine federation). When injured, you don't necessarily have to stop training – what hurts when running may not hurt when cycling. Indeed, the injury may only affect one aspect of the sport, for example it may hurt running up hills, but not on the flat. The best practical guide is whether the pain is persistent and/or it increases during or after a workout.

A good sports doctor, or physiotherapist, should be able to tell you how to manage your injury. *Don't try and train through an injury without expert guidance.* If you do try and train through an injury, it may result in damage that cannot be repaired properly. Generally, however, you can still train when injured as long as the injury management programme is properly set up. Such a programme might include:

- medical consultations
- physiotherapy
- chiropractic work
- rehabilitation work at home or in a gym
- massage
- talking to an experienced coach
- a properly constructed training programme that allows for training improvements without aggravating or compounding the injury. For example: exercise in water (aqua jogging); break your routine into two parts, morning and evening, to allow more recovery between sessions and give you time to assess what you can do in the evening; use an alternative 'like' sport to replace or bolster your specific training (runners may cycle, for instance).

Try to establish why you became injured – was it due to overtraining, too much intensity, too much speedwork, too much hill work? If you can discover the answer, you can set up your training programme so it doesn't happen again.

Chapter 7

How to Write Your Own Programme

◆ Set realistic training ◆ goals

Goal setting improves motivation, but only if the goal is realistic and achievable. When planning your training programme set yourself realistic intermediate and long-term goals in terms of how much and how fast. It is always tempting to set training goals that you would like to achieve rather than those you can achieve at this point in your sporting career. Unattainable goals may look good on paper, but they can lead to overtraining and decrease motivation as you fail to achieve them. Of course, if you have already been training for several seasons and have been keeping a training log, then you should have a good idea of what you can handle when it comes to races, training volume and training intensity. Use this hard-earned knowledge to establish effective training seasons and periods.

For most athletes, increases in training volume should not exceed 10 or, at the most, 15 per cent over a season. Remember, there is a limit to how much training you can do no matter how much time and motivation you have at your disposal! So, set goals you can achieve, be patient and don't become a slave to your programme. If in doubt, back off and regroup. You'll be a happier, healthier athlete for doing so.

◆ The three levels of your ◆ training programme

When planning a training programme three levels are used. These are:

1 Blueprint – the plan, what you would like to do
2 Working programme – what you actually do; 'the real world'
3 Log book – what happened

1 Blueprint

The blueprint outlines your overall training plan for the year (or longer), including specific details about build-up and racing. This blueprint is your ideal plan and as such will prove almost impossible to follow to the letter. Fatigue, illness, lack of time, work, family, study, and so on can, and will probably, all have an adverse effect on training type, intensity and duration at some stage during the year. Don't worry. The blueprint is only a guide as to how to approach your training programme and achieve training goals. It is not your definitive training programme.

2 Working programme

A working programme is the weekly programme recorded at the end of each week. It takes into account:

- Blueprint
- Next week's commitments
- You and/or your coach's requirements for the week
- Your experience
- Information from the log book and any other relevant information from the previous week's training

Combined, these elements are used to determine each week's programme (*see* fig. 7.1). It's called the working programme because it's the programme that actually 'works'. It almost certainly won't follow the blueprint exactly and will include subtle changes and refinements from week to week as circumstances change and your experience grows. For a step-by-step guide on how to complete your working programme *see* page 127.

3 The log book

The log book is a combination of the previous year's blueprint, past weekly training programmes, monthly summaries and post-peak analysis summaries (summary of complete build-up). The log book is used to see exactly what happened in previous build-ups, what effect the training had on performance, and to identify long-term trends in

training. The log book, therefore, is used to develop the next blueprint, including the week-to-week programme.

◆ How to set up your ◆ blueprint

Training programmes must be set up in a logical order. This involves setting up the blueprint first.

Step 1: Set up your 'seasonal programme'

Your seasonal programme includes: off-season, pre-season, in-season. To set up the programme you will need to decide the exact dates of the races you wish to compete in, and the length of those races (longer races require longer build-ups, meaning fewer races can be raced in a season). Once you have these dates, set out your seasonal programme using Template 1 (*see* appendix 13). An example is given in figure 7.2, page 104. To work out how long your seasons should be refer to the relevant sections earlier in the book.

Step 2: Set up your microcycle

Now you need to set up your microcycle (the format for a standard training week), i.e. what training you do on each day. To do this you first need to work out your 'peak-mileage week'.

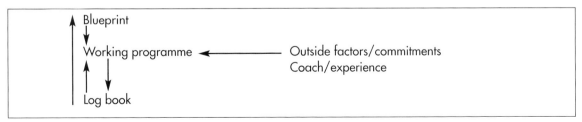

Figure 7.1 Working programme

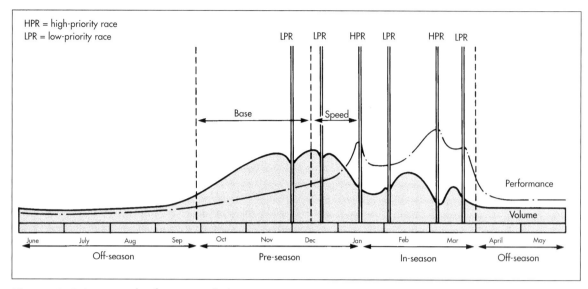

HPR = high-priority race
LPR = low-priority race

LPR   LPR   HPR   LPR   HPR   LPR

Base

Speed

Performance

Volume

June   July   Aug   Sep   Oct   Nov   Dec   Jan   Feb   Mar   April   May

Off-season   Pre-season   In-season   Off-season

Figure 7.2 An example of a seasonal plan

Your peak-mileage week

Your peak-mileage (or duration) week is the week in your build-up in which you do the greatest volume (hours or kilometres) of training. This is *not* a weekly average. It is the mileage for one week only. You may only do this week once or twice in your entire build-up (near the end of base, or early in speed-work), as it is the culmination of a gradual build-up of volume over a long time.

To work this out, simply calculate the biggest weekly mileage you think you could cope with, given your experience, commitment, time and ability to avoid injury, in all the disciplines you intend to compete in. For example, let's imagine you are an elite runner with ten years' experience of high training loads. You might decide that your peak-mileage week will be 160 km. Alternatively, you might be a novice triathlete in your second season of competing, who also works full-time. You might decide that you can only cope with a maximum of six hours' training per week spread across swimming, cycling and running. If training for a multi-disciplinary sport, such as triathlon, generally you are better off to establish training mileages or durations for each discipline.

You can determine your own 'peak-mileage week', or if you need help Section A (*see* pages 111–12) provides guidelines to work out your peak-mileage week based on your sport, the distance you intend to race, and your level of training commitment (explained more fully in 'Levels of training commitment' on page 105–6). Whatever you decide, remember it is best to be cautious. Fill in your peak-mileage week total (or totals if you plan to compete in more than one discipline) using Template 2 (*see* appendix 14).

Now you have to decide how to spread that peak mileage (or duration) throughout the week. In other words, what training you will do on each day. When making your decision take account of work, study, family and social factors, as well as availability of resources, such as pool times, daylight for cycling, training partners, and so on. Also take account of the need for a rest day or a day that is very easy. For many people, Friday fits the bill nicely as it comes at the end of the working week and provides a chance to socialise and regroup before the weekend, when much of your mileage work is likely to be done.

Here's an example of how a triathlete might spread 211.5 km (swim 5.5 km, bike 160 km, run 46 km) of training across a week:

M	T	W	T	F	S	S
S 2 km		S 2 km		DAY OFF	S 1.5 km	
	B 40 km		B 40 km			B 80 km
R 16 km		R 20 km			R 10 km	

Key: S = swim; B = bike; R = run

If you are an experienced athlete, you will probably have a good idea as to how to set up your microcycle for a peak-mileage week. When setting up a microcycle, work it out in the following order:

1 Day or days off
2 Workout days
3 Long or medium long workouts
4 Speed workouts
5 Hill workouts
6 Other easy workouts

If you need help, there are pre-set peak-mileage week microcycles for a range of sports and distances in Section B (*see* pages 112–20). The peak-mileage weeks in Section A have numbers next to them which correspond to the training weeks in Section B. If using Section B, remember to select a pre-set programme based on your sport, the distance you intend racing over, and the level of training that suits you. These programmes are set up in terms of daily workouts, experience levels, number of workouts per week, and mileage for each workout during your *peak-mileage week* only. The programmes can be converted to duration rather than mileage by using Section D (*see* page 126). The times are only approximate, however, and you will need to adjust them according to your ability and experience.

As your peak-mileage week represents the most training you think you can handle in one week, it equates to your 100 per cent week. All other training weeks are based on this week. If you are not experienced in your sport, make sure you select a programme that is realistic in terms of your training experience and non-training commitments. If you have limited time available, you may want to choose a programme based simply on the number of workouts per week. Select a programme based on what you think you can do, not based on what you would like to be doing or what your friends/clubmates are doing. Dreams are free but overtraining is costly. Select wisely!

Levels of training commitment

You need to select your level from the categories below before choosing peak-mileage and training weeks from Sections A and B.

1 Recreational/novice
- You want to get the most out of little training time because you can't commit to too much training.
- You are in your first year of the sport.

2 Semi-competitive
- You are prepared to invest a moderate level of commitment. You are serious about training but you have other commitments and interests. You are interested in becoming competitive but you aren't aiming at coming first.
- You are in your second year of competing and happy to remain at this level of commitment.
- Having fun is more important than doing 'really well'.

3 Elite

- You are either a top young athlete, a talented athlete new to the sport, or a top athlete who works 40 hours per week. You are serious about your sport and want to place well.
- You have been competing for three or more years and you are placing well (top 10 or better in most races).

4 Elite-plus

- You are a very serious athlete who trains full-time in order to win!
- You have been competing for over four years and have already won big races.

Once you have chosen the programme from Section B that you think suits you best, complete Template 2 by filling in each day's training mileage/duration for each of the disciplines you plan to compete in. Figure 7.3 illustrates a peak-mileage week based on Template 2 and using the example given on page 105. You may need to juggle the days around your personal and work schedule. In figure 7.3 for instance, you might not be able to do a long run on Wednesdays because of a weekly meeting. Swap it with one of the other running days, but make sure it doesn't upset the balance of the programme. Remember, this is only your peak-mileage week and the basis for working out all other weeks.

You have now filled out Template 1, showing your seasonal plan (including race dates), and Template 2, showing your peak-mileage week total and how much mileage (duration) you are going to do on each day of this week.

Your weekly and daily workouts

You now need to go to Template 3 (*see* appendix 15) or Template 4 (*see* appendix 16). On these templates, you will need to count back from your 'Full Peak' race day and fill in the date for Monday of each week during your training build-up.

You now need to work out how much mileage you do each week in your race build-up based on a percentage of your peak-mileage (100 per cent) week. For example, if week two is a 50 per cent week, that means all your workouts in week two are 50 per cent of

Sport	Mon	Tues	Wed	Thurs	Fri	Sat	Sun	Total
Swim	Swim 2 km		Swim 2 km		D A Y	Swim 1.5 km		5.5 km
Bike		Bike 40 km (speed)		Bike 40 km (hills)	O F F		Bike 80 km (long)	160 km
Run	Run 16 km (hills)		Run 20 km (long)			Run 10 km (speed)		46 km

Figure 7.3 An example of a peak-mileage week

the distance/duration of those workouts in your peak-mileage week. To find these percentages use Section C (*see* pages 121–5). Even if you have set up the rest of your programme by yourself, it's worth looking at Section C to get an idea of how you can use it. You will see that it provides training percentages based on:

1 Number of weeks of speedwork (four, six or eight)
2 Mesocycle (hard/easy week ratio: 2:1; 3:1; 4:1)
3 Percentage of training volume increase (7 per cent or 10 per cent)
4 Race distance (short or long)

You now need to select an option for each of these variables. To help you make your selection, consider the following:

1 Number of weeks of speedwork. Four weeks is recommended for beginners and eight weeks for experienced elite athletes. Most athletes will lie in the four-to-six week range. Section C offers three blocks (A, B, C). Block A = four weeks of speedwork; block B = six weeks of speedwork; block C = eight weeks of speedwork. Select the number of weeks that you feel suits you best.

2 Mesocycle (hard/easy weeks). Remember, a mesocycle is the number of hard weeks (high volumes of distance/duration in base, high volumes of intensity in speed) in a row you can cope with before a recovery or compensation week. A ratio of two hard/one easy is recommended for beginners and four hard/one easy for elite athletes. Choose the option you feel comfortable with (if in doubt, be conservative). You will see that each block offers a mesocycle option. Choose the mesocycle from the block you selected in (1) above.

Ideally, although this option isn't shown in these basic tables, mesocycles change during a build-up, going from smaller cycles (two hard/one easy) to larger cycles (four hard/one easy) in base as you become better conditioned. Then as you move into speedwork the cycle gets smaller again to accommodate the increasing training intensity. You need to be particularly careful at this time that your programme allows you sufficient recovery.

3 Percentage increase per week. If you are experienced, 10 per cent is acceptable, but if you are less experienced, then 7 per cent is the best option. Ideally, and again this option isn't shown in these tables, your programme will start off with smaller increases (as you get used to training), with larger increases in the middle, and then smaller increases again at the end (you can't keep increasing mileage indefinitely!). Select the percentage option from the block you chose earlier (A, B, or C).

4 Race distance. A race is long if it is over three-and-a-half hours, short if it is under. Choose short or long from the block you have chosen.

Here's an example using Section C of how these choices determine your daily training distances or durations:

1 Number of weeks of speedwork = 6
Go to Block B

2 Mesocycle = 2 hard/1 easy
Go to lines A–D

3 Percentage increase per week = 10 per cent
Go to line C or D

4 Race distance = short
Go to line D.

Line D gives you the percentages you will use to calculate your weekly training distances through build-up and speedwork.

You will notice the programme allows for a base of up to 18 weeks (plus the six weeks of speedwork chosen in this example). You will also notice that some of the weeks indicate your 100 per cent or peak-mileage week, upon which all other weekly mileages are based.

You can start anywhere in the programme. If you do not wish to do a structured eighteen-week build-up, or are unable to, then start your build-up in later weeks, e.g. start in week seven. Just make sure you give yourself enough time to prepare adequately for the speedwork to come.

If you are not starting a programme at the beginning, make sure your first week of the programme corresponds to current training volumes. You can't just jump into the middle of a programme unfit and expect it to work! The best approach is to determine the number of weeks until you race and then count back until you reach the week you are currently in. If the mileages in the programme equate to what you are doing now, start there. If they are greater than you are doing now, you may need to make some programme adjustments (*see* page 110).

Okay, so you've made your personal choices concerning speedwork, mesocycle and percentage increase. Now go back to Template 3 or 4 and fill in the percentage lines using section 2 of the sample in figure 7.4 as a guide, although it is only a 16-week programme. Note that in most instances the lines in the percentage ranges at the end of build-up – weeks 23 or 24 – in Section C are excluded, as you should use the taper programmes presented in the sport-specific programmes discussed in chapter 14.

Now complete Template 3 or 4 for each week, and each discipline by multiplying your peak-mileage week total by the percentage you wrote for each week, e.g. bike 160 km × 72% (0.72) = 115 km. This gives you the mileage you will do each week for each discipline. Write these totals on the appro-

priate lines. For example, in figure 7.4 (based on the earlier example on page 105 of 160 km cycling, 46 km running, 5.5 km swimming) the percentage in week 1 is 72 per cent. If you then go to section 3 you will see that this means in base week 1 you would do: 4 km swimming, 115 km cycling, 33 km running. *Note*: Seventy-two per cent would not be an appropriate starting point for a novice; 40 per cent would be more appropriate.

Once you have got mileages (or durations) for each week, you can graph them at the top of the page of Template 4 (see section 4 of fig. 7.4). This will give you a good idea of the increasing and decreasing training volumes throughout build-up and speedwork.

Now go back to Template 2 where you wrote in your daily workouts based on your peak-mileage week. This will show you how you structured your maximum training volume week. Then, using Template 4 and starting with week 1, simply write in each day's workout based on the peak-mileage week workout. For example, again using base week 1 and 72 per cent (*see* section 5, figure 7.4) the week would look like this:

Swimming
Monday and Wednesday: 2 km (workout in peak-mileage week) × 72% = 1.4 km
Saturday: 1.5 km × 72% = 1.1 km

Cycling
Tuesday and Thursday: 40 km × 72% = 28.8 km
Sunday: 80 km × 72% = 57.6 km

Running
Monday: 16 km × 72% = 11.5 km
Wednesday: 20 km × 72% = 14.4 km
Saturday: 10 km × 72% = 7.2 km

You then repeat this process for each week.

Race: Olympic triathlon
Race date: 20 April
Training starts: 30 December

Maximum distance for the 100% week
Swim: 5.5 km
Bike: 160 km
Run: 46 km

Mileage profile

Subphase

| Easy ❶ | Load ❷ | High load ❸ | Load/speed ❹ | Low speed ❺ | High speed ❻ |

Base   Speed

Race

Week	1	2	3	4	5	6	7	8	9	10	11	12	13	14	15	16
	30 Dec	6 Jan	13 Jan	20 Jan	27 Jan	3 Feb	10 Feb	17 Feb	24 Feb	3 Mar	10 Mar	17 Mar	24 Mar	31 Mar	7 Apr	14 Apr
	Base	Base	Base	Base	Base	Base	Base	Base	Base	Base	Base	Base	Speed	Speed	Speed	Speed
	Hard	Hard	Easy	Hard	Hard	Easy	Hard	Hard	Easy	Hard	Hard	Easy	Hard	Hard	Easy	Easy
%	72	79	72	79	86	79	86	93	86	100	86	72	86	79	65	—
Weekly mileage (km)																
Swim	4.0	4.3	4.0	4.3	4.7	4.3	4.7	5.1	4.7	5.5	4.7	4.0	4.7	4.3	3.6	2.0
Bike	115	126	115	126	138	126	138	149	138	160	138	115	138	126	104	46
Run	33	36	33	36	40	36	40	43	40	46	40	33	40	36	30	12
Daily mileage																
Mon	km	km	km	km	km	km	km	km	km	km	km	km	km	km	km	km
Swim	1.4_1	1.6_1	1.4_1	1.6_1	1.7_1	1.6_1	1.7_1	1.9_1	1.7_1	2.0_1	1.7_1	1.4_1	1.7_1	1.6_1	1.3_1	1.0_1
Bike																
Run	11.5_1	12.6_1	11.5_1	12.6_2	13.8_2	12.6_1	13.8_{2-3}	14.9_{2-3}	13.8_1	16_{2-4}	13.8_{2-4}	11.5_1	13.8_{2-4}	12.6_{2-4}	10.4_{2-4}	6.0_{5-6}
Tues																
Swim																
Bike	28.8_1	31.6_2	28.8_1	31.6_3	34.4_3	31.6_1	34.4_4	37.2_4	34.4_1	40.0_5	34.4_5	28.8_1	34.4_{5-6}	31.6_{5-6}	26.0_{5-6}	26.0_1
Run																
Wed																
Swim	1.4_1	1.6_1	1.4_1	1.6_2	1.7_2	1.6_1	1.7_{2-3}	1.9_{2-3}	1.7_1	2.0_{2-4}	1.7_{2-4}	1.4_1	1.7_{2-4}	1.6_{2-4}	1.3_{2-4}	1.0_1
Bike																
Run	14.4_1	15.8_1	14.4_1	15.8_1	17.2_1	15.8_1	17.2_1	18.6_1	17.2_1	20.0_1	17.2_1	14.4_1	17.2_1	15.8_1	13.0_1	6.0_1
Thu																
Swim																
Bike	28.8_1	31.6_1	28.8_1	31.6_1	34.4_2	31.6_1	34.4_{2-3}	37.2_{2-3}	34.4_1	40.0_{2-4}	34.4_{2-4}	28.8_1	34.4_{2-4}	31.6_{2-4}	26.0_{2-4}	20.0_1
Run																
Fri																
Swim																
Bike	D/O	D/O	D/O	D/O	D/O	D/O	D/O	D/O	D/O	D/O	D/O	D/O	D/O	D/O	D/O	D/O
Sat																
Swim	1.1_1	1.2_2	1.1_1	1.2_3	1.3_3	1.2_1	1.3_4	1.4_4	1.3_1	1.5_5	1.3_5	1.1_1	1.3_{5-6}	1.2_{5-6}	1.0_{5-6}	
Bike																D/O
Run	7.2_1	7.9_2	7.2_1	7.9_3	8.6_3	7.9_1	8.6_4	9.3_4	8.6_1	10.0_5	8.6_5	7.2_1	8.6_{5-6}	7.9_{5-6}	6.5_{5-6}	
Sun																
Swim																
Bike	56.4_1	63.2_1	57.4_1	63.2_1	68.8_1	63.2_1	68.8_1	74.4_1	68.8_1	80.0_1	68.8_1	57.4_1	68.8_1	63.2_1	52.0_1	RACE
Run																

Figure 7.4 Sample Training programme

Step 3: Set up subphases

To make your training programme more specific more experienced athletes may wish to set up training subphases (*see* chapter 4). To set up subphases in your programme:

1 Identify which subphases are appropriate to your sport by using the information in figure 4.3 on page 39.

2 Place the subphases into your programme (each subphase should start, if possible, at the first hard week of a mesocycle). The sample programme in figure 7.4 includes subphases and is an example of how to set up training subphases (1 = preparation, 2 = load, 3 = high load, 4 = load/speed, 5 = low speed, 6 = high speed). See also the programme examples in chapter 14.

You may choose to emphasise a weakness by spending more time on it, i.e. more than one mesocycle. Sometimes you may not have enough time to cover all the subphases by training one subphase per mesocycle. So you may need to compress more than one subphase into a mesocycle or leave one or two subphases out.

3 Make sure the subphases are placed and applied in the correct order.

4 Maintain all subphases continually after the first build-up.

Programme adjustments

1 Make sure that the training mileages/durations you have worked out are similar to those you are currently doing. If they are higher, make small adjustments in your blueprint over a four- to eight-week period to gradually bring you up to your planned mileages. The first example below shows how you can start at 40 per cent instead of 60 per cent, but still build up to the same percentage over an eight-week period.

If the mileages you have worked out are too low in comparison to what you are presently doing, it's better to cut back and follow your programme.

2 If you have races scheduled before your peak race, you will have to make slight adjustments to the programme in order to taper in and taper out of the low-priority race(s). Remember, each race will affect your training mileages and too many races can reduce your ability to peak for 'the big one'. In the second example below, if you have a race scheduled at the end of a 75 per cent week you need to adjust the percentage by reducing it to 60 per cent.

Programme adjustment examples

Week	1	2	3	4	5	6	7	8
Scheduled %	60	65	70	60	75	80	85	90
Adjusted %	40	50	60	40	65	75	85	90
						R		
						A		
						C		
						E		

Week	1	2	3	4	5	6	7	8
Scheduled %	40	50	60	40	65	75	85	90
Adjusted %	40	50	60	40	65	60	70	90

3 Approximate 'in-season' adjustments. In-season involves manipulation of base and speed training. Ideally, your peak races need to be six to eight weeks apart to enable you to peak effectively (100 per cent potential). In such cases, the approximate plan would be two to four weeks of base immediately after the race, including a recovery week, with a little speedwork after the recovery week. The build-up to moderate to high mileage is gradual. Following this, three to five weeks of full speedwork should be implemented to make up the six to eight weeks. A longer race would best suit five weeks of base and three weeks of speed (because of the race distance), while a short race would involve three weeks of base and five weeks of speed (because speed is more important in a shorter race).

For adjustments to training if you have less than six weeks between races, *see* 'How to manage training during the 'in-season'' on page 58. Remember to use the sport-specific programmes outlined previously so you can work out your requirements for speedwork, long workouts, hills etc., and appropriate tapers.

The basic programme is now in place. Remember that the blueprint is a guide only; it is designed to provide you with a framework to build your training around. And it is this training that gives you the working programme, which we look at in the next chapter.

◆ Section A ◆
Peak-mileage weeks

Use this as a guide to work out your peak-mileage week. *Note*: 2×, 3×, 4× etc. are the number of times you train in each discipline each week; S = swim, B = bike, R = run, K = kayak.

Triathlon		**S** (km)	**B** (km)	**R** (km)
Sprint distance triathlon *(700 m/20 km/6 km)*				
1 Novice	2×	3	70	16
2 Semi	3×	5.5	120	22
3 Elite	4×	10	180	34
Standard distance triathlon *(1.5 km/40 km/10 km)*				
4 Novice	2×	3	100	25
5 Semi	3×	5.5	160	46
6 Elite	4×	10.5	280	49
7 Elite +	5×	12.5	310	55
Half-Ironman triathlon *(2 km/90 km/21 km)*				
8 Semi	3×	8	220	62
9 Elite	4×	11	320	69
10 Elite +	5×	13	350	75
Ironman triathlon *(3.8 km/180 km/42 km)*				
11 Semi	3×	9	280	66
12 Elite	4×	11	380	79
13 Elite +	5×	13	410	89
Duathlon				
4 km/20 km/4 km				
14 Novice	3×		90	24
15 Semi	4×		160	38
16 Elite	5×		250	45
10 km//60 km/10 km				
17 Novice	3×		170	42
18 Semi	4×		260	63
19 Elite	5×		320	69

Multisport		R (time)	B (km)	K (time)
Coast to Coast				
Day one: 2.8 km run/58 km cycle/26 km mt run				
Day two: 15 km cycle/67 km kayak/70 km cycle				
20 Semi	3×	4 hr 30 min	160	6hr
21 Elite	4×	5 hr 50 min	240	8 hr
22 Elite +	5×	6 hr 20 min	270	9 hr
Mountains to Sea				
Day one: 23 km run/61 km cycle/35 km kayak				
Day two: 87 km kayak				
Day three: 30 km run/54 km cycle				
23 Semi	3×	5 hr 30 min	130	8 hr
24 Elite	4×	7 hr	190	9 hr
25 Elite +	5×	7 hr 30 min	220	10 hr

Cycling and mountain biking		km
40 km		
26 Novice	3×	160
27 Semi	4×	220
28 Semi	5×	260
29 Semi	6×	350
30 Elite	6×	400
80 km		
31 Novice	4×	240
32 Semi	5×	280
33 Semi	6×	390
34 Elite	6×	470
160 km		
35 Novice	4×	280
36 Semi	5×	380
37 Semi	6×	450
38 Elite	6×	560
39 Elite +	6×	700
Tour		
40 Semi		560
41 Elite		680
42 Elite +		850

Rowing		km
Coxed 4 (2000 m)		
43 Novice	5×	42
44 Semi	6×	57
45 Elite	6×	100

Distance running		km
10 km		
46 Novice	3×	32
47 Novice	4×	42
48 Semi	5×	58
49 Semi	6×	64
50 Elite	6×	87
Half-marathon		
51 Novice	4×	53
52 Semi	5×	70
53 Semi	6×	84
54 Elite	6×	92
Marathon		
55 Novice	4×	66
56 Semi	5×	88
57 Semi	6×	94
58 Elite	6×	113

♦ Section B ♦
Peak-mileage week microcycles

Use this section as a guide to work out how you will spread your training during your 'Peak-mileage week' (100%). The daily workouts for each discipline are listed, top to bottom, in the order they should be done; in the case of duathlon training programmes this may involve a run/bike/run format. When referring to the elite programmes in Section B, the underlined workouts are kept if you are doing the elite+ programme, and eliminated if you are doing the elite programme.

Sprint distance triathlon (700 m/20 km/5 km)

1 Novice 2×

M	T	W	T	F	S	S
S 2 km	DAY OFF	B 10 km R 10 km	DAY OFF	S 1 km R 6 km	B 60 km	

2 Semi-competitive 3×

M	T	W	T	F	S	S
S 2 km R 6 km	B 30 km	S 2 km R 10 km	B 30 km	DAY OFF	S 1.5 km B 60 km R 6 km	

3 Elite 4×

M	T	W	T	F	S	S
S 3 km R 10 km	B 40 km	S 3 km R 15 km	B 40 km	S 3 km B 20 km R 6 km	S 1 km B 80 km R 3 km	

Standard distance triathlon (1.5 km/40 km/10 km)

4 Novice 2×

M	T	W	T	F	S	S
S 1.5 km	DAY OFF	B 40 km	R 15 km	DAY OFF	S 1.5 km R 10 km	B 60 km

5 Semi-competitive 3×

M	T	W	T	F	S	S
S 2 km R 16 km	B 40 km	S 2 km R 20 km	B 40 km	DAY OFF	S 1.5 km B 80 km R 10 km	

6 Elite 4× / 7 Elite+ 5×

M	T	W	T	F	S	S
S 3 km R 16 km	S <u>2 km</u> B 60 km	S 3 km B <u>30 km</u> R 20 km	B 60 km R <u>6 km</u>	S 3 km	S 1.5 km B 40 km R 10 km	B 120 km R 3 km

113

Half-Ironman (2 km/90 km/21 km)

8 Semi-competitive 3×

	M	T	W	T	F	S	S
S	3 km		3 km		DAY OFF	2 km	
B		60 km		60 km			100 km
R	16 km		26 km			20 km	

9 Elite 4× /10 Elite+ 5×

	M	T	W	T	F	S	S
S	3 km	2 km	3 km		3 km	2 km	
B		60 km	30 km	80 km		40 km	140 km
R	16 km		30 km	6 km		20 km	3 km

Ironman (3.8 km/180 km/42 km)

11 Semi-competitive 3×

	M	T	W	T	F	S	S
S	3 km		3 km		DAY OFF	3 km	
B		40 km		60 km			180 km
R	20 km		30 km			16 km	

12 Elite 4× /13 Elite+ 5×

	M	T	W	T	F	S	S
S	3 km	2 km	3 km		3 km	2 km	
B		80 km	30 km	60 km		60 km	180 km
R	20 km		36 km	10 km		20 km	3 km

Duathlon (4 km/20 km/4 km)

14 Novice 3×

M	T	W	T	F	S	S
DAY OFF	R 6 km	B 30 km	R 10 km	DAY OFF	R 4 km B 20 km R 4 km	B 40 km

15 Semi-competitive 4×

M	T	W	T	F	S	S
R 10 km	B 40 km	R 18 km	B 40 km	DAY OFF	R 4 km B 20 km R 4 km	R 2 km B 60 km

16 Elite to Elite+ 5×

M	T	W	T	F	S	S
R 10 km	B 40 km	R 18 km B 30 km	R 6 km B 60 km	DAY OFF	R 4 km B 20 km R 4 km	R 3 km B 100 km

Duathlon (10 km/60 km/10 km)

17 Novice 3×

M	T	W	T	F	S	S
DAY OFF	R 20 km	B 40 km	R 10 km	DAY OFF	R 6 km B 30 km R 6 km	B 100 km

18 Semi-competitive 4×

M	T	W	T	F	S	S
R 15 km	B 40 km	R 25 km	B 40 km	DAY OFF	R 10 km B 60 km R 10 km	R 3 km B 120 km

19 Elite to Elite+ 5×

M	T	W	T	F	S	S
R 15 km	B 60 km	R 25 km B 30 km	R 6 km B 50 km	DAY OFF	R 10 km B 60 km R 10 km	R 3 km B 120 km

Multisport (Coast to Coast)

20 Semi-competitive 3×

	M	T	W	T	F	S	S
R	2 hr 30 min		1 hr		DAY OFF	1 hr	
B		40 km		80 km		40 km	
K	1 hr	1 hr					4 hr

21 Elite 4× / 22 Elite+ 5×

	M	T	W	T	F	S	S
R	3 hr		1 hr 30 min	20 min		1 hr	30 min
B	40 km	60 km		100 km	40 km	30 km	
K		1 hr	2 hr		1 hr	1 hr	4 hr

Multisport (Mountains to Sea)

23 Semi-competitive 3×

	M	T	W	T	F	S	S
R	2 hr 30 min		1 hr 30 min		DAY OFF	1 hr 30 min	
B		40 km		60 km		30 km	
K	1 hr	2 hr					5 hr

24 Elite 4× / 25 Elite+ 5×

	M	T	W	T	F	S	S
R	3hr		1 hr 30 min	1 hr		1 hr 30 min	30 min
B	40 km	40 km		80 km	DAY OFF	30 km	30 km
K		1 hr	2 hr		1 hr	1 hr	5 hr

Note: Friday is a day off for Elite 4× only.

Cycling and mountain biking (40 km)

26 Novice 3×

M	T	W	T	F	S	S
DAY OFF	40 km	DAY OFF	40 km	DAY OFF	DAY OFF	80 km

27 Semi-competitive 4×

M	T	W	T	F	S	S
DAY OFF	40 km	DAY OFF	60 km	DAY OFF	40 km	80 km

28 Semi-competitive 5×

M	T	W	T	F	S	S
DAY OFF	50 km	30 km	60 km	DAY OFF	40 km	80 km

29 Semi-competitive 6×

M	T	W	T	F	S	S
30 km	60 km	40 km	60 km	DAY OFF	40 km	120 km

30 Elite to Elite+ 6×

M	T	W	T	F	S	S
40 km	60 km	40 km	80 km	DAY OFF	40 km	140 km

Cycling (80 km)

31 Novice 4×

M	T	W	T	F	S	S
DAY OFF	40 km	DAY OFF	60 km	DAY OFF	40 km	100 km

32 Semi-competitive 5×

M	T	W	T	F	S	S
DAY OFF	50 km	30 km	40 km	DAY OFF	40 km	120 km

33 Semi-competitive 6×

M	T	W	T	F	S	S
30 km	60 km	40 km	60 km	DAY OFF	60 km	140 km

34 Elite to Elite+ 6×

M	T	W	T	F	S	S
40 km	80 km	50 km	80 km	DAY OFF	60 km	160 km

Cycling (160 km)

35 Novice 4×

M	T	W	T	F	S	S
DAY OFF	40 km	DAY OFF	60 km	DAY OFF	40 km	140 km

36 Semi-competitive 5×

M	T	W	T	F	S	S
DAY OFF	60 km	40 km	80 km	DAY OFF	40 km	160 km

37 Semi-competitive 6×

M	T	W	T	F	S	S
30 km	80 km	40 km	80 km	DAY OFF	60 km	160 km

38 Elite 6×

M	T	W	T	F	S	S
40 km	100 km	60 km	80 km	DAY OFF	80 km	200 km

39 Elite+ 6×

M	T	W	T	F	S	S
80 km	160 km	40 km	130 km	DAY OFF	90 km	200 km

Cycling (Tour)

40 Semi-competitive 6×

M	T	W	T	F	S	S
40 km	100 km	60 km	100 km	DAY OFF	80 km	180 km

41 Elite 6×

M	T	W	T	F	S	S
60 km	160 km	40 km	130 km	DAY OFF	90 km	200 km

42 Elite+ 6×

M	T	W	T	F	S	S
80 km	160 km	130 km	160 km	DAY OFF	120 km	200 km

Rowing coxed four (2000 m)

43 Novice 5×

M	T	W	T	F	S	S
DAY OFF	6 km	10 km	6 km	DAY OFF	10 km	10 km

44 Semi-competitive 6×

M	T	W	T	F	S	S
6 km	10 km	6 km	10 km	DAY OFF	10 km	15 km

45 Elite to Elite+ 6×

M	T	W	T	F	S	S
12 km	17 km	12 km	17 km	DAY OFF	23 km	19 km

Distance running (10 km)

46 Novice 3×

M	T	W	T	F	S	S
DAY OFF	6 km	DAY OFF	10 km	DAY OFF	DAY OFF	16 km

47 Novice 4×

M	T	W	T	F	S	S
DAY OFF	10 km	DAY OFF	10 km	DAY OFF	6 km	16 km

48 Semi-competitive 5×

M	T	W	T	F	S	S
DAY OFF	16 km	6 km	10 km	DAY OFF	6 km	20 km

49 Semi-competitive 6×

M	T	W	T	F	S	S
6 km	16 km	6 km	10 km	DAY OFF	6 km	20 km

50 Elite to Elite+ 6×

M	T	W	T	F	S	S
6 km	18 km	10 km	16 km	DAY OFF	12 km	25 km

Distance running (half-marathon)

51 Novice 4×

M	T	W	T	F	S	S
DAY OFF	10 km	DAY OFF	16 km	DAY OFF	6 km	21 km

52 Semi-competitive 5×

M	T	W	T	F	S	S
DAY OFF	14 km	6 km	18 km	DAY OFF	6 km	26 km

53 Semi-competitive 6×

M	T	W	T	F	S	S
6 km	16 km	10 km	20 km	DAY OFF	6 km	26 km

54 Elite to Elite+ 6×

M	T	W	T	F	S	S
8 km	16 km	10 km	20 km	DAY OFF	12 km	26 km

Distance running (marathon – 42 km)

55 Novice 4×

M	T	W	T	F	S	S
DAY OFF	20 km	DAY OFF	16 km	DAY OFF	10 km	30 km

56 Semi-competitive 5×

M	T	W	T	F	S	S
DAY OFF	20 km	10 km	16 km	DAY OFF	12 km	30 km

57 Semi-competitive 6×

M	T	W	T	F	S	S
6 km	20 km	10 km	16 km	DAY OFF	12 km	30 km

58 Elite to Elite+ 6×

M	T	W	T	F	S	S
6 km	25 km	10 km	20 km	DAY OFF	16 km	36 km

◆ Section C ◆
Percentage Ranges

These tables give the percentages used to calculate training distances based on:

- number of weeks of speedwork
- hard/easy week ratio (mesocycle)
- percentage of training volume increase
- race distance

Key:
Long race = over 3.5 hours; short race = under 3.5 hours
H = hard week (high volume in base and high intensity in speedwork)
E = easy week

See chapter 14 for sport-specific programmes for tapers for weeks 23 and 24.

Block A – four weeks speedwork

Mesocycle: 2 hard weeks, 1 easy week
A = 7% training volume increase for a long race
B = 7% training volume increase for a short race
C = 10% training volume increase for a long race
D = 10% training volume increase for a short race

								Base												Speed			
Week 1	2	3	4	5	6	7	8	9	10	11	12	13	14	15	16	17	18	19	20	21	22	23	24
E	E	H	H	E	H	H	E	H	H	E	H	H	E	H	H	E	H	H	E	H	H	E	E
A 44	51	58	65	58	65	72	65	72	79	72	79	86	79	86	93	86	93	100	86	100	86	—	—
B 44	51	58	65	58	65	72	65	72	79	72	79	86	79	86	93	86	93	100	72	79	72	65	—
C 35	40	45	50	40	50	60	50	60	70	60	70	80	70	80	90	80	90	100	90	100	80	—	—
D 35	40	45	50	40	50	60	50	60	70	60	70	80	70	80	90	80	90	100	70	80	70	60	—

Mesocycle: 3 hard weeks, 1 easy week

E = 7% training volume increase for a long race

F = 7% training volume increase for a short race

G = 10% training volume increase for a long race

H = 10% training volume increase for a short race

	Base																				Speed			
Week	1	2	3	4	5	6	7	8	9	10	11	12	13	14	15	16	17	18	19	20	21	22	23	24
	E	H	E	H	H	H	E	H	H	H	E	H	H	H	H	E	H	H	H	E	H	H	E	E
E	44	51	44	51	56	58	51	58	65	72	58	72	79	86	72	86	93	100	86	93	100	93	—	—
F	44	51	44	51	56	58	51	58	65	72	58	72	79	86	72	86	93	100	72	86	79	72	65	—
G	40	45	40	45	55	60	45	60	70	80	60	80	85	90	80	90	95	100	90	95	100	90	—	—
H	40	45	40	45	55	60	45	60	70	80	60	80	85	90	80	90	95	100	70	90	80	70	60	—

Mesocycle: 4 hard weeks, 1 easy week

I = 7% training volume increase for a long race

J = 7% training volume increase for a short race

K = 10% training volume increase for a long race

L = 10% training volume increase for a short race

	Base																				Speed			
Week	1	2	3	4	5	6	7	8	9	10	11	12	13	14	15	16	17	18	19	20	21	22	23	24
	E	H	H	E	H	H	H	E	H	H	H	H	E	H	H	H	H	E	H	H	H	H	E	E
I	44	48	51	44	54	56	58	51	58	65	72	79	58	79	86	93	100	79	100	93	100	86	—	—
J	44	48	51	44	54	56	58	51	58	65	72	79	58	79	86	93	100	79	93	86	78	72	65	—
K	45	50	55	45	55	60	65	55	65	70	75	80	65	85	90	95	100	70	100	90	100	90	—	—
L	45	50	55	45	55	60	65	55	65	70	75	80	65	85	90	95	100	70	90	85	80	70	60	—

Block B – six weeks speedwork

Mesocycle: 2 hard weeks, 1 easy week

A = 7% training volume increase for a long race
B = 7% training volume increase for a short race
C = 10% training volume increase for a long race
D = 10% training volume increase for a short race

	Base																				Speed			
Week	1	2	3	4	5	6	7	8	9	10	11	12	13	14	15	16	17	18	19	20	21	22	23	24
	E	E	H	H	E	H	H	E	H	H	E	H	H	E	H	H	E	H	H	E	H	H	E	E
A	44	51	58	65	58	65	72	65	72	79	72	79	86	79	86	93	86	100	93	86	100	93	—	—
B	44	51	58	65	58	65	72	65	72	79	72	79	86	79	86	93	86	100	86	72	86	79	65	—
C	40	45	50	55	50	55	60	55	60	70	60	70	80	70	80	90	80	100	90	80	100	90	—	—
D	40	45	50	55	50	55	60	55	60	70	60	70	80	70	80	90	80	100	80	70	80	70	60	—

Mesocycle: 3 hard weeks, 1 easy week

E = 7% training volume increase for a long race
F = 7% training volume increase for a short race
G = 10% training volume increase for a long race
H = 10% training volume increase for a short race

	Base																				Speed			
Week	1	2	3	4	5	6	7	8	9	10	11	12	13	14	15	16	17	18	19	20	21	22	23	24
	E	H	E	H	H	H	E	H	H	H	E	H	H	H	E	H	H	H	E	H	H	H	E	E
E	44	51	44	51	56	58	51	58	65	72	58	72	79	86	72	86	93	100	86	93	100	93	—	—
F	44	51	44	51	56	58	51	58	65	72	58	72	79	86	72	86	93	100	72	86	79	72	65	—
G	40	45	40	45	55	60	45	60	70	80	60	80	85	90	80	90	95	100	90	95	100	90	—	—
H	40	45	40	45	55	60	45	60	70	80	60	80	85	90	80	90	95	100	70	90	80	70	60	—

Mesocycle: 4 hard weeks, 1 easy week

I = 7% training volume increase for a long race

J = 7% training volume increase for a short race

K = 10% training volume increase for a long race

L = 10% training volume increase for a short race

	Base																		Speed					
Week	1	2	3	4	5	6	7	8	9	10	11	12	13	14	15	16	17	18	19	20	21	22	23	24
	E	H	H	E	H	H	H	E	H	H	H	H	E	H	H	H	H	E	H	H	H	H	E	E
I	44	48	51	44	54	56	58	51	58	65	72	79	58	79	86	93	100	79	100	93	100	93	—	—
J	44	48	51	44	54	56	58	51	58	65	72	79	58	79	86	93	100	79	93	86	78	72	65	—
K	45	50	55	45	55	60	65	55	65	70	75	80	65	85	90	95	100	70	100	90	100	90	—	—
L	45	50	55	45	55	60	65	55	65	70	75	80	65	85	90	95	100	70	90	85	80	70	60	—

Block C – eight weeks speedwork

Mesocycle: 2 hard weeks, 1 easy week

A = 7% training volume increase for a long race

B = 7% training volume increase for a short race

C = 10% training volume increase for a long race

D = 10% training volume increase for a short race

	Base																		Speed					
Week	1	2	3	4	5	6	7	8	9	10	11	12	13	14	15	16	17	18	19	20	21	22	23	24
	E	E	H	H	E	H	H	E	H	H	E	H	H	E	H	H	E	H	H	E	H	H	E	E
A	51	58	65	72	65	72	79	72	79	86	79	86	93	86	93	100	79	93	100	79	100	86	—	—
B	51	58	65	72	65	72	79	72	79	86	79	86	93	86	93	100	72	93	86	72	79	72	65	—
C	40	45	50	60	50	60	70	60	70	80	70	80	90	80	90	100	80	90	100	80	100	80	—	—
D	40	45	50	60	50	60	70	60	70	80	70	80	90	80	90	100	80	90	80	70	80	70	60	—

Mesocycle: 3 hard weeks, 1 easy week

E = 7% training volume increase for a long race
F = 7% training volume increase for a short race
G = 10% training volume increase for a long race
H = 10% training volume increase for a short race

										Base											Speed			
Week	1	2	3	4	5	6	7	8	9	10	11	12	13	14	15	16	17	18	19	20	21	22	23	24
	E	H	E	H	H	H	E	H	H	H	E	H	H	H	E	H	H	H	E	H	H	H	E	E
E	44	51	44	51	58	65	51	65	72	79	65	79	86	93	79	100	93	100	86	93	100	93	—	—
F	44	51	44	51	58	65	51	65	72	79	65	79	86	93	79	100	93	86	79	86	79	72	65	—
G	50	55	50	60	65	70	60	70	75	80	70	80	85	90	80	100	90	100	80	90	100	90	—	—
H	50	55	50	60	65	70	60	70	75	80	70	80	85	90	80	100	90	80	70	90	80	70	60	—

Mesocycle: 4 hard weeks, 1 easy week

I = 7% training volume increase for a long race
J = 7% training volume increase for a short race
K = 10% training volume increase for a long race
L = 10% training volume increase for a short race

										Base											Speed			
Week	1	2	3	4	5	6	7	8	9	10	11	12	13	14	15	16	17	18	19	20	21	22	23	24
	E	H	H	E	H	H	H	E	H	H	H	H	E	H	H	H	H	E	H	H	H	H	E	E
I	44	48	51	44	54	56	58	51	58	65	72	79	58	79	86	93	100	86	100	93	100	93	—	—
J	44	48	51	44	54	56	58	51	58	65	72	79	58	79	86	93	100	86	93	86	79	72	65	—
K	45	50	55	45	55	60	65	55	65	70	75	80	65	85	90	95	100	80	100	90	100	90	—	—
L	45	50	55	45	55	60	65	55	65	70	75	80	65	85	90	95	100	70	85	80	75	70	60	—

◆ Section D ◆
Approximate mileage to duration conversion

Cycling Based on 30 kph		Running Based on 5 min/km		Kayaking Based on 10 kph		Swimming Based on 60 m/min		Rowing Based on 12 kph	
Dist (km)	*Time (hr/min)*	*Dist (km)*	*Time (hr/min)*	*Dist (km)*	*Time (hr/min)*	*Dist (m)*	*Time (hr/min)sec)*	*Dist (km)*	*Time (hr/min)*
20	40	2	10	6	36	250	4 10	2	30
30	1	3	15	10	1	500	8 20	10	50
40	1 20	4	20	12	1 12	750	12 30	12	1
50	1 40	6	30	15	1 30	1000	16 40	15	1
60	2	10	50	16	1 36	1250	20 50	16	1 20
80	2 40	12	1	17	1 42	1500	25	17	1 25
90	3	15	1 15	19	1 54	1750	29 10	19	1 36
100	3 20	16	1 20	20	2	2000	33 20	23	1 56
120	4	18	1 30	23	2 18	2250	37 30		
130	4 20	20	1 40	25	2 30	2500	41 40		
140	4 40	25	2 05	30	3	2750	45 50		
160	5 20	26	2 10	35	3 30	3000	50		
180	6	30	2 30	40	4	3250	54 10		
200	6 40	36	3	50	5	3500	58 20		
						3800	1 03 20		

You can test yourself to make the duration conversions more accurate by the following method.

- Do a short workout at your average cruising pace (LSD)
- Record 1 Time: ....
    2 Distance: ....
- Use the calculations in appendix 8 to determine your speed.
    3 Speed: ....

You can use further calculations in appendix 8 to determine durations for all workouts. This will help to refine and personalise your training duration estimates.

♦ How to use the blueprint ♦ to get your working programme

A working programme template is provided in appendix 9. You can use this, following the three steps below, to complete your weekly working programme.

1 Using your previous week's experience (and suggestions from your coach if you have one), you would put your calculated mileages from the relevant week in the blueprint into the working programme in *pencil*. Using pencil allows you to change the workout if you need to – remember, adjustments will be made as illness, fatigue, work commitments, etc. have an effect on your training.

2 As you complete each workout, write it down in pen over the top of the figures you have written in pencil, and then fill in the rest of the data. Filling in this data is very important because the questions in the working programme are similar to the sorts of questions a good coach would ask. How you answer provides a clear picture of how your training is going and how it might be modified to optimise performance.

Complete the questions in the performance analysis by circling the appropriate answers. This way you fill out all the specific information quickly and in a set order, which makes it easy to refer to. The circles also allow you to assess your training very quickly because they clearly show up patterns (good and bad) in training. Other relevant specifics (if required) can be filled out in the log book in the standard way.

3 Once you have completed your training week, complete the weekly summary. Look for patterns and errors that harm your training. Record these in the training notes. And look for ways to refine and improve your training. You won't find something every week, of course, but it may happen often enough to make a real difference in the way you train. Ways of picking up training faults and strengths are described in the next chapter, on training analysis. Once the working programme has been completed and summarised, it then becomes your log book. This is then used in conjunction with the blueprint to help you write and refine each week's new working programme.

♦ Important points when ♦ using your training programme

1 Don't do every workout, every week, every month, regardless of how you feel. This will not work, and you will end up overtrained. Listen to your body. Remember the principles we have discussed so far in this book. You will probably miss 5 to 20 per cent of your workouts. This is normal, and you shouldn't worry about it. If you are missing more than 10 to 20 per cent of your workouts you may need to reassess how much training you have set yourself – it may be too much.

2 If you miss a workout, it is gone. Never try to 'bring it back', as this will destroy the balance of your programme and you may end up overtrained.

3 Don't develop 'accountancy mentality'. You should not try to balance your log book numbers.

4 Listen to your body!!

Chapter 8

Analysis of Training

♦ The benefits of sports ♦ analysis

Training and coaching is really an experiment. The key to experimentation is making sure you only manipulate one variable at a time. You then check to see whether that manipulation has produced a good result or a bad result. If the result is good, then the manipulation (or change) is kept. If not, the variable reverts to its former state and another variable is manipulated, and so on. This is how experimentation works, and this is how coaching an athlete works. Through changing training variables and then receiving feedback on whether that change was effective, training becomes more efficient and performance improves.

In analysing your sport the two most important questions you need to ask yourself are: What are the variables or parts that make up my sport? How do these parts contribute to the sport and in what proportions? For example, let's have a look at some of the parts of cycle training:

1 Duration of workout
2 Average speed of workout
3 Distance of workout
4 Topography (terrain) and locality of workout
5 Training intensity (heart rate) and training load (watts)
6 Subjective feeling of workout
7 Stress during the day
8 Sleep
9 Weather conditions
10 Nutrition
11 Warm-up/warm-down
12 Cycle set-up
13 Use of equipment not often used, e.g. disk wheel
14 Cumulative mileage during current or previous week
15 Illness/injury
16 Resting heart rate
17 Weight goal and pre- and post-workout weight
18 Training load/stress and training effectiveness
19 Cadence (pedal rpm)

These are all parts of cycle training and racing that should be considered, as any number of them can have an impact (good or bad) on performance.

Think about what happened after each workout!

By making a note after each workout of the elements that influence training you will quickly be able to identify a problem. Or better still, identify a workout that seemed to really improve your performance potential – most elite athletes have two or three favourite workouts they know work for them. By optimising and personalising your training programme in this way, you will gain confidence that what you are doing is right for you as you chase your goals.

The other thing you should note is how much each element contributes to performance. What is the most important element, and the next most important? For instance, distance is generally more important than intensity for a tour cyclist because the primary aim of a tour cyclist is to complete the tour! So, distance work will provide the foundation for training. The secondary element is speed/intensity. A track cyclist, on the other hand, is more interested in speed than volume training. Decide how much each variable contributes to your sport and take this into account in your programme.

Where's the fun in analysis?

Some people will suggest that by analysing your training in great detail you risk taking the fun out of your sport. This is true, if you forget the reason you are training in the first place. Think of analysis as a tool to help you recreate yourself, as a means by which you can become a faster, stronger, healthier person. Not only is the challenge of perfecting your training fun in itself, but by paying attention to detail you optimise training and perform better. And let's face it, it's much more fun to succeed than to be frustrated because the work you did has failed to produce the result you wanted. And, finally, all that planning doesn't mean you can't get plenty of fun out of individual workouts, such as a long run through a forest with friends, or some fartlek – it's not called speed play for nothing – along a beach.

◆ The log book ◆

It cannot be stressed enough that a log book is an essential way of refining your programme. *Always use a log book.* A lot of people say: 'Why should I waste my training time writing things into a log book?' The answer is simple: 'How could you train without one?'

Part of the problem may be that few athletes understand how to use a log book correctly. You don't just write in it. You also read it. You use it to optimise your training. Most people would laugh at a businessperson who didn't keep accounts – how do they know if their business is performing, that they are maximising resources? What's the difference between that and training? If you train an average of eight hours per week in an 18-week build-up, that equates to 144 hours of effort. That's a lot of time to invest in your fitness. Using a log book correctly will make sure that time isn't wasted.

Of course, recording and analysing training is an ongoing process from build-up to build-up. You continually refine your training to further improve your response, and your performance at peak. See appendix 9 for more practical advice on how to use a log book.

♦ Working programme ♦ analysis

How to use your log book

Figures 8.1 and 8.2 (*see* pages 132–5) are two examples of a cyclist's working programme with training errors added, then detected through analysis.

- Average resting heart rate: 45 bpm
- Average base training heart rate: 150–155 bpm
- Speedwork interval training heart rate: 175–180 bpm

Training errors that would be rectified in the following week's programme:

Example one (Figure 8.1)

1 During the week: diet is poor and should be improved.

2 During the week: more sleep required.

3 On Wednesday: training too hard. This is adversely affecting training on Thursday. This is indicated by elevated training heart rate despite a normal resting heart rate.

The normal resting heart rate indicates that the athlete was fully recovered from the previous day's workout. The elevated training heart rate was due to training at too high an intensity (*see* average training heart rate). This is also indicated by a tired subjective feeling on Thursday combined with an elevated resting heart rate.

A slower than usual 30 kph training speed also showed that some fatigue was present. Friday also indicated the cyclist was fatigued.

In summary, it took two days to recover (Thursday/Friday) from the mistake of training too hard on Wednesday. This wasted valuable time and energy.

4 Saturday training affecting Sunday: the same error occurred on the Saturday. (Note the elevated resting heart rate on Sunday.)

Example two (Figure 8.2)

1 Tuesday and Wednesday: either too many intervals were performed on Tuesday, or they were performed too hard, or doing intervals two days in a row was too tough (most likely).

To solve this problem, the number of intervals should be reduced or the second interval session should be moved from Wednesday to Thursday to allow a recovery day. (*See* elevated resting heart rates on the Wednesday and Thursday following intervals, indicating insufficient recovery.)

2 Monday and Tuesday: the legs were overworked with the hill training on Monday and the speedwork on Tuesday. This made Wednesday's speedwork totally wasted. Either reduce the hillwork or reduce the speedwork depending on which is most important during the current training phase.

If hillwork and speedwork are equally important, then the two training sessions will need to be moved further apart. Clearly, the cyclist's legs were tired before Wednesday's session started as target heart rate could not be reached.

3 Wednesday/Thursday/Friday/Saturday: if the cyclist was 'tired', he/she should have had an easy day, and if 'very tired', a day off.

The hills on Monday followed by two days of speedwork placed too much stress on the body. The weekly programme needs to be restructured. Doing 'hard' workouts three days in a row was totally ineffective.

4 Thursday/Friday/Saturday/Sunday: the athlete became ill on Thursday, probably due to overtraining Monday through Wednesday. If you are ill, stop training! Training through an illness will be ineffective and may prolong the illness.

The resting heart rate was a good indicator of lack of recovery due to illness. Thursday's workout with elevated resting and training heart rates and a slower average speed should have indicated it was time to go home and rest!

5 Saturday: never race when ill or over-trained. It's dangerous and a waste of time.

In summary, this athlete's programme needs a lot of restructuring. There is no balance between exercise and rest. Remember, exercise plus rest equals improvement! Following hills on Monday with interval training (speedwork) on Tuesday and Wednesday was totally ineffective. The athlete became over-trained and workouts were wasted. Training through illness delayed recovery and resulted in twelve hours and three minutes of training time that came to nothing. If the athlete had rested as soon as the overtraining indicators showed up, he/she might not have become ill and might not have wasted so much training time. More is not better!

♦ Time trials ♦

Time trials are used to find out how effective your training programme is. Generally, they are done over 33 to 50 per cent of your race distance. If training for a 10 km run, doing a 5 km time trial around a 1 km circuit is excellent as this allows you to gauge your fitness adequately and get lap times as well as a final time. Getting lap times is particularly helpful as they may pinpoint weaknesses or strengths in your training and pace judgement. Here are some guidelines concerning time trials.

1 A plateauing of time trial times is a good indicator of where your training is at, as long as they are not adversely affected by the rest of your training. If, after a period of weeks, your time trial times cease to improve, then in most cases you have achieved your training objective – time to start speedwork if this happens at the end of base; time to race if this happens at the end of speedwork. The other possibility is that your training is not working – time to check out your programme and log book.

2 If your time trial times start to drop, you may be ill or overfatigued. If it is the latter, make sure this doesn't lead to overtraining by reducing volume and/or intensity in the following days or weeks. See an experienced coach if you can. Expect lap times to slow after you peak, though. You then slowly build to your next peak.

3 If your lap times become progressively faster in your time trial, this indicates either:

• your warm-up was inadequate, or
• you started too slowly.

4 If lap times become progressively slower during your time trial, this indicates your speedwork is adequate but you need more aerobic work or you started too fast.

5 If you cannot complete or have difficulty completing a time trial, this indicates either:

• you require a lot more base training (you're unfit!);
• you are ill;
• a previous workout has overfatigued you;
• you are overtrained.

Time trials are demanding and should only be done by experienced athletes, and then only every two to four weeks. Elite athletes may be able to time trial every one to two weeks, but the time trial should replace a speed session. If you use a heart rate monitor during your time trials, this will help you establish your approximate race pace (*see* page 34 for more details on time trials and heart rate monitor use). Appendix 5 provides a record sheet and speed calculations for time trial tests.

DAY	ACTIVITY	PERFORMANCE ANALYSIS
MON **DATE** 6|4 **H.R.** 45 **WGHT** 70	SPORT Cycling SPORT SPORT TIME: 1hr 15min TIME: TIME: DIST: 38 Km DIST: DIST: AV SPEED: 30.4 AV SPEED: AV SPEED: AV H.R. 170·175 AV H.R. AV H.R. SPECIFICS: SPECIFICS: SPECIFICS: TOTAL TIME: _____ Stretching/Injury/Illness GYM: Weights– Strength/Circuit Aerobics/Flex	FELT: Excellent/(Good)/Average/Tired/V.Tired STRESS: (Mellow)/Moderate/High/V.High BENEFIT: Excellent/(Good)/Average/Poor/☺☹ SLEEP: 11,10,9,8,7,6,5,4,3 Good/(Average)/Broken NUTRITION: (Good)/Average/Poor/Binge Day AIM: (Base)→Long/Hills 1 2 3/(Easy)/Technique Speed – Race/Time Trial/(Intervals)/Sprint 1 2 3 INTENSITY: >100%,100%,90%,80%,(70%),60%,50% WEATHER: Calm/(Moderate)/Windy/Wet/Cold/Hot WATER: Calm/Moderate/Rough COMMENTS: Post Exercise Weight: 70
TUES **DATE** 7|4 **H.R.** 44 **WGHT** 70.5	SPORT Cycling SPORT SPORT TIME: 2hr 30min TIME: TIME: DIST: 76Km DIST: DIST: AV SPEED: 30.4 AV SPEED: AV SPEED: AV H.R. 170·175 AV H.R. AV H.R. SPECIFICS: SPECIFICS: SPECIFICS: TOTAL TIME: _____ Stretching/Injury/Illness GYM: Weights– Strength/Circuit Aerobics/Flex	FELT: Excellent/(Good)/Average/Tired/V.Tired STRESS: (Mellow)/Moderate/High/V.High BENEFIT: Excellent/(Good)/Average/Poor/☺☹ SLEEP: 11,10,9,8,7,6,5,4,3 Good/(Average)/Broken NUTRITION: Good/Average/(Poor)/Binge Day AIM: (Base)→Long/(Hills 1 2) 3/Easy/Technique Speed – Race/Time Trial/Intervals/Sprint 1 2 3 INTENSITY: >100%,100%,90%,80%,(70%),60%,50% WEATHER: (Calm)/Moderate/Windy/Wet/Cold/(Hot) WATER: Calm/Moderate/Rough COMMENTS: Post Exercise Weight:
WED **DATE** 8|4 **H.R.** 44 **WGHT** 70	SPORT Cycling SPORT SPORT TIME: 1hr 7min TIME: TIME: DIST: 38 Km DIST: DIST: AV SPEED: 34 AV SPEED: AV SPEED: AV H.R. 185·190 AV H.R. AV H.R. SPECIFICS: SPECIFICS: SPECIFICS: TOTAL TIME: _____ Stretching/Injury/Illness GYM: Weights– Strength/Circuit Aerobics/Flex	FELT: Excellent/(Good)/Average/Tired/V.Tired STRESS: (Mellow)/Moderate/High/V.High BENEFIT: Excellent/(Good)/Average/Poor/☺☹ SLEEP: 11,10,9,8,(7),6,5,4,3 (Good)/Average/Broken NUTRITION: Good/Average/(Poor)/Binge Day AIM: (Base)– Long/Hills 1 2 3/(Easy)/Technique Speed – Race/Time Trial/Intervals/Sprint 1 2 3 INTENSITY: >100%,(100%),90%,80%,70%,60%,50% WEATHER: Calm/(Moderate)/Windy/Wet/Cold/Hot WATER: Calm/Moderate/Rough COMMENTS: Post Exercise Weight:
THUR **DATE** 9|4 **H.R.** 53 **WGHT** 69.5	SPORT Cycling SPORT SPORT TIME: 2hr 10min TIME: TIME: DIST: 57 Km DIST: DIST: AV SPEED: 26.3 AV SPEED: AV SPEED: AV H.R. 115·180 AV H.R. AV H.R. SPECIFICS: SPECIFICS: SPECIFICS: TOTAL TIME: _____ Stretching/Injury/Illness GYM: Weights– Strength/Circuit Aerobics/Flex	FELT: Excellent/Good/Average/(Tired)/V.Tired STRESS: Mellow/(Moderate)/High/V.High BENEFIT: Excellent/Good/Average/(Poor)/☺☹ SLEEP: 11,10,9,8,7,6,5,4,3 Good/Average/(Broken) NUTRITION: Good/(Average)/Poor/Binge Day AIM: (Base)/(Long)/Hills 1 2 3/Easy/Technique Speed – Race/Time Trial/Intervals/Sprint 1 2 3 INTENSITY: >100%,100%,(90%),80%,70%,(60%),50% ? WEATHER: Calm/Moderate/Windy/Wet/Cold/(Hot) WATER: Calm/Moderate/Rough COMMENTS: Not a good day Post Exercise Weight:

Figure 8.1 Example of working programme (1)

ACTIVITY			PERFORMANCE ANALYSIS	DAY

FRI

SPORT	SPORT	SPORT
TIME:	TIME:	TIME:
DIST:	DIST:	DIST:
AV SPEED:	AV SPEED:	AV SPEED:
AV H.R.	AV H.R.	AV H.R.
SPECIFICS:	SPECIFICS:	SPECIFICS:

DAY OFF

TOTAL TIME: _____ Stretching/Injury/Illness
GYM: Weights– Strength/Circuit Aerobics/Flex

FELT: Excellent/Good/(Average)/Tired/V.Tired
STRESS: (Mellow/Moderate/High)/V.High
BENEFIT: Excellent/Good/Average/Poor/☺☹
SLEEP: 11,10,9,8,7,(6),5,4,3 Good/(Average)/Broken
NUTRITION: Good/Average/Poor/Binge Day
AIM: Base – Long/Hills 1 2 3/Easy/Technique
    Speed – Race/Time Trial/Intervals/Sprint 1 2 3
INTENSITY: >100%,100%,90%,80%,70%,60%,50%
WEATHER: Calm/Moderate/Windy/Wet/Cold/Hot
WATER: Calm/Moderate/Rough
COMMENTS:
    I need this!!
Post Exercise Weight:

DATE 10|4
H.R. 56
WGHT 70

SAT

SPORT	SPORT	SPORT
Cycling		
TIME: 1hr 5min	TIME:	TIME:
DIST: 40 km	DIST:	DIST:
AV SPEED: 36.9	AV SPEED:	AV SPEED:
AV H.R. 190-195	AV H.R.	AV H.R.
SPECIFICS:	SPECIFICS:	SPECIFICS:

TOTAL TIME: _____ Stretching/Injury/Illness
GYM: Weights– Strength/Circuit Aerobics/Flex

FELT: Excellent/(Good)/Average/Tired/V.Tired
STRESS: (Mellow)/Moderate/High/V.High
BENEFIT: Excellent/(Good)/Average/Poor/☺☹
SLEEP: 11,10,9,8,7,6,5,4,3 Good/(Average)/Broken
NUTRITION: Good/Average/Poor/(Binge Day)
AIM: (Base) – Long/Hills 1 2 3/Easy/Technique
    Speed – Race/Time Trial/Intervals/Sprint 1 2 3
INTENSITY: >100%,100%,(90%),80%,70%,50%
WEATHER: Calm/Moderate/(Windy)/Wet/Cold/Hot
WATER: Calm/Moderate/Rough
COMMENTS:
Post Exercise Weight:

DATE 11|4
H.R. 43
WGHT 70

SUN

SPORT	SPORT	SPORT
Cycling		
TIME: 4hr 5min	TIME:	TIME:
DIST: 115 km	DIST:	DIST:
AV SPEED: 28.2	AV SPEED:	AV SPEED:
AV H.R. 170-175	AV H.R.	AV H.R.
SPECIFICS:	SPECIFICS:	SPECIFICS:

TOTAL TIME: _____ Stretching/Injury/Illness
GYM: Weights– Strength/Circuit Aerobics/Flex

FELT: Excellent/Good/Average/(Tired)/V.Tired
STRESS: (Mellow)/Moderate/High/V.High
BENEFIT: Excellent/Good/Average/Poor/(☺)☹
SLEEP: 11,10,9,8,7,6,5,4,3 Good/(Average)/(Broken)
NUTRITION: Good/Average/Poor/(Binge Day)
AIM: (Base) – Long/Hills 1 2 3/Easy/Technique
    Speed – Race/Time Trial/Intervals/Sprint 1 2 3
INTENSITY: >100%,100%,90%,(80%),70%,(60%),50%
WEATHER: (Calm)/Moderate/Windy/Wet/Cold/Hot
WATER: Calm/Moderate/Rough
COMMENTS:
Post Exercise Weight:

DATE 12|4
H.R. 57
WGHT 69.8

WEEKLY SUMMARY

WEEK NO: 8
WEIGHT (AV): 70
REST PULSE (AV): 48.9 (45.8 av)
SLEEP (AV): 4.5 (5b)
TRAINING TIME/DIST (AV): 2 hr 20 min
TOTAL TRAINING TIME/DIST: 12 hr 12 min
LAST WEEK'S TOTAL: 10 hrs
% INCREASE/DECREASE: + 22%
PHYSICAL CONDITION: Excellent/Good/(Average)/Groan!
STRESS: (Mellow)/Moderate/High
EFFECTIVENESS: Excellent/Good/(Average)/☺☹
NUTRITION: Good/Moderate/(Poor)

TRAINING NOTES

Diet poor.
Need more sleep.
Got a bit excited on
Wednesday & Saturday.
Keep training intensity
low.

133

DAY	ACTIVITY			PERFORMANCE ANALYSIS
MON **DATE** 8|6 **H.R.** 45 **WGHT** 70	SPORT Cycling TIME: 1hr 15min DIST: 38 Km AV SPEED: 30·4 AV H.R. 150-155 SPECIFICS: hills TOTAL TIME: GYM: Weights– Strength/Circuit Aerobics/Flex	SPORT TIME: DIST: AV SPEED: AV H.R. SPECIFICS:	SPORT TIME: DIST: AV SPEED: AV H.R. SPECIFICS: Stretching/Injury/Illness	FELT: Excellent/(Good)/Average/Tired/V.Tired STRESS: (Mellow)/Moderate/High/V.High BENEFIT: Excellent/(Good)/Average/Poor/☺☹ SLEEP: 11,10,9,(8),7,6,5,4,3 (Good)/Average/Broken NUTRITION: (Good)/Average/Poor/Binge Day AIM: (Base) – Long/(Hills) 1 2 3/Easy/Technique Speed – Race/Time Trial/Intervals/Sprint 1 2 3 INTENSITY: >100%,100%,90%,80%,(70%),60%,50% WEATHER: Calm/Moderate/Windy/(Wet)/(Cold)/Hot WATER: Calm/Moderate/Rough COMMENTS: Post Exercise Weight:
TUES **DATE** 9|6 **H.R.** 44 **WGHT** 71	SPORT Cycling TIME: 2hr 30min DIST: 76 Km AV SPEED: 30·4 AV H.R. 150-155 SPECIFICS: Intervals 175-180 HR 40 Kph 4 x 6 at AT; 3 min rest btwn TOTAL TIME: GYM: Weights– Strength/Circuit Aerobics/Flex	SPORT TIME: DIST: AV SPEED: AV H.R. SPECIFICS:	SPORT TIME: DIST: AV SPEED: AV H.R. SPECIFICS: Stretching/Injury/Illness	FELT: Excellent/(Good)/Average/Tired/V.Tired STRESS: (Mellow)/Moderate/High/V.High BENEFIT: (Excellent)/Good/Average/Poor/☺☹ SLEEP: 11,10,9,(8),7,6,5,4,3 (Good)/Average/Broken NUTRITION: (Good)/Average/Poor/Binge Day AIM: Base – Long/Hills 1 2 3/(Easy)/(Technique) (Speed) – Race/Time Trial/(Intervals)/Sprint 1 2 3 INTENSITY: >100%,100%,(90%),80%,(70%),60%,50% WEATHER: Calm/(Moderate)/Windy/(Wet)/Cold/Hot WATER: Calm/Moderate/Rough COMMENTS: Post Exercise Weight:
WED **DATE** 10|6 **H.R.** 53 **WGHT** 70	SPORT Cycling TIME: 1hr 7min DIST: 38 Km AV SPEED: 34 AV H.R. 160-165 SPECIFICS: Intervals: 165·170 HR 37 Kph 3 x 8 min at AT, 3 min rest btwn TOTAL TIME: GYM: Weights– Strength/Circuit Aerobics/Flex	SPORT TIME: DIST: AV SPEED: AV H.R. SPECIFICS:	SPORT TIME: DIST: AV SPEED: AV H.R. SPECIFICS: Stretching/Injury/Illness	FELT: Excellent/Good/Average/(Tired)/V.Tired STRESS: (Mellow)/Moderate/High/(V.High) BENEFIT: Excellent/Good/Average/(Poor)/☺☹ SLEEP: 11,10,(9),8,7,6,5,4,3 Good/(Average)/Broken NUTRITION: (Good)/Average/Poor/Binge Day AIM: Base – Long/Hills 1 2 3/Easy/Technique (Speed) – Race/Time Trial/(Intervals)/Sprint 1 2 3 INTENSITY: >100%,100%,90%,(80%),70%,60%,50% WEATHER: Calm/(Moderate)/Windy/Wet/Cold/Hot WATER: Calm/Moderate/Rough COMMENTS: Legs tired !! Post Exercise Weight:
THUR **DATE** 11|6 **H.R.** 60 **WGHT** 70	SPORT Cycling TIME: 2hr 10min DIST: 57 Km AV SPEED: 26·3 AV H.R. 160-165 SPECIFICS: TOTAL TIME: GYM: Weights– Strength/Circuit Aerobics/Flex	SPORT TIME: DIST: AV SPEED: AV H.R. SPECIFICS:	SPORT TIME: DIST: AV SPEED: AV H.R. SPECIFICS: Stretching/Injury/Illness	FELT: Excellent/Good/Average/Tired/(V.Tired) STRESS: (Mellow)/Moderate/High/V.High BENEFIT: Excellent/Good/Average/(Poor)/☺☹ SLEEP: 11,(10),9,8,7,6,5,4,3 Good/Average/(Broken) NUTRITION: (Good)/Average/Poor/Binge Day AIM: (Base) – Long/Hills 1 2 3/(Easy)/Technique Speed – Race/Time Trial/Intervals/Sprint 1 2 3 INTENSITY: >100%,100%,90%,80%,70%,(60%),50% WEATHER: Calm/Moderate/(Windy)/Wet/(Cold)/Hot WATER: Calm/Moderate/Rough COMMENTS: Sick ! Post Exercise Weight:

Figure 8.2 Example of working programme (2)

ACTIVITY	PERFORMANCE ANALYSIS	DAY

FRI

SPORT / SPORT / SPORT
TIME: / TIME: / TIME:
DIST: / DIST: / DIST:
AV SPEED: / AV SPEED: / AV SPEED:
AV H.R. / AV H.R. / AV H.R.
SPECIFICS: / SPECIFICS: / SPECIFICS:
DAY OFF
TOTAL TIME: _____ Stretching/Injury/Illness
GYM: Weights– Strength/Circuit Aerobics/Flex

FELT: Excellent/Good/Average/Tired/(V.Tired)
STRESS: Mellow/Moderate/(High)/V.High
BENEFIT: Excellent/Good/Average/Poor/☺☹
SLEEP: 11,(10),9,8,7,6,5,4,3 Good/Average/(Broken)
NUTRITION: Good/(Average)/Poor/Binge Day
AIM: Base – Long/Hills 1 2 3/Easy/Technique / Speed – Race/Time Trial/Intervals/Sprint 1 2 3
INTENSITY: >100%,100%,90%,80%,70%,60%,50%
WEATHER: Calm/Moderate/Windy/Wet/Cold/Hot
WATER: Calm/Moderate/Rough
COMMENTS: Sick !
Post Exercise Weight:

DATE 12/6
H.R. 59
WGHT 70

SAT

SPORT cycling / SPORT / SPORT
TIME: 56 min
DIST: 40 km
AV SPEED: 42.9
AV H.R. 190-195
SPECIFICS: Race !
TOTAL TIME: _____ Stretching/Injury/Illness
GYM: Weights– Strength/Circuit Aerobics/Flex

FELT: Excellent/Good/Average/(Tired)/V.Tired
STRESS: Mellow/Moderate/(High)/V.High
BENEFIT: Excellent/Good/Average/(Poor)/☺☹
SLEEP: 11,10,9,(8),7,6,5,4,3 Good/(Average)/Broken
NUTRITION: (Good)/Average/Poor/Binge Day
AIM: Base – Long/Hills 1 2 3/Easy/Technique / (Speed) – (Race)/Time Trial/Intervals/Sprint 1 2 3
INTENSITY: >100%,100%,(90%),80%,70%,60%,50%
WEATHER: Calm/(Moderate)/Windy/Wet/Cold/Hot
WATER: Calm/Moderate/Rough
COMMENTS: Not feeling the best – maybe still sick.
Post Exercise Weight:

DATE 13/6
H.R. 54
WGHT 70.5

SUN

SPORT cycling / SPORT / SPORT
TIME: 4 hr 5min
DIST: 115 km
AV SPEED: 28.2
AV H.R. 150-155
SPECIFICS:
TOTAL TIME: _____ Stretching/Injury/Illness
GYM: Weights– Strength/Circuit Aerobics/Flex

FELT: Excellent/Good/(Average)/Tired/V.Tired
STRESS: (Mellow)/Moderate/High/V.High
BENEFIT: Excellent/Good/(Average)/Poor/☺☹
SLEEP: 11,10,9,(8),7,6,5,4,3 Good/(Average)/Broken
NUTRITION: (Good)/Average/Poor/Binge Day
AIM: (Base) – Long/Hills 1 2 3/(Easy)/Technique / Speed – Race/Time Trial/Intervals/Sprint 1 2 3
INTENSITY: >100%,100%,90%,80%,(70%),60%,50%
WEATHER: (Calm)/Moderate/Windy/(Wet)/Cold/Hot
WATER: Calm/Moderate/Rough
COMMENTS:
Post Exercise Weight:

DATE 14/6
H.R. 52
WGHT 70

WEEKLY SUMMARY
WEEK NO: 12
WEIGHT (AV): 70.2
REST PULSE (AV): 52.4 (45.8 av.)
SLEEP (AV): 61 (56)
TRAINING TIME/DIST (AV): 2 hrs
TOTAL TRAINING TIME/DIST: 12 hr 3 min
LAST WEEK'S TOTAL: 11 hr 40min
% INCREASE/DECREASE: + 3.3%
PHYSICAL CONDITION: Excellent/Good/Average/(Groan!)
STRESS: Mellow/(Moderate)/High
EFFECTIVENESS: Excellent/Good/Average/(☺☹)
NUTRITION: (Good)/Moderate/Poor

TRAINING NOTES
Hills on Monday, Intervals Tuesday & Wednesday wasn't a good idea.
Illness was a bummer! Shouldn't have raced.

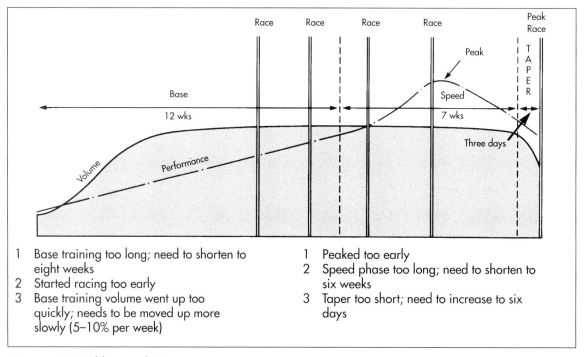

1 Base training too long; need to shorten to eight weeks
2 Started racing too early
3 Base training volume went up too quickly; needs to be moved up more slowly (5–10% per week)

1 Peaked too early
2 Speed phase too long; need to shorten to six weeks
3 Taper too short; need to increase to six days

Figure 8.3 Build-up analysis

♦ Peak-to-peak analysis ♦

Peak-to-peak or post-peak analysis is a review of your entire training from beginning of build-up through to your 'peak' or big race. After this race, it is time to sit down, analyse your training and, with hindsight, ask some specific questions. What worked? What was ineffective? What could have been changed slightly? What was done at the wrong time?

The aim is to identify errors and strengths in your training so that your training programme and training itself is refined from build-up to build-up (*see* fig. 8.3). This allows you to optimise your training and should stop you making the same errors over and over again.

Athletes, coaches, clubs and national squads should always be in search of the best possible results. If the season went badly, look at the programme and all its parts. Keep the programme's good points and eliminate the bad points. And the same applies if the season went well.

Post-peak analysis should be done as soon as the season finishes, while ideas on the previous season's training are still fresh in your mind. Both the athlete and the coach should have input into the review.

Chapter 9

The Coach

♦ The value of the coach ♦

If you possibly can, get a coach or experienced athlete to help you with your training, even if it is just now and again. Most experienced athletes and coaches are only too happy to share their knowledge. Coaching is an invaluable aid. The experience and knowledge of a good coach allows you to progress faster because pitfalls and mistakes are avoided. They also provide an objective opinion on your training, and are very good for motivation as they tend to push you to greater efforts when required. Good technique can also be taught by the coach, which can have a huge effect on performance, and his/her advice on the choice of equipment and its set-up can significantly help performance.

♦ The relationship between ♦ athlete and coach

Communication is vital between the coach and the athlete and the communication must always be two-way! The coach is a guide and consultant, not a dictator. He or she needs to know how the athlete is feeling and responding to training. This requires a thorough dialogue. It is also important to know whether the athlete is 'picking up' aspects of training which may require work, for example in rowing this may include things like slide control, movement of the boat at the catch, complete unity of the crew in leg drive.

When writing the next training programme the coach should use data from previous training logs and input from the athlete. (Inexperienced athletes will obviously need to rely more on the coach's experience than experienced athletes.)

The key to good coaching is the coach's knowledge of the sport, his/her experience, the ability to relate to many personality types, an understanding of how to get the most out of an athlete, communication with the athlete based on equality, the desire and need to continue learning, and a willingness always to put the athlete's welfare first.

♦ Level of coach ♦ involvement

Coaching an inexperienced athlete requires a high level of coach involvement. The coach needs to explain the hows and whys of training, including the reason it is structured the way it is. In this way, the athlete will gain a better understanding of training and will be able to have a greater input into the programme.

Initially, the coach is a benevolent dictator when it comes to training. As the athlete's training knowledge increases, however, and they become more self-sufficient, the coach takes on more of a consultancy role, more concerned with fine tuning than designing the programme entirely.

A coach should always accept that they can learn from the athlete, and there is a philosophy which suggests the coach has done a good job if the athlete surpasses the achievements of the coach (this makes it tough if you are coached by an Olympic champion!).

♦ Responsibilities of the ♦ athlete, coach, and administrator

The athlete's responsibilities

- To have fun
- To have self-discipline, dedication and self-motivation
- To learn to understand his/her own training
- To be realistic
- To respect and listen to the coach/administrators
- To set his/her own goals (short and long-term)
- To be able to take disappointments
- To have humility when successful
- To take full responsibility for his/her own performance
- To be professional in dealing with coaches, administrators, the public, the media and sponsors

The coach's responsibilities

- To encourage the athlete
- To ensure the athlete's welfare always comes first
- To ensure the goals set are primarily the athlete's goals

- Not to push the athlete too hard
- To let the athlete make her/his own decisions
- To help the athlete's training in every way possible
- To make sure the athlete develops athletically and socially
- To ensure the athlete learns from and understands her/his training
- To make sure the athlete enjoys training
- To teach and allow the athlete self-sufficiency

The administrator's responsibilities

- To make sure the athlete's (and coach's) welfare comes first
- To look after the best interests of the sport
- To ensure the athlete is freed from internal politics and administration and is able to train freely
- To ensure administration is effective and set up to help the athlete and coach
- To ensure the athlete can train and compete without administrative interference
- To encourage the athlete
- To provide opportunities that the athlete is unable to create for her/himself
- To provide organisational and developmental support for the athlete and coach
- To set up racing, training and coaching at the best times for the athlete
- To help raise funds for the athlete
- To ensure the sport's image is a positive one that provides plenty of opportunities for participation and enjoyment

♦ Coaching young athletes ♦

Don't bury a young athlete under a mountain of work. A critical aspect of coaching young athletes is an understanding of their athletic development. It is important to realise that improvement will take place over many seasons and that the first few years of an athlete's career are somewhat akin to an apprenticeship.

The emphasis early on should be on fun and learning, not on results. Let the young athlete gain some experience and establish a training pattern. Don't burden them with expectations of success and records. Let them gain an understanding of their training and how it will develop them as an athlete.

Success in endurance sports takes many years to achieve at the highest level, and trying to 'bring on' a young athlete too soon may see them lose interest in the sport long before they have had a chance to enjoy all the sport has to offer (and any success that may have come their way). Too many coaches seem prepared to sacrifice an athlete's long-term prospects and short-term enjoyment for the sake of records and championships that may mean more to the coach than the athlete. With young athletes it can be tempting to create a junior champion through sheer volume of training. This often amounts to a coach abusing his/her power and feeding his/her ego, both at the expense of the athlete.

Fun and learning – those are the twin pillars upon which young athletes should be supported.

Chapter 10

The Environment – Altitude, Heat, Cold and Travel

You may have had a perfect training build-up, and you may be at the absolute peak of your performance potential, but a mistake in how you acclimatise to the racing climate or travel to the race venue can mean all your good preparatory work is wasted. It is very important, therefore, that you understand how climate and travel can disrupt performance. Acclimatisation can be defined as physiological compensation to environmental stress over a period of time.

♦ Altitude training ♦

Altitude training is one of the most controversial areas in sports science today. Does it work or doesn't it? Researchers around the world continue to study the issue, but as yet there is no universal agreement within the scientific community as to the value of altitude training for endurance athletes. Similarly, athletes and coaches can't agree on the effect of altitude training on performance. Everyone agrees that altitude training is beneficial for racing at altitude; the heated discussions occur when considering altitude training and sea-level performance.

There is a lot of anecdotal evidence to support the theory that altitude training enhances sea-level performance, but first-hand reports by athletes and coaches make it equally clear that it doesn't work for everyone. As you increase altitude, barometric pressure drops and the air becomes thinner (decreased oxygen per volume of air). This means there is less oxygen to bind with haemoglobin (the part of blood that transports oxygen from the lungs to the muscles). As a result, the working muscles don't function as well during exercise because they don't receive as much oxygen.

Aerobic ability begins to decline at approximately 1524 metres (5000 feet) above sea level. Initially, a 3 per cent decrease in aerobic ability occurs every 300 metres (1000 feet). At higher altitudes, however, the rate of decrease is much greater, for example, exercising at 3050 metres (10,000 feet) is more than twice as difficult as exercising at 1500 metres (5000 feet). Very simply, at altitude there is a reduction in aerobic ability. This in turn reduces performance in endurance sports.

Altitude	Aerobic ability
0 m	100%
1976 m (6500 ft)	90%
4286 m (14,100 ft)	75%
6992 m (23,000 ft)	50%

Performance changes (by percentage) at altitude for various distances
- 100–400 m: enhanced 1 to 2 per cent
- 3000 m steeplechase to 5000 m: impaired by 5 to 6 per cent
- 10,000 m to marathon: impaired 6 to 7 per cent

The body adapts to altitude stress by increasing haemoglobin and red blood cell production. At 4500 metres red blood cell levels increase by 20 per cent in three to four weeks. This means the oxygen-carrying capacity is increased and more oxygen theoretically gets to the muscles. Performance potential at that altitude is then increased from the initial unadapted state. After the first three to four weeks the increase in red blood cell level becomes more gradual, although it may continue for up to a year. Acclimatisation to altitude is therefore associated with red blood cell production.

The magnitude of the increase is not only altitude-dependent, but is also influenced by the way your training is organised (more on that soon). If you return to sea level after altitude adaptation, the adaptation remains briefly, possibly allowing a level of performance that could not have been achieved if you had stayed at sea level. However, the amount of blood that your heart pumps per minute is reduced by altitude acclimatisation – not only at rest but during exercise. This largely offsets the advantage of increased red blood cell numbers, so that the capacity for the transport of oxygen to the muscles remains virtually the same.

But maybe it is some other factor, or an aspect of the same factor, that promotes performance enhancement. It is known that 'blood doping' (an infusion of the athlete's own blood back into her/his body – more blood means more red blood cells which means a higher oxygen-carrying capacity) works, although there are other factors involved. A drug called EPO (erythropoietin) is used (illegally) by some endurance athletes because it is considered to increase red blood cell levels. Increased blood cell levels mean more oxygen can be carried in the blood, boosting endurance performance. Unfortunately these performance enhancers also increase your chance of a heart attack as the increased blood cell levels thicken the blood to the point where the heart becomes overloaded and cannot pump it adequately.

Although the jury is still out on the benefits of training at altitude to enhance sea-level performance, plenty of athletes would like to find out for themselves if it works. So, let's assume that you want to train at altitude. How would you go about it?

How to train at altitude

The most effective altitude for endurance training is around 1500 to 2000 metres, although recent research suggests 2200 to 3000 metres. Below these levels there appears to be no significant effect, while higher altitudes impede training too much. Some athletes, thinking 'more is better', have made the mistake of training at too high an altitude. This can lead to a lot of training time being wasted waiting for adaptation to occur. It can also lead to overtraining due to the greater training stress.

The higher above 1500 metres you go, the longer adaptation takes. The question is: Can you afford that time? You might be better off spending the seven to ten days it takes to acclimatise at 1500 to 2000 metres on training. Seven to ten days is the minimum time needed for adaptation to take place; two to four weeks is the generally accepted optimal adaptation time. This adaptation will supposedly last approximately two weeks upon returning to sea level, and is reputed to be greatest in the first week.

Recent thinking suggests the timing of your sea-level race upon returning from altitude may be critical. It is believed now that a slight delay between your return from altitude and your sea-level race is most effective. For intense sports (anaerobic sprint sports), 10 to 14 days and maybe even up to three weeks may be necessary to improve performance, but reports are conflicting. Most endurance sports, on the other hand, seem only to require a few days' delay although, once again, reports are conflicting.

A lot of elite US athletes live at altitude, with Boulder, Colorado (1626 metres/5350 ft) being very popular. Most athletes do, however, alternate altitude and sea-level training.

The first two days of altitude training create no real problems except shortness of breath. In the following days the athlete begins to feel very tired. A drop of 15 per cent in VO$_2$max may occur the second day after arriving at 2200 metres. This is the time to be careful. In fact, a mistake during this time could be very costly in terms of performance. It is easy to overtrain at this time and damage your build-up. It is a good idea, therefore, to lower training intensity and volume during this period, and then to gradually build training levels back up. You may want to come down to lower altitudes during the first week to do speedwork (the time during which the effects of altitude are most keenly felt). Or you may choose to do all your training at lower altitude during this period – remember, just living at altitude takes a bit of getting used to. Alternatively, you can gradually adapt to altitude by using a stepped approach, so as not to hinder your training (*see* 'When is it best to go to altitude?', later in this chapter).

If you can't drop down in altitude to do your speedwork, it is best not to do any speedwork during your first week.

Heart rate monitors and altitude

Heart rate monitors are very useful for avoiding training errors at altitude. Uses include:

1 Measuring degree of adaptation to altitude: In the first few hours at altitude, heart rate will drop. After this it will begin to rise. At 2000 metres your heart rate will be about 10 per cent above your sea-level heart rate. At 4500 metres, it will be about 50 per cent higher (until you begin to acclimatise). As you acclimatise, resting and training heart rates will return to normal, or even lower. At this point, acclimatisation is complete. By measuring the time it takes (i.e. the number of days) for heart rate to return to sea-level rates, the length of adaptation can be calculated.

2 Matching altitude and sea-level intensities: It is easy to overdo initial training at altitude. The tendency is to push too hard because you are going so slowly (you may be faster on the bike, however, because of the reduction in air resistance). By using your heart rate monitor you can train at the same intensities that you would at sea level, without succumbing to the desire to increase your speed. (For example, an athlete running at altitude at his/her usual intensity will be performing at a slower pace due to the 'thin' air's effects on aerobic ability.) Once adaptation has taken place, training workloads similar to those carried out at sea level will be possible.

3 Setting correct rest periods between intervals: If you are doing speedwork at altitude, particularly intervals, rest periods need to be longer because recovery takes longer. To ensure your rest periods are not too short (or too long), make sure you don't begin exercising until your heart rate has dropped the same amount it would at sea level (40 to 60 bpm for most athletes). During the adaptation phase it will take longer for your heart rate to drop than it would at sea level at the same intensity.

Factors to consider about altitude training

Dehydration seems to be amplified when training at altitude, so it is particularly important that you consume large quantities of water/fluid before, during and after workouts. Weight should be checked before and after workouts and any weight loss should be overcome by adequate hydration. If weight loss has occurred through a workout, try to drink more the next time.

While altitude training has been promoted as a way to enhance performance in endurance athletes, there are a number of factors that need to be considered before heading up the mountain to train.

1 The time loss that occurs through adaptation to altitude. As athletes often go to altitude in the last two to six weeks before racing, it is important that any time lost during this training phase is allowed for in the programme. If you can't afford to lose this time, don't go!

2 During the adaptation period, endurance athletes can't train as effectively at altitude even though they can reach the same relative percentage of maximum heart rate. For example, for the same effort, a runner will not be able to run as fast at altitude as at sea level. Muscular strength and motor patterns are therefore not developed in the way they would be at sea level. This can be overcome by doing speedwork at a lower altitude or by running intervals on a slightly downhill slope. (Sprinting and cycling – and other sports affected strongly by wind resistance – will be faster in the 'thin' air though.)

3 Altitude training does not work for everyone, especially for those athletes who already naturally possess high haemoglobin levels. Higher blood viscosity (thickness) due to greater haemoglobin may also counteract any performance gains made through altitude training. The amount of blood your heart pumps per minute is reduced, which may offset the increase in red blood cells.

4 There is a school of thought that suggests altitude training is overrated and that some of the gains may be due to factors other than altitude per se, for example, a good training environment, plenty of time to train and rest because you are often away from home and work, and the opportunity to train with other highly competitive athletes.

5 Any slight mistake at altitude (intensity too high, too much volume) is punished severely.

6 Asthmatics may have trouble acclimatising.

Recovery at altitude

It appears that training at altitude is not the major cause of altitude adaptation – recovery from altitude training is. In other words, where you train may not be as important as where you spend the rest of your time. This is because it is during recovery that red blood cells (haemoglobin) are produced. This does not occur during training sessions to any great extent. It is more beneficial, therefore, to live/sleep at altitude than to simply train at altitude. An athlete may get good results by living at 2000 to 3000 metres, doing long slow distance at 1500 to 2000 metres and doing speedwork below 1000 metres.

One drawback to this approach, however, is that during the adaptation phase the athlete may need to live/sleep and train at different altitudes. You may benefit from living/sleeping below 1000 metres after a hard training session because recovery is slower if done at altitude. This speeds up recovery from this workout. You may live/sleep at higher altitudes after an easy workout where recovery is not so important. Therefore, during the adaptation phase, you may 'sleep high' if the scheduled workout is easy and 'sleep low' if the scheduled workout is intense.

Speedwork and altitude

Speedwork is affected during adaptation to altitude. For a distance runner, as we have said, speed is slower compared to similar intensities at sea level. This means the cardio-vascular effect of training is the same, but the muscular and biomechanical effects are different. Similarly, for cyclists, even though the lower air resistance may mean greater speeds, the muscular effect is lower because the cyclist can't push as hard on the pedals. This may affect the cyclist's hill-climbing and sprint ability. For both runners and cyclists, speedwork is best carried out at lower altitudes until full adaptation has occurred.

When is it best to go to altitude?

This is a difficult question to answer. When planning your 'altitude programme' – when to 'go up', when to 'come down' – you need to remember it takes a minimum of seven to ten days to acclimatise at around 1500 metres above sea level, longer if you go higher. Well before going to altitude you should have blood tests to ensure your iron stores are adequate.

Once you return from altitude, the benefits will disappear in about two weeks. It is best for endurance athletes, therefore, to race as soon as possible after returning to sea level (within a few days). This means, of course, that unless you are aiming at peaking for an event, there is little point in simply going to altitude to train.

Six approaches to adapting to training at altitude

1 *You do the whole build-up at altitude*
This is one of the traditional options, and the most expensive. In this situation your body is better able to adapt, and there are no sudden changes in the training environment in the middle of build-up.

2 *Stepped adaptation to altitude*
This allows you to adjust gradually to the change in altitude. A stepped approach may be preferable to going to altitude the traditional three weeks before a race because seven to ten days of that three weeks is lost through acclimatisation, and about a week is used for tapering. This leaves only one week of useable training time at a critical stage in the programme. Stepped adaptation takes a little longer (approximately four to six weeks), and should follow this pattern:

Step one
Week one is spent alternating training between low altitude (below 1000 metres) and medium altitude (1000–1500 metres). Living and sleeping is alternated between medium altitude (800–1200 metres) and medium – high altitude (1500–2000 metres). Sleep low after speedwork and alternate sleeping high and low for the other workouts.

Step two
Week two is spent alternating training between medium altitude (1000–1500 metres) and medium to high altitude (1500–2000 metres). Speedwork is performed at low altitude (below 1000 metres). Living and sleeping is alternated between medium to high altitude (about 1500 metres) and high altitude (2000–2500 metres). Once again, sleep low after speedwork and alternate sleeping high and low after other workouts.

Step three

Weeks three and four involve training at between 1500 metres and 3000 metres, with speedwork below 1000 metres. The athlete lives and sleeps at 2500–3000 metres. After step three the athlete returns to sea level to race. However, if the athlete is racing at altitude, step four is added.

Step four

Weeks five and six (posssibly seven as well) are spent gradually moving speedwork up to altitude. Speedwork may be alternated between high altitude and sea level at this time. You need to be able to perform well at altitude if that is where you are going to compete. Follow the philosophy 'simulate racing conditions and intensities' in training.

The stepped approach to altitude adaptation is an expensive exercise, no question, but if it means the difference between first and third it might be worthwhile!

3 *Go to altitude at the end of base and begin speedwork without 'stepping'*

This commonly occurs three to five weeks before a race. Minimum acclimatistaion is seven to ten days.

For the 1993 Tour de France, cyclist Tony Rominger was told to avoid the usual European race build-up, go to altitude in Colorado and largely train by himself with a heart rate monitor. This was unheard of in European professional cycle racing. Rominger went to Colorado five weeks before the Tour and trained for three weeks at altitude before returning to Europe for two weeks of racing. He came second in the Tour, and although he is a very good cyclist, he was not expected to perform at this level. In the final week of the Tour de France Rominger was very strong, and some say that given a few more days he might even have won. This performance has made a few athletes and coaches think very hard about altitude training.

4 *Alternate brief stays at altitude (2300 metres) with similar periods at sea level*

During one study, six champion distance runners alternated training at altitude with training at sea level. During the study period they recorded a total of fourteen personal bests including two world records.

5 *Go to altitude twice each year*

Frank Dick, ex-Director of Coaching for the British Athletics Federation and top international fitness consultant, suggested the following:

> Athletes would spend three weeks at a time at altitude. This would be long enough to get the 'altitude effect' but short enough so overall fitness didn't deteriorate. Each stay would be at approximately 2000 m. The first stay would be at the end of the off-season/early pre-season after winter training. The second would be during the final preparation for your major event and peak competition should be scheduled to take place 15 to 24 days after returning from altitude.

The report did not indicate which specific events this might apply to. The recovery period was suggested because it took the athletes 8 to 11 days to reacclimatise to sea level after altitude training, and therefore peak performance would not occur until 15 to 24 days after returning from altitude. Tony Rominger scheduled his racing of the 1993 Tour de France to fall 20–40 days after returning from altitude.

6 *Live at altitude, train at sea level*

A lot of people are excited by this theory. It is based on the idea that it's not when you train that you get improvement, it's when you recover. If you train at lower altitudes you don't have to put up with all the problems that training at altitude produces. And because your recovery is at altitude, more red blood cells are created. Maybe the answer is to live at sea level and sleep in an altitude chamber, something a number of top endurance athletes now do.

So which approach is likely to be the most effective? Alternating altitudes, going to altitude twice a year, living high and training low, and stepped adaptation seem to be the best. Going to altitude for three weeks or a minimum of seven to ten days before competing may be less effective as it will probably disrupt your training. Going to altitude less than seven days before competition definitely gets the thumbs down. Approaches 1, 2 and 3 apply for competition at altitude. All apply for competition at sea level.

Competing at altitude

If you are competing at altitude and cannot go there early to adapt, what should you do?

Compete within 24 hours of arriving at altitude (essentially, the sooner the better) for a one-day event. The cumulative effects of altitude will not be fully felt immediately but you will still perform at a lower level due to the fact that you are not altitude adapted. It is by no means the best way to do things but it is better than the tiredness you will feel within 24 to 48 hours as your body fatigues and starts the adaptation process.

Variations between preparing for racing at altitude and at sea level

1 *Racing at altitude*
You must do speedwork at altitude in order to adapt to racing in 'thin' air. During a three-week adaptation plan, an element of speedwork still needs to be done at lower altitudes, in order to maintain the muscular effects of speedwork that cannot be simulated at altitude. The speedwork done at altitude needs to be done at the same altitude at which you are racing.

2 *Racing at sea level*
You should do all speedwork at lower altitudes. A lot of information suggests that there may be no benefits to be gained from doing speedwork at altitude. If you do speed training at altitude, it seems that a combination of short interval, high-intensity exercise and distance training works best.

Summary

Avoid too much training volume and intensity during the first 7 to 14 days. If you decide to do speedwork at altitude, initially do shorter intervals with longer rests and keep the session shorter. You should have regular blood tests before going to altitude and while at altitude; ferritin and iron studies are particularly important.

Remember that altitude acclimatisation does not include the taper period, when you should be recovering.

On arrival at altitude
1 Don't sit around in the first few days at altitude. Light exercise stimulates breathing and circulation, slightly quickening your adjustment. Train lightly during the first few days.

2 Even if you have trouble sleeping, get plenty of rest.

3 You may want to use a humidifier to help combat the dry air at altitude.

4 Eat smaller meals but more of them, since digestion can be difficult at altitude. Emphasise carbohydrates for recovery.

5 Avoid alcohol in the first three days at altitude and drink plenty of water.

Clearly, altitude training is a very complex issue. You don't just go up there, train a bit and hang out. And to top it all off, we can't even say that it works for competition at sea level. A lot of studies that have shown altitude training works have used carefully supervised athletes. It may be the careful supervision of the athletes' training programmes that enhanced performance. So, should you rush off and train at altitude? Maybe a more effective training programme at home would be better (and cheaper).

In summary, the benefits of altitude training have yet to be proven. Any improvements made by elite athletes exercising at their maximum capacity while on a very comprehensive and carefully supervised training programme may not necessarily be due to altitude. Alternatively, there is some excitement over the living high, training low theory.

♦ Heat ♦

Any athlete competing in an environment that is not conducive to heat loss is at risk of heat injury and a drop in performance. It takes between seven and ten days to acclimatise to hot, humid climates. When travelling to any country where ambient temperature is above 25.6°C, acclimatisation is necessary. Heat acclimatisation does not include the taper period, when you should be fully rested. Even if the temperature is below 25.6°, but hotter than where you normally train, some form of acclimatisation is advisable. The fitter you are, the better you will adapt to the heat.

The key to full acclimatisation is to get used to exercising in the heat. It is not good enough to simply live in the hot environment. You should train in the heat (same environmental conditions, same training intensity and a similar training duration). Again, the rule of specificity is important. The exercise intensity should be at least 70 to 75 per cent of VO_2max to evoke adaptation (heart rate at 155 to 160 bpm for a 25-year-old). If you race in the middle of the day and it is very hot, you need to be conditioned to racing in that kind of environment. Be very careful, though, not to do too much when you arrive at the competition venue. This can overtire you and impair the following workouts.

When you first arrive in a hot environment you will be very susceptible to fatigue, so reduce training volumes and intensities. Start with short, low-intensity workouts and do them in the cooler times of the day (early morning and evening). Over the next seven to ten days gradually return to normal training volumes and intensities. This may be a little difficult for triathletes in Hawaii for the Ironman, when acclimatisation occurs during a major race taper. Ideally, three weeks is required in this situation (eleven days' acclimatisation, ten taper days). If you can't do this, artificially acclimatise before you arrive (*see* page 149).

A basic acclimatisation schedule looks like this:

Day	% of normal training volume
1	50
2	60; early a.m. and p.m. workouts, lower intensities
3	70
4	80
5	90; start training at the time of day that you will race. Small amounts of speed-work early a.m. and late p.m.
6	100
7	100
8	100
9	100; gradual progression to usual speed-work, moving it to the time of day when you will race
10	100

It is important to understand the relationship between temperature and humidity. Temperatures up to 25°C are safe even in high humidity. However, when the temperature climbs to 27°C an increase in humidity can be very dangerous. High humidity (water vapour in the air) will not allow adequate evaporation of sweat from the body. Sweating is the body's way of reducing its core temperature. If the core temperature gets too high, you begin to experience the first symptoms of heat stress. If it continues to climb, you may suffer from potentially fatal heat injury.

Temperature is not the only contributing factor to heat stress. Other factors include dehydration, lack of sleep, infection and glycogen depletion.

It is important that you understand the symptoms of heat stress. Early symptoms are excessive sweating or cessation of sweating, dizziness, goose pimples, headaches, nausea and vomiting.

Exercising in the heat when not fully acclimatised will initially raise heart rate. If you have a heart rate monitor use it to stay within your heart rate training zone as pace will be slower due to the heat. A heat acclimatised athlete will have a slightly lower resting heart rate and submaximal heart rate than normal and will tend to sweat more.

If you are doing speedwork in hot conditions, initially do shorter intervals with longer rests. Alternatively, do your speedwork in the cooler parts of the day.

In hot conditions, as all athletes know, the body loses a lot of fluid. This is particularly so during the first four days of training in a hot environment. It is critical, therefore, that you replenish fluid supplies in order to avoid dehydration. Drink before, during and after workouts, and steadily throughout the day. This may seem excessive but thirst is not a good indicator of the need for fluids – if you feel thirsty, dehydration has begun – so it is best to establish a regular drinking pattern.

It is a good idea in hot climates to weigh yourself before and after workouts to keep a check on fluid loss. Any weight loss is fluid loss! Drink one litre of fluid for every kilogram of body weight lost during exercise, and keep a full water bottle beside your bed during the night. A 2 per cent loss in body weight after a workout or race (1.4 kg loss for a 70 kg athlete) represents a fluid loss due to thermal or exercise-induced dehydration. This decreases muscular strength and endurance considerably (*see* fig. 10.1).

Weight (kg)	Fluid Loss (% of total body weight)	Physiological effect
70	0	
68.6	2	Impaired temperature regulation but not athletic performance
67.9	3	Decreased muscular endurance
67.2–65.8	4–6	Decreased muscular strength
<65.8	>6	Heat stress injuries
		Heat cramps
Increasing dehydration		Heat exhaustion
		Heat stroke
		Coma
		Death

Figure 10.1 Physiological effects of fluid loss

Dehydration can affect training for 24 to 36 hours as it takes time to rehydrate completely. Urine colour should be clear if you are well hydrated (unless you are taking vitamin pills). Try alternating water and sport drinks to avoid losing too much salt and potassium. If you are going to compete in a race that supplies a particular kind of sport drink during the event, try to get used to that drink well before race day to avoid stomach upsets. Avoid drinks that contain caffeine (tea, coffee, colas), and alcohol, as they have a dehydrating effect.

If you are flying to an event, drink plenty of fluids while travelling and, again, avoid alcohol. Wear loose-fitting clothing so that the air circulates around your body. This helps sweat evaporation and cooling.

When in hot climates wear light-coloured clothing that reflects sunlight, rather than dark clothing that absorbs the heat. Clothing that 'wicks' sweat away from the skin is also good for evaporation, for example polypropylene, cotton. Wearing a light-coloured hat in hot conditions can also help cooling. Materials impermeable to water or that hold water and become damp affect the cooling mechanism of sweating and increase the chance of heat injury.

When racing (particularly running) constantly check wind conditions. In headwinds and sidewinds the cooling effect of the wind is greater. A following wind will not have the same cooling effect as the evaporation of sweat is reduced (the speed of the wind passing over the body is slower as you are moving with the wind). In races where this occurs, sponge yourself down. The extra water on the skin will evaporate and have a cooling effect. Putting water on the head is particularly good for cooling. Before a race it pays to check for wind-sheltered areas (for example in the Hawaii Ironman the first 6 km of the marathon) and areas where the wind will be blowing (on the Queen K' highway). And check on the prevailing winds – some races, such as the Hawaii Ironman, will include a change of wind direction during the event. Sheltered parts of the course and areas with a following wind will increase your core temperature due to a decrease in evaporation. This means more sponging is required on these sections of the course.

Artificial heat acclimatisation

Artificial heat acclimatisation can help if you cannot get to the competition venue early enough. This form of heat training has been carried out in heat chambers, greenhouses and heated training rooms. For many athletes, however, these techniques may not be available. Exercising in a bathroom with both the shower and a heater full-on is a good home-made alternative. Another technique for inducing hot conditions artificially involves wearing excessive layers of clothing while exercising, especially layers on the head. Acclimatising to hot conditions in these ways is often necessary for athletes living in one hemisphere and racing in another. Alternating techniques for different workouts is acceptable but combining two techniques may overwhelm the body's temperature-regulating mechanism and lead to problems.

If using these techniques, gradually increase the heat stress (add layers of clothing or increase the room temperature), over the seven to ten days prior to competition. Do not overdo it! Training in the same temperature as the race will be run in is sufficient. Hotter is not better! Finally, if training in a heated room, use a fan to aid evaporation of sweat from the body.

♦ Cold ♦

The metabolic heat generated during exercise means that cold temperatures tend not to pose quite the same threat to performance as do hot, humid conditions. Nevertheless, severe exposure to low temperatures can lead to hypothermia and even death, so it pays to be prepared.

When training and racing in cold conditions it is best to dress in layers that provide an insulating barrier of air that helps retain body heat. Ideally, the clothing should allow for the evaporation of sweat while still providing added protection against the cold. Clothing closest to the skin should be polypropylene as this helps 'wick' sweat away from the skin. On top of this, a woollen shirt and/or a sweater is useful as it is warm and to some extent water resistant. Finally, an outer waterproof coat (one that breathes is best) is advisable.

If clothing becomes wet due to sweat or weather, the insulating qualities are decreased and body heat is lost. Manufacturers are now producing lightweight clothing with good insulation, freedom of movement and evaporation qualities, making training and racing even in harsh conditions both possible and enjoyable. The primary aim in low temperatures is to prevent cold exposure and to avoid damp clothing. Cold weather, wind chill and wet clothing can be a deadly combination.

Alcohol consumption can also increase the rate of heat loss and a drop in blood glucose levels, resulting in a decrease in energy.

Triathletes with low body fat need to be particularly careful during the swim sections to avoid hypothermia. If stopping and starting during training, put on warm clothing during the breaks otherwise body temperature will drop, muscle function will be impaired and performance will decline.

Warm-ups are extremely important during cold conditions. Warm up longer and more thoroughly in cold conditions to prevent injury and drops in performance.

♦ Transmeridian travel ♦ and jet lag

You may have to travel long distances to a competiton venue and this may involve flying across many time zones. This leads to a disruption in the normal daily rhythm of body functions. These rhythms are known as circadian rhythms and represent your 'body clock'.

Our internal 'clock' controls physiological and psychological systems on a 24-hour day/night cycle. Cues allow this clock to function correctly. For instance, the presence/absence of light, meal times, physical activity and sleep all contribute to the maintenance of the circadian rhythm. Factors that follow regular rhythms include sleep, body temperature, heart rate, blood pressure and metabolic rate. Performance factors that also appear to have rhythms are strength, power and reaction time.

Rapid travel across time zones leads to the desynchronisation of circadian rhythms and results in the feeling known commonly as 'jet lag'. The symptoms of jet lag include malaise, tiredness during the day, appetite loss and disturbed sleeping patterns. Even travelling through one time zone will affect your body clock, but effects only become significant after a time change of three or more hours. The greater the distance travelled and the more time zones crossed, the greater the jet lag.

Direction of travel is also important. North/south travel has little effect. Travelling westward takes 30 to 50 per cent less time to adjust to than travelling eastward. To work out how long it may take to overcome jet lag, allow one day for every time zone crossed when travelling eastward, and eighteen hours (0.75 of a day) for every time zone crossed when travelling westward. It seems easier for the body clock to adapt to longer days while travelling rather than shorter days. This may be due to the effects of sleep. Of course, not all people react the same way to transmeridian travel. 'Night people' tend to react better to westward travel than 'morning people'. Morning people are better travelling eastward.

Jet lag affects the athlete's body in many ways. The body's daily high and low points are altered, which in turn affect energy systems, reaction times and concentration levels. This is partly due to the disruption of the production of those hormones involved in controlling body function. This results in a greater likelihood of muscle cramps, tiredness, headaches, digestive disorders and kidney dysfunction. When you are jet lagged strength decreases, particularly at high speed, and muscle endurance also declines. Psychological effects include a reduced feeling of well being, low arousal, low motivation to train, and increases in malaise and irritability.

The low humidity in an aircraft cabin can lead to a dry mouth, sore throat and mild dehydration. The high altitude in the cabin (equivalent to 1000 to 1500 metres) can create mild effects of oxygen deficiency, promoting lethargy.

A major cause of jet lag is the disruption of sleep/wake patterns. A possible way to overcome this is to pre-adapt to the new time zone. Deliberately desynchronise your circadian rhythm before the flight and align it with that of your destination. This will enable you to adjust more quickly to your new environment. This pre-adaptation should be gradual and progressive. Alter sleep times one to two hours per day several days before the flight (advance if travelling eastward and delay if travelling westward). Unfortunately, this does not work for everyone (that would be too easy!).

If possible, get a departure time that permits you to leave at a reasonable hour so that you are not forced to rise too early or stay up too late. If you are travelling east, make sure you leave in daylight hours and leave early in the day. If travelling westward, leave late in the day and try to arrive as close to your normal retiring hour as possible. If your journey crosses more than ten time zones, consider travelling westward as the adaptation will be easier and worth the extra travelling time.

Athletes respond differently to jet lag and in a team situation it may be preferable to send some athletes to the competition venue earlier than others. Recovery durations do not include the taper period, when you should be fully rested. Learn as much as you can about the destination before you get there: facilities, transport, customs, climate. This removes much of the uncertainty associated with new places and countries.

During the flight
Set your watch to the destination time and alter your daily routine as soon as you enter the plane to correspond to this time. Increase fluid intake (water, fruit juices), and avoid alcohol, coffee and the smoking areas of the plane. Try to keep yourself entertained throughout the flight, wear loose-fitting clothes and do simple exercises to relieve stiffness and to alleviate fatigue – walk around a little, contract/relax muscles, and stretch to reduce the swelling in your feet.

After the flight
Try to adapt immediately to the new time and sleep patterns. Do not attempt difficult or complex tasks. It is also best to taper training slightly due to the effects of jet lag.

Get out of your hotel room but keep activity levels low. If you arrive in the morning, stay active throughout the day, but don't train hard. If you arrive in the evening, train lightly and then go to sleep.

Try to make sure your hotel room is quiet, comfortable and dark. Avoid naps as they upset the resynchronisation process of your body clock. If you start to get insomnia, use relaxation exercises, such as slow, deep breathing, and learn to disassociate the bed from wakefulness, for example avoid the bedroom unless sleeping.

Hold on to your resynchronisation regime – if you wake too early, stay in bed and try to sleep until it is time to get up. If you can't get back to sleep, however, get up.

Diet and jet lag

Only eat what you are used to as altering your normal diet can have dire consequences. Using alcohol to induce sleep is ineffective as it has a negative effect on the amount of deep sleep.

Drugs and jet lag (chronobiotics)

There are drugs available that can aid resynchronisation by lengthening or shortening your natural body rhythm in accordance with the direction in which you are travelling. If you decide to use them, ensure that the tablet suits you by trying it at home before you travel.

Drug restrictions and testing make it inadvisable for sportspeople to use drugs. It is also the opinion of the authors that 'natural is better' most of the time.

Environmental factors and acclimatisation time before a race

Example 1:

Environmental factors	Environmental specifics
Travel	Cross 4 time zones
	Travel westward (add 18 hr or 0.75 of a day per time zone)
Altitude	2000 m
Temperature	10°C

Environmental factors	Acclimatisation (before taper)		
	Minimum	Acceptable	Optimal
Travel	0	2–3 days	3+ days
Altitude	0	7–10 days	3 weeks or stepped adaption (4–6 weeks)
Temperature	0	0	0

Total acclimatisation time (taking the environmental factor that requires the greatest acclimatisation time):

Arrival at race venue:	Minimum	—	0 days
(no. of days before race day)	Acceptable	—	7–10 days
	Optimal	—	3–6 weeks

Example 2:

Environmental factors	Environmental specifics
Travel	Cross 9 time zones
	Travel eastward (add 24 hr or 1 day per time zone)
Altitude	500 m
Temperature	27°C

Environmental Factor	Acclimatisation (before taper)		
	Minimum	Acceptable	Optimal
Travel	0	7–9 days	9–14 days
Altitude	0	0	0
Temperature	0	7–10 days	10–21 days

Total acclimatisation time (taking the environmental factor that requires the greatest acclimatisation time):

Arrival at race venue	Minimum	—	0 days
(no. of days before race day)	Acceptable	—	10 days
	Optimal	—	21 days

Acclimatisation time does not include taper, which is a recovery from training period, not a time for adaptation to altitude, heat or a new time zone. If, for example, the time required to adapt to a hot climate is 7–10 days, and the taper period is 5 days, you should arrive there 10 + 5 days (acclimatisation plus taper) before competition.

Chapter 11

Medical Matters

Dr Dene Egglestone

A sports medicine doctor trained at the London Hospital, Whitechapel, Dr Egglestone was Medical Director of the New Zealand Institute of Sport and Corporate Health for four years. He has a specific interest in exercise physiology, injury prevention and rehabilitation and has been involved with top athletes in a number of sports including rugby, athletics, triathlon, cricket, soccer, netball, gymnastics, yachting and karate.

Many of the problems seen in endurance athletes are preventable, and the following discussion is designed to highlight some of these problems and offer ways to manage them. Most problems can be prevented by adequate preparation in fitness, flexibility and acclimatisation, and care with rehydration.

♦ Pre-season medicals ♦

Having a pre-season medical helps to pick up those people who are at risk from exercise. This is especially true for those over 35 years of age. It is also important at the medical to do baseline blood tests. If problems occur during training, then further blood tests will give more information, and interpretation of the trends is helpful. Discussion on the use of some of the blood tests follows under specific problem areas.

♦ Temperature control ♦

When muscles are used for activity they generate heat. This heat is used to keep the body's temperature at 37°C. With exercise more heat is created than is needed, and the body needs to remove this by cooling the blood. This happens principally over the head and the extremities like hands and feet. Cooling the body is achieved by convection and evaporation.

Convection is the loss of heat from the warmer skin into the cooler air around the body. The closer the air temperature gets to 33°C (our skin temperature), the less effective convection becomes, and if the air temperature is greater than the skin temperature this may lead to the body heating up. Wind speed assists convection and the greater the relative wind speed to us, the more effective it becomes.

Evaporation is the loss of sweat from the skin as a vapour, and this process cools the skin. In conditions of high humidity there is a lot of water vapour in the air and evaporation is less effective. Wind also aids evaporation.

Apart from the air temperature, wind speed and humidity, other factors such as dehydration can also affect heat loss. When exercising vigorously in hot conditions athletes can lose up to two litres of fluid per hour. If this is not replaced then there is less blood to go to the working muscles and even less to go to the other organs and the skin.

With less blood going to the skin less heat can be removed by convection. When dehydrated we also sweat less, which means evaporation is less effective. If we lose 1 per cent of body weight of fluid, thirst is usually noted; by 2 per cent we get impaired temperature regulation, and by 3 per cent athletic performance drops off (*see* also fig. 10.1, page 148).

The symptoms of heat stress are:
- thirst
- cessation of sweating
- headaches
- nausea and vomiting
- dizziness
- goose pimples
- confusion and disorientation
- eventual collapse

The best treatment for heat stress is prevention with adequate rehydration and preparation. Replacement of the electrolytes and fluid lost will maintain performance. Training is important – if training has been carried out in similar conditions for about ten days, the body can acclimatise to the conditions experienced.

Just as overheating is a cause for concern, heat loss can occur if the temperature is too low or the relative wind speed is high. The heat loss is greatest from the head and extremities.

The symptoms of hypothermia are:
- shivering initially
- poor co-ordination
- muscle cramps
- lethargy
- confusion

Treatment is to stop the heat loss with appropriate clothing, and gradually warm the person up with blankets, dry clothes and warm drinks. Acclimatisation to cold conditions can also be done, but use of appropriate clothing such as hats and gloves to reduce heat loss is very important.

♦ Electrolyte problems ♦

With prolonged exercise fluid loss occurs through breathing and sweat. The sweat has more water than sodium in it compared to blood, but if this sodium is not replaced through replacement fluids then water intoxication or sodium depletion can occur in long races, although this is rare. Sodium and other electrolytes are important for the function of cells in the body and muscles, and disturbances of the electrolytes can cause problems.

The symptoms of sodium deficiency are:
- nausea and cramps
- disorientation
- fitting
- coma

Prevention of the condition is by the use of electrolyte replacement fluids, as well as water and carbohydrates for longer events. Replacement fluid should have a carbohydrate concentration of 5 to 10 per cent, and a sodium concentration of 20–30 mmol/l. It should be taken in quantities of about 600–1200 ml/hr.

♦ Cold and flu ♦

Colds and influenza are viral infections. Colds usually cause a blocked nose, sore throat, headache and cough. The flu viruses are often more severe and cause sore throats, headaches, muscle aches and pains, and usually fever.

If you have a fever from a viral illness or any other infection, training can lead to serious complications from the infection or to hyperthermia. During an infection the body is trying to remove the virus and repair damaged cells. Training in this situation leads to more cell damage and will not improve fitness.

Athletes who train during an infection can continue to feel tired for some time after the cold or flu symptoms go. This is similar to overtraining and a reduction in training may be necessary to allow the body to fully recover. Some atypical infections can lead to the same problems – glandular fever is an example. It may take several months, training only on the good days, before the energy returns and symptoms settle.

If there is no fever, training should be done at a much reduced intensity and duration until the symptoms have reduced. Monitoring of early morning pulse rate, temperature and general feelings of fatigue are good estimates of when you can go back to normal training. Generally, the early morning pulse rate will rise at times of infection, fatigue and stress, and when it has returned to your normal rate training can continue.

Listening to one's body is important, and a general feeling of fatigue can be an early warning of infections, overtraining, stress and other problems, and should not be ignored. Consulting a doctor with an interest in sports medicine may help find the problem and mean an early return to training.

◆ Stitch ◆

Stitch is common with runners and is a sharp pain felt at the bottom edge of the ribs on either or both sides. The exact cause is not known, although several ideas have been put forward. The most likely is cramp or spasm of the diaphragm, the large muscle between the chest and the abdominal cavity. Another idea is that stitch is related to bowel spasm from oxygen debt or repeated jostling from the running action. Factors relating to the onset of stitch are often oxygen debt from vigorous exercise, and the breathing pattern.

Stitch can be helped by slowing down and improving the breathing pattern by breathing deeply and regularly. Another helpful manoeuvre is to lift both arms above the head while breathing in and lower them when breathing out for several breaths.

◆ Runners' diarrhoea ◆

Diarrhoea has many causes, and most people have experienced the need to go to the toilet prior to the start of a race as a result of nerves. This is usually easily dealt with by ensuring you empty the bowel as part of the pre-race preparation and warm-up. Eating a low-fibre diet for several days before the race may help this situation.

The true runners' diarrhoea is a much more difficult problem, which occurs with every race or training run and comes later in the run, not usually at the start. It is thought to be caused by poor blood supply to the gut when the exercising muscles demand more of the blood. The mechanical movement of the gut when running may also contribute. Other factors which may aggravate the problem and should be avoided are electrolyte replacement fluids which are too strong, and a high-fibre diet. If diluted electrolyte fluids and low-fibre diets have been tried and have not helped then seeking medical advice to exclude food allergies or other problems may be beneficial. If there is no other problem, then some medication for diarrhoea is available, such as Lomotil or Immodium, which are safe and effective but should be used sparingly to avoid making the bowel lazy.

◆ Iron deficiency ◆

Iron is important for an athlete as it is one of the chief components of haemoglobin which is the red oxygen-carrying particle in blood. With less haemoglobin we get less oxygen to our muscles, which affects performance. Iron is lost with menstruation but also through the bowel, bladder and kidneys, and through broken red blood cells passing through capillaries in our feet when we run.

Iron is poorly absorbed from the gut and poor dietary habits or being vegetarian can lead to iron deficiency and anaemia. Vegetarian athletes need to make a special effort to eat foods with a high iron content, such as tofu, spinach, beetroot, peas, beans, fruit and bran cereal. The taking of vitamin C-rich foods or supplements with meals will aid the absorption of the iron.

The symptoms of anaemia and iron deficiency are:
- tiredness
- difficulty in concentrating
- feeling cold
- getting colds and infections
- poor performance

If these symptoms are occurring, then a simple blood test can be done to check for haemoglobin and ferritin (which shows the level of iron stores). If these are low, iron supplements may be required. (*see* also 'Iron' on page 165).

◆ Cramp ◆

Cramp is the sudden involuntary contraction or spasm of a muscle, which is often painful. It can be brought on by electrolyte depletion, especially in longer races, and dehydration. Proper fluid replacement during a race can help to prevent this. Deficiencies of calcium and magnesium can also lead to cramp, and if the cramps persist then see a doctor.

Minor injuries, such as a muscle strain, can be present and training on these may lead to cramping. Examination of the affected muscle for an injury will detect this problem, and this is best treated with stretching and massage of the affected muscle. Training is very important in reducing the likelihood of cramp as untrained muscle cramps more easily than trained muscle.

If cramps persist and the above problems have been checked, then adding salt to your food for a few days before the race can be tried. The use of calcium and magnesium supplements can also be tried if abnormalities in the blood levels of these minerals have been excluded. Quinine sulphate is a safe, effective medication for the problem if everything else has been tried and tests have been done to exclude more serious problems.

◆ Chafing ◆

Chafing and blisters are common ailments with athletes. They result from friction between clothing or shoes and the skin. If the skin gets wet, then chafing tends to be worse. The common problem areas are the feet, crotch and under the arms.

Never break in new shoes with a race or a long workout; they need to be used for shorter runs until they are comfortable. Socks should be thick and snug fitting to prevent chafing and blisters.

Early blisters or chafed areas should be taped and further friction avoided until the area is healed. Larger blisters can have the fluid removed by puncturing them with a sterile needle and leaving the skin in place. These can be taped or padded to avoid further friction. Open blisters need clean sterile dressings to prevent infection and avoid further friction. Areas prone to chafing may benefit from the use of powder or petroleum jelly to reduce the friction.

◆ Injuries ◆

Injuries can be broken down into two groups: traumatic and overuse. The traumatic group are usually unexpected and not preventable. However, the severity of the injury can often be minimised with good preparation, stretching exercises, the use of proper equipment and rapid first aid treatment. Good preparation and stretching can help reduce muscle tears, strains and ligament damage, and the first aid known as the RICE treatment will minimise the bleeding into the tissues which only causes more swelling and inflammation. RICE stands for Rest, Ice, Compression and Elevation, and should be used for the first 48 hours, then followed by heat and gentle use for more minor injuries. More severe injuries may need physiotherapy or a sports doctor's attention.

Overuse injuries are related to the repetitive use of an area, often when an unusually high level of activity has been carried out. Injuries are likely to occur when you change your programme and increase certain activities. Changes in equipment such as shoes or bike settings can also lead to injuries. Many of these injuries can be helped using the RICE management, and certainly by reducing the levels of the exercise causing the problem. These injuries tend to be more difficult to treat and may require physiotherapy, anti-inflammatory medication or a sports doctor's attention.

Chapter 12

Sports Nutrition, Race Rehydration and Refuelling

Shona Goldsbury

Shona Goldsbury (Dip HSc, RD) is a consultant dietitian specialising in sports nutrition. She was one of the first practitioners to be employed in the fitness industry in New Zealand in the mid 1980s, and now runs her own private practice. She has been an advisor to many athletes and teams in different sports, working at all levels, from school and club to elite. As a competitive tennis player she knows the difference that nutrition can make to a performance.

Nutrition plays a key role in the optimal health and performance of all athletes. Many athletes have realised that unless they refuel their bodies with the right foods their training becomes difficult and their performance drops. Sports nutrition is not about magic pills, potions or special foods. It is about sound nutritional principles that help all athletes keep healthy, train hard, recover well and enjoy life. The New Zealand Food and Nutrition Guidelines provide the nutritional basis that all athletes (and non-athletes) should follow. These guidelines are:

1 Eat a variety of food each day from each of the four major food groups: fruit and vegetables; bread and cereals; milk and milk products (especially low-fat varieties); lean meat, fish, poultry, eggs, nuts or legumes.

2 Prepare meals with minimal added fat (especially saturated fat) and salt.

3 Choose pre-prepared foods and snacks that are low in fat, salt and sugar.

4 Maintain a healthy body weight by regular physical activity and by healthy eating.

5 Drink plenty of liquids each day.

6 If you drink alcohol, do so in moderation.

♦ The role of nutrients ♦ during exercise

'Fuel' supply

Our muscles require energy to exercise and this energy comes from the food we eat. The two major fuel sources are carbohydrate and fat. Carbohydrate (CHO) is regarded as the 'premium' fuel as it is the only nutrient used when exercising anaerobically (without oxygen) or at a high intensity. Fats can only be used under aerobic conditions, so it becomes an important fuel source for endurance events, but less important for shorter events or high-intensity exercise.

Protein is only used as an energy source under 'extreme' conditions, such as when carbohydrate levels become low. Carbohydrate is the central fuel for the body. Once our body's stores of carbohydrate (muscle glycogen) are exhausted, our ability to use fat and protein is diminished and intensity has to decrease.

159

Fuel provided by nutrients

1 g CHO	=	17 kJ
1 g protein	=	17 kJ
1 g fat	=	38 kJ
*1 g alcohol	=	25 kJ

*not an essential nutrient but does have an energy value.

Estimated energy expenditure in kilojoules (kJ)/minute

Discipline	Body weight (kg)				
	50	60	70	80	90
Running					
7 min/km	29	34	42	46	50
5 min/km	46	55	63	71	76
3.5 min/km	63	76	88	97	109
Cycling					
15 kph	19	24	28	31	35
25 kph	34	41	47	53	60
30 kph	49	60	69	79	88
Swimming					
freestyle	32	39	46	52	59

Source: adapted from Melvin H. Williams, *Nutrition for fitness and sport*, William C. Brown Publishers, Iowa, 1988.
Note: to convert kJ to kCal divide by 4.2.

The ratio of fuels metabolised to provide energy depends on four main factors:

1 Intensity: The harder we train the more carbohydrate we use.

2 Duration: This depends on the intensity at which we train and the amount of carbohydrate in the body. As our body's store of glycogen becomes low, protein is used more as an energy source. Branched-chain amino acids in the muscles can be broken down to glucose. Endurance athletes get approximately 10 per cent of their energy from protein whereas other athletes get only one to two per cent.

3 Diet: A high carbohydrate diet helps restore glycogen storage and minimises lean tissue loss by decreasing protein usage. Dietary manipulation through carbohydrate loading can also increase glycogen storage. Higher glycogen stores enable an athlete to exercise for longer and sustain intensity levels.

4 Fitness Level: Well-trained athletes have a better nutritional status. They have an increased ability to store glycogen, metabolise fats and sustain high-intensity exercise.

Therefore, the fuel supply is crucial to performance. Carbohydrate is the most important 'fuel' for athletes. Inadequate levels will compromise the training programme and, ultimately, the performance of all athletes (*see* fig. 12.1).

Vitamins and minerals

Vitamins and minerals are needed for the proper functioning of many body processes. If you choose your foods well, 5000 kJ will provide all the nutrients you need. Many athletes have been led to believe that vitamin and mineral supplements will enhance sporting performance, yet scientific research has failed to substantiate this, except in cases where an athlete has an inadequate diet. Taking large amounts of some of these supplements has been shown to harm the health of athletes and impair their performance.

It is also important to put these nutrients into perspective next to our 'fuel supply'. For example, an 80 kg male triathlete training two hours daily requires:

1	Carbohydrate:	600–700 g	=	38–44 oranges
	Vitamin C:	40 mg	=	1 orange
2	Protein:	120–160 g	=	550 g beef
	Iron:	10 mg	=	350 g beef
3	Fat:	100–110 g	=	3.2 l whole milk
	Calcium:	800 mg	=	700 ml whole milk

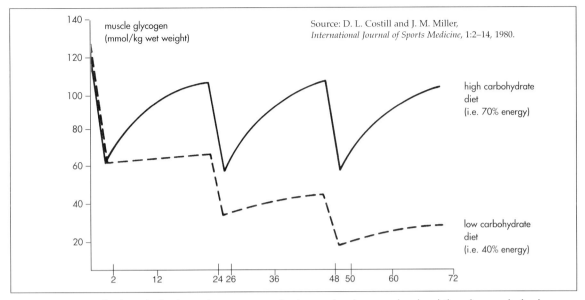

Figure 12.1 A high carbohydrate diet maintains high muscle glycogen levels while a low carbohydrate diet depletes glycogen stores rapidly

Fluid

Water makes up approximately two-thirds of our body weight and is second only to oxygen in sustaining life. Without it we can only survive a few days. Dehydration has the biggest impact on the working capacity of muscles and temperature control of the body.

Dehydration occurs when fluid loss exceeds 1 per cent of body weight. Studies have shown that at 2 per cent body weight loss, VO$_2$max has decreased 10 per cent and endurance 22 per cent.

Failure to replace fluid during exercise can lead to heat stroke, heat coma and, eventually, death. The need for athletes to have an adequate fluid intake before, during and after exercise is critical to preventing dehydration and a decline in performance. Water is considered the nutrient most essential to athletes. *See* figure 10.1, page 148, for the effects of fluid loss.

◆ The training diet ◆

The most important role nutrition has is to support the training and conditioning programme of athletes. A poor training diet leaves you feeling tired and lethargic, and unable to achieve desired or expected success. A good quality diet is essential to maximise your potential. No matter what success or level you have achieved as an athlete, if you know your diet is inadequate you could achieve more!

Nutritional considerations

Energy
Total energy needs are based on your weight, and the amount and intensity of exercise. The following is a relatively simple method of calculating energy needs.

161

Calculating energy needs

(a) Determine normal or ideal weight for you (kg).

(b) Multiply this by: 168 if adult and active; 252 if adolescent and active.

(c) Calculate total kJ cost of exercise. (Guidelines to use: 1 km swimming, 2 km running, 4 km biking = 525 kJ)

(d) Add (b) and (c) to get an approximate level of energy needed to maintain body weight.

For example: woman, age 35, height 165 cm, 16% body fat

(a)	Ideal weight	=	57 kg
(b)	Adult active	=	57 × 168
		=	9576 kJ

(c) Weekly training schedule of 200 km cycling, 50 km running, 5 km swimming
Energy expenditure:

Cycling	=	26,250 kJ
Running	=	13,125 kJ
Swimming	=	2625 kJ
Total	=	42,000 kJ
Average per day	=	6000 kJ

(d) Energy needed daily = 15,500 kJ

Carbohydrate

The 'premium' fuel for the body and the limiting nutrient for endurance athletes. The athlete who fails to replenish glycogen stores on a daily basis will end up with chronic carbohydrate depletion and an inability to cope with training. The key to a successful training diet is ensuring adequate carbohydrate intake daily. Carbohydrate requirements are usually quoted as a percentage of energy. Endurance athletes should aim to get at least 55 per cent of their energy from carbohydrate, more if training for over two hours. The training diet should be made up of the following energy components:

CHO: 55–60%
Protein: 15–20%
Fat: 25–30%

For example, an active woman aged 35 and weighing 57 kg requires 15,500 kJ daily. If she trains for less than two hours daily, her carbohydrate requirement will be 55–60 per cent CHO. This will be 55–60 per cent of 15,500 kJ, or 8525–9300 kJ, which is 500–550g CHO (1 g CHO = 17 kJ).

The major disadvantage of using percentages is that they are too vague and although athletes often know percentages of carbohydrate to include, they are unable to convert that to the meals they actually prepare and eat. A more recent method of calculating carbohydrate requirements uses body weight and time spent exercising.

(a) Training less than 60 min: 5–6 g CHO per kg body weight per day

(b) Training 60–120 min: 7–8 g CHO per kg body weight per day

(c) Training more than 120 min: 9–10 g CHO per kg body weight per day.

For example, a 57 kg woman training 2.5 hours per day requires 9–10 g CHO × 57 kg = 510–570 g CHO.

Work out a meal pattern to suit you, taking into account your training schedule and food habits. Spread your carbohydrate intake throughout the day, for example:

Breakfast and morning tea	=	150 g
Lunch and afternoon tea	=	200 g
Dinner	=	150 g

Meal pattern supplying 550 g carbohydrate (CHO)

	CHO	Protein	Fat
Breakfast			
Before training			
200 ml weak fruit juice	10	—	—
200 g low-fat yoghurt	25	8	4
After training			
200 ml fruit juice	20	—	—
3 Weetabix, 250 ml			
skimmed milk	50	12	4
2 toast, jam, margarine	35	4	8
Lunch			
Filled roll (or 3 bread)			
and margarine	40	6	12
75 g salmon, salad	—	20	6
2 tsp salad dressing	2	3	3
1 large banana, 1 other fruit	35	—	—
Pre-training			
500 ml 5–10% CHO drink	35	—	—
Low-fat muesli bar	25	2	4
During training			
Minimum 500 ml CHO drink	35	—	—
Post-training			
200 ml 20% CHO drink	40	—	—
Large banana	25	—	—
Dinner			
Fruit juice, 200 ml	20	—	—
200 g pasta with sauce	75	12	2
100 g broccoli, cauliflower,			
tomato	5	—	—
100 g peas, corn, carrot	10	4	—
100 g lean beef	—	23	16
225 g fruit salad	25	—	—
125 ml custard	15	4	4
Supper			
Cup of Horlicks, skimmed milk	6	1	3
2 fruit biscuits	15	1	1
Milk in 4 cups tea and coffee	6	4	4
Total (g)	**554**	**104**	**71**

Total Energy (kJ):
CHO: 554 × 17   = 9418: 68% total energy
Protein: 104 × 17 = 1768: 13% total energy
Fat: 71 × 38   = 2698: 19% total energy
Total energy   = 13,884

Common foods supplying 50 g carbohydrate

Breads, Cereals	Fruit, Vegetables
4 wholemeal bread	2 large bananas
2 English muffins	3 other fruit
1⅓ medium bread rolls	300 g tinned fruit
6 rice cakes	75 g dried fruit
20 water crackers	9 dried apricots
100 g cereal	2 medium potatoes
60 g porridge oats	2 large kumara
100 g muesli	300 g corn
1½ muffins, scones	

Pasta, Grains	Juices
170 g pasta, rice	600 ml fruit juice
400 g baked beans	500 ml soft drink
300 g kidney beans	700 ml sports drink
	(5–10%)
	200 ml sports drink
	(20–25%)

Snacks, Confectionery	Milk and Milk Products
7 plain biscuits	500 ml semi-skimmed
5 chocolate biscuits*	milk
2 long or 4 small	2 200 g low-fat yoghurt
muesli bars*	400 ml custard*
150 g chocolate*	225 g creamy rice*
50 g sugar, boiled sweets	225 g fruit dessert*
100 g potato crisps,	3½ scoops ice cream
corn chips*	(210 g)*
5 tbsp honey, jam	

*Use lower fat options; if none, limit usage.
Source: NZ Food Composition Tables, 1993

Protein

Although it is not considered a good fuel source, endurance athletes use considerable amounts of protein due to the length of time spent exercising and the resulting low glycogen levels. Protein's prime function is to repair, build and maintain tissue and the more training an athlete does, or the higher the intensity they work at, the more tissue damage that is done. It is essential that athletes consume enough good quality protein to aid in their recovery from hard training. With much of the emphasis in meal plans on adequate carbohydrate intake, athletes can unintentionally have marginal protein intakes.

The protein requirement for endurance athletes has been established at 1.5–2.0 g per kg body weight per day. For example, a woman weighing 57 kg requires 85–115 g of protein each day.

Protein needs can be achieved quite easily with a well-balanced diet. There is little need for protein supplement for most athletes.

Protein content of common foods

Weight	g protein
Beef, lamb 150 g	40–45 g
Venison, pork 20 g slice	5 g
Chicken, fish 150 g	30–35 g
Ham 50 g	10 g
Bacon 1 rasher	6 g
Eggs 1 medium	6 g
Baked beans 125 g	6 g
Peas, corn 125 g	3 g
Potato, kumara 1 medium	2 g
Peanut butter 1 tbsp	5 g
Peanuts 50 g	10 g
Walnuts 25 g	4 g
Muesli bar	2 g
Muesli small bowl	10 g
Pasta, rice, cooked 200 g	5 g
Bread roll long	7 g
Bread 2 slices	4 g
Cereal 50 g	2 g
Milk 225 ml	9 g
Yoghurt 150 g	7 g
Cheese 50 g	12 g
Ice cream 1 cup	6 g
Cheese scone medium	6 g
Plain biscuits 2	2 g
Muffin 1	6 g
Sports bar 1	10 g

Source: NZ Food Composition Tables, 1993

Fat

Most athletes could lower the fat content of their diet. There are several good reasons for doing this.

1 Fat often replaces carbohydrate. Fat contains twice as much energy as carbohydrate, leaves you feeling fuller for longer and depresses your desire to eat. This can be detrimental to an athlete with a high carbohydrate need. For example, 50 g of potato crisps has 25 g carbohydrate, 18 g fat. The fat content of the crisps is providing 62 per cent more energy than if you ate one large banana.

2 Fat is not good for your health. Many of the chronic age-related diseases (obesity, heart disease, some cancers) may be related to high-fat diets.

Nutritional tips to lower fat intake

1 Keep high-fat foods to a minimum. Examples of high-fat foods include: most takeaway meals, pies, pastries, chocolate, potato crisps, many snack bars, cakes, biscuits, salad and oil dressings, luncheon sausage, salami, sausages, croissants, most desserts. If you can eliminate these foods from your diet most of the time, you will better manage your fat intake. It is important to read food labels. Use 3 g fat per 100 g or 30 kJ per 100 kJ as a guide as to what is satisfactory.

2 Replace high-fat foods with low-fat options. For example, replace whole milk with skimmed or semi-skimmed; replace cheddar cheese with Edam, mozzarella, Slimiz, reduced fat cheese, cottage cheese, quark, ricotta, fromage frais; replace ice cream with low-fat varieties of frozen yoghurt; replace butter and margarine with low-fat spread; make sure meats are lean or low-fat processed meats. Always be on the lookout for new products when shopping.

3 Use low-fat cooking methods. Grill, bake, steam or microwave when you can, and do not add unnecessary oil or butter (if you do have to use them, do so in minimal amounts).

4 Modify common recipes. For salad dressing, use plain low-fat yoghurt, or add a small amount of ordinary dressing and flavour with lemon juice and herbs. For mashed potato use skimmed or semi-skimmed milk and a small amount of low-fat spread. For white sauces use a low-fat spread, skimmed or semi-skimmed milk, and a small amount of cheese. For cream sauces for pasta use low-fat yoghurt or fromage frais. For meat dishes try decreasing the meat content by adding beans, pasta, rice, vegetables and sauces.

Fat content of common foods

Weight	g fat
Butter, margarine and oil 1 tbsp	12 g
Cream 100 ml	40 g
Milk, whole 225 ml	9 g
Skimmed milk 225 ml	1 g
Yoghurt 100 g	3–5 g
Ice cream 100 g	11 g
Cheese 100 g	34 g
Edam or lower fat 100 g	25 g
Cottage cheese 100 g	4 g
Eggs 1	6 g
Peanuts 50 g	20 g
Peanut butter 1 tbsp	8 g
Chocolate bar 60 g	12–14 g
Scone 1	8 g
Beef, lamb, poultry 100 g	12–15 g
Fish 100 g	10 g
Salami 100 g	45 g
Grilled sausage 1	15 g
Meat pie, average	24 g
Big Mac hamburger	32 g
Potato fries serving	20–30 g
Sausage roll	23 g
Pizza 1 slice	6 g
Avocado ¼	10 g
Muffin 1	5 g
Muesli 100 g	6 g
Muesli bar	4–6 g
Potato crisps 100 g	33 g

Source: NZ Food Composition Tables, 1993

Vitamins and minerals

A diet that supplies enough energy, carbohydrate, protein and fat has plenty of variety and should meet all vitamin and mineral requirements. As already mentioned, in most cases the use of supplements is unwarranted. But if you decide to use supplements, use a multivitamin and mineral supplement in the dosages recommended.

There are two minerals that are of concern to the athlete, for reasons of both performance and health: iron and calcium.

Iron

This mineral is an integral part of the oxygen supply system. It is found in the haemoglobin of red blood cells, which transport oxygen around the body. Low haemoglobin levels resulting from iron deficiency anaemia will seriously affect aerobic training. A blood test which measures serum ferritin (the body's iron store) should be done regularly (at least annually by athletes, especially endurance-trained athletes training two hours a day or more). For athletes who have been anaemic or who have marginal iron levels, checks should be done several times a year. At particular risk of low iron stores are women athletes, teenage athletes, endurance athletes, athletes with low energy intake and athletes not eating red meat.

Iron deficiency is fairly common among endurance athletes. It is, in fact, the most common mineral deficiency in the Western world. Athletes, especially menstruating females, are at more risk of iron loss through exercise than most of the population. Inadequate dietary intake and food choices can also reduce iron absorption and contribute to iron deficiency. When iron deficiency is first diagnosed, iron supplementation is required. But it must be remembered that diet is the key to achieving a satisfactory and sustainable iron status in the long term.

Iron content of common foods

Haem sources
(well absorbed by body)

Liver, 100 g	11.5 mg
Kidney, 100 g	11.0 mg
Beef, 100 g	3.2 mg
Lamb, 100 g	2.1 mg
Poultry, 100 g	0.75 mg
Fish, 100 g	0.5–3 mg

Non-haem sources
(poorly absorbed by body)

Legumes, 100 g	1.2 mg
Cereal, 50 g	2.0–4 mg
Bread, 1 medium slice	1.0 mg
Egg, 1	0.9 mg
Dried Fruit, 40 g	0.6 mg
Spinach, cooked 50 g	1.0 mg
Peas, 100 g	1.1 mg

Source: NZ Food Composition Tables, 1993

Nutritional tips for adequate iron intake
1 Eat a variety of lean red meat at least three to four times per week; approximately 150 g per serving.

2 Eat cereals with a high iron content, wholegrain breads, pasta and rice.

3 Include vitamin C-rich food at each meal to enhance absorption of non-haem stores, for example citrus fruit and juice, kiwifruit, strawberries, green peppers, tomatoes.

4 Keep tea to a minimum (two cups daily!) as the tannic acid in tea reduces iron absorption by 50 per cent. Try to drink it between meals rather than at meals.

5 Polyphenols in coffee inhibit iron absorption about 20 per cent. The oxalic acid in silverbeet and spinach also reduces iron absorption.

See also 'Iron Deficiency' page 157.

Calcium
The risks associated with calcium deficiency are more to do with long-term health problems than short-term performance. Studies have shown that low calcium intake increases the risk of osteoporosis (thinning of the bones) in later life, particularly in females. To help prevent osteoporosis it is important to have a good calcium intake throughout life, but especially in the teenage years and early twenties. The importance of this as a health maintenance strategy for athletes and non-athletes alike cannot be emphasised enough.

Many athletes have reduced their consumption of dairy products under the mistaken assumption that these products will greatly increase their fat intake. Instead, they increase their risk of developing osteoporosis and stress fractures, despite the increased calcium absorption associated with weight-bearing exercise.

Some female athletes, because of training levels, low energy intake and low body fat content, also develop a condition known as 'amenorrhoea' (they stop normal menstrual functioning). This increases the risk of osteoporosis and negates the effects of increased calcium absorption through exercising.

Daily calcium requirements are:
Adults: 600 mg
Teenage females: 800 mg
Amenorrhoeic females: 1200–1600 mg

The richest sources of calcium are dairy products; plant-based sources are not as well absorbed. Where athletes are unable to eat dairy products, a calcium supplement is recommended, especially for amenorrhoeic female athletes.

Common food sources of calcium

Weight	mg calcium
Milk, whole 200 ml	230 mg
Yoghurt 200 g	250 mg
Ice cream 100 g	140 mg
Cheese 25 g	175 mg
Cottage cheese, 25 g	15 mg
Sardines 4 large	190 mg
Salmon 100 g	190 mg
Almonds 25 g	60 mg
Soya milk, 100 ml	100 mg
Tofu, 100 g	105 mg
Bread, 2 slices	20–25 mg
Dried apricots, 5	30 mg
Egg, 1	25 mg
Broccoli, 100 g	100 mg
Legumes, 100 g	50 mg
Orange, 1	55 mg

Source: NZ Food Composition Tables, 1993

Fluid

Fluid is of prime concern to athletes as dehydration will compromise training. A hydration plan must involve fluid before, during and after all training and racing.

Recommended training hydration plan

2 hours before exercise: 800 ml

30 to 0 min before exercise: 300–500 ml

Every 20 to 30 min during exercise: 150–200 ml

After exercise: minimum 800 ml

Fluid balances should be worked out for training sessions so requirements can be established. Aim for a 100 per cent replacement of fluid lost during exercise. 1 kg weight loss = 1 litre fluid.

For example: woman, 57 kg, normal weight
After 1 hour swimming – weight 55 kg
She needs to drink 2000 ml to restore fluid balance.

What to drink?

Variety is important as fluid needs are so high.

- During the day: water, fruit juice, milk, milk drinks, soft drink, tea and coffee (4 cups total), herbal teas, caffeine-free coffee
- Two hours before exercise: water, diluted fruit juice (1:2), low percentage carbohydrate drink (4–8 per cent)
- During exercise: plain water or low percentage carbohydrate drink (4–8 per cent) if exercising more than one hour
- Immediately after exercise: 200 ml 20–25 per cent carbohydrate drink with electrolytes, especially sodium, 600 ml plain water (minimum)
- One hour later: 200 ml 20–25 per cent carbohydrate drink with electrolytes or solid food containing 50 g carbohydrate

Research has established that sports drinks containing 4 to 8 per cent carbohydrate and 20–30 mmol sodium and 3–5 mmol (120–195 mg) potassium per litre are more rapidly absorbed during exercise than plain water, thus decreasing the risk of dehydration and providing carbohydrate to sustain high-intensity endurance training.

No drink has the perfect combination of ingredients but the better ones for taking during exercise appear to be Exceed Fluid and Energy, Gatorade, Carboblast, FRN Enduro Booster, and PowerAde. For recovery the better ones appear to be Exceed High CHO Source, Gatorlode and Lucozade. The final choice will come down to personal preference in taste, suitability and cost (*see* page 168, 'Carbohydrate (CHO) and sodium content per 500 ml for common sports drinks').

Nutrition diary

A nutrition diary should be kept along with your training programme. It provides a guideline for you to check when training performance drops off or an endurance event goes badly. A week of low carbohydrate intake, inadequate fluid and too much alcohol can explain an unexpected poor performance.

◆ The pre-race fuelling ◆

The two major nutritional considerations for athletes before the race are 'carbohydrate loading' and the 'pre-race meal'. Both of these dietary techniques are short term and do not in any way compensate for poor training diets.

Carbohydrate (CHO) and sodium content per 500 ml for common sports drinks

Product	CHO (g)	CHO (%)	Sodium (mg)	Main ingredients
Exceed Fluid and Energy Replacement (Abbott)	34	7	100	glucose polymers (GP), fructose
Exceed High CHO Source (Abbott)	118	23	235	GP, sucrose, glucose
Gatorade (Gatorade Co)	32	6.5	250	sucrose
Gatorlode (Gatorade Co)	93	18.5	135	maltodextrin (Md), dextrose
Maxim (Advanced Sport Management)	100	10	—	
Carboblast (Nutralife)	40	8	155	GP, fructose, glucose
Carboplex (Nutralife)	74	15	—	Md, fructose, dextrose
Nutra-sport Restore	37	7.5	425	GP, fructose, glucose
Nutra-sport Energy (Nutralife)	78	15.5	—	GP, fructose, dextrose
FRN Enduro booster (Leppin)	50	10	170	GP
FRN Carbo booster (Leppin)	100	20	—	GP
FRN Squeezy Sachets (Leppin)	25	100	30	GP (recommend drinking with 250–350 ml water)
Lucozade 90 (Reckitt & Colman)	18	146		glucose
PowerAde (Coca-Cola)	40	8	78	Md, sucrose

Carbohydrate loading

This is a technique that developed in the 1950s to supersaturate the muscles with glycogen. With the greater emphasis on athletes having a high carbohydrate training diet, this technique is of limited value. A highly trained endurance athlete has muscle glycogen levels almost at capacity. However, it may still be of use to the athlete training less than two hours daily, an athlete consuming inadequate carbohydrate during training or an athlete changing from short-course events to long-distance events.

Procedure for carbohydrate loading

A tapered training programme is followed by a carbohydrate loading diet of 10 g per kg body weight, or 75–85 per cent carbohydrate content for three days prior to the event.

Points to remember with carbohydrate loading

1 The athlete must be endurance trained and taking part in a race lasting more than 90 minutes.

2 Exercise must be tapered.

3 Weight gain may occur as for every gram of carbohydrate stored 3 g water is stored as well. This can be minimised by decreasing food intake but ensure carbohydrate is sufficient (fat low, protein moderate).

4 You will often feel sluggish and heavy at the start of the race – carbohydrate loading means you have more fuel so that you are able to maintain intensity for longer.

5 Always try out carbohydrate loading during training to see that it suits you and does help your performance. Don't do it too often – no more than one to three times a year.

An example of a carbohydrate loading meal pattern for person weighing 65 kg

	CHO (g)
Breakfast	
250 ml high CHO sports drink	60
1 cup cereal, 250 ml trim milk	35
2 toast, large banana	50
Morning tea:	
English muffin with jam	60
Lunch:	
250 ml high CHO sports drink	60
200 g fruit yoghurt	25
Large banana, 3 other fruit	75
Afternoon tea:	
Fruit muffin	30
Dinner:	
250 ml high CHO drink	60
450 g cooked rice	75
Chicken and vegetables	
1 large roll	40
1 cup fruit salad	25
Supper:	
Horlicks, trim milk	15
2 crumpets, honey	35
Total	645 g

(*See* 'Common foods supplying 50 g carbohydrate', page 163, to exchange foods so the three-day pattern is varied.)

Notes:
1 High carbohydrate drinks add substantial amounts of carbohydrate to the diet without increasing the bulk of food.
2 All alcohol should be avoided in the days leading up to a race.

Pre-race meal

Ideally this meal should be eaten two to three hours before the race. Even early morning races need a 'pre-event' meal.

Nutritional tips

1 The pre-race meal should be enjoyable and familiar – this is no time for surprises!

2 The main aim is to prevent hunger and weakness during the race.

3 It should be high in carbohydrate, low in fibre, and include plenty of fluid.

4 It should be low in protein and fat (these take too long to digest and could cause gastrointestinal upsets).

5 Avoid gaseous or spicy foods that may cause indigestion.

6 Use 'liquid' foods (fruit smoothies and commercial liquids such as Exceed, Gatorpro) if you suffer from pre-race nerves. These can be eaten within two hours of the race as they leave the stomach more quickly.

Commercial ready-to-drink pre-event meals

	CHO (g)	protein (g)	fat (g)
Exceed Sports Nutrition Supplement, 1 can, 237 ml	54	14	9.5
Gatorade Co. Gatorpro	58	16	7.0

There are also several powered products such as Sustagen Sports, Stamin R, that can be made up to liquid meals.

Examples of pre-race meals

Breakfast
diluted fruit juice
low-fibre cereal, low-fat milk
white toast, honey
pancakes with golden syrup

Evening
fruit juice
pasta with low-fat sauce and vegetables, small serving chicken, fish, lean red meat
broccoli, cauliflower, mushrooms

Supper
Milo, low-fat milk drink
English muffin or crumpet with honey

Other nutritional pre-race considerations

1 If you are not carbohydrate loading two days before the race, place special emphasis on carbohydrate and fluid intake. Consume limited alcohol, if at all.

2 The last big meal should be twelve to sixteen hours before the race.

3 Two hours before the start of the race, begin your pre-hydration regime – 800 ml of water, diluted fruit juice or low carbohydrate drink.

4 Fifteen minutes before the start, drink another 300–500 ml of fluid – for races an hour or longer use only plain water. Immediately before the race you can have 200 ml of low carbohydrate drink. Early in these races fat metabolism should be promoted. For races under an hour, 500 ml of low carbohydrate drink can be used with no side effects.

♦ Race fuelling ♦

The two crucial nutrients for racing are fluid and carbohydrate. During the race the primary need is for *fluid*. It is important to drink plenty *early* because once you are dehydrated it is too late. Never use thirst as a guideline for fluid need – by then you are already dehydrated.

Fluid should be supplied at minimum rate of 500 ml up to maximum 1600 ml per hour. The more hot and humid conditions are and the more you sweat, the greater the fluid needed to be consumed. The rate at which the stomach processes fluids (gastric emptying) depends on a number of factors, such as quantity, concentration and temperature of fluids. Some recommendations are:

- 150–200 ml of cold (4–10°C) fluid should be taken every 20–30 minutes of exercise.
- For races under an hour plain water is fine.
- For races over an hour take a 4–8 per cent carbohydrate drink with 460–720 mg sodium and 120–195 mg potassium per litre. Diluted fruit juice and soft drinks can be used (1 part drink:2 parts water) although they are not as suitable as they contain no sodium to aid absorption.
- If the concentration is too high or too much is drunk, it can cause gastrointestinal upsets and retard both the gastric emptying rate and carbohydrate absorption.
- For races over three hours you probably need to have a combination of fluid and solid food to provide variety.
- Check what carbohydrate drink is provided during the race. If it is not a drink you have used, start using it in training to familiarise yourself with it. If you are using a different carbohydrate drink during the event, you will need to organise yourself to have it placed at the aid stations.

What type of solid food should be eaten?

Foods high in carbohydrate and low in fat which are easy to chew and easy to digest are best. Remember to try out any dietary changes or new foods during training first.

At present there is some interesting research being done on the glycaemic index of carbohydrate foods and how this glycaemic index may help the athlete. The glycaemic index measures how much glucose levels rise in the blood after eating carbohydrates. High glycaemic foods have a value greater than 85. Moderate glycaemic foods rate from 60–85 and low glycaemic foods rate below 60.

Foods with a high glycaemic index cause blood sugar levels to rise quickly after eating, whereas those with a low glycaemic index provide a steady supply of glucose over several hours.

Initial results show that using low to moderate glycaemic foods before long workouts, and high glycaemic foods during long workouts and for recovery, could help optimise your training and race fuelling. The following is a list of foods belonging to the three categories.

High glycaemic foods
Bread
Rice
Bananas
Raisins
Carrots, corn, potatoes
Exceed sports drinks
Gatorade sports drinks
Honey, glucose

Moderate glycaemic
Grapes
Oranges
Pasta
Sweet plain biscuits
Oatmeal, oatmeal biscuits
Potato chips
Ice cream

Low glycaemic
Apples, peaches, plums
Dates, figs
Legumes
Fructose
Milk
Yoghurt
Cornflakes, muesli, Weetabix

How much carbohydrate should be eaten?

Approximately 60 g carbohydrate per hour or 1–1.5 g per kg body weight per hour has been established as sufficient to prevent glycogen depletion. For example: a 57 kg woman in endurance events needs 60–80 g CHO per hour. With 500 ml of low CHO drink supplying 35 g, a further 25–50 g would need to be eaten.

For a more detailed estimate of fluid and carbohydrate requirements *see* appendices 6 and 7.

Nutrition tips

1 Consume drink and food early. Drinking and eating small amounts often decreases the chance of gastrointestinal upsets.

2 Do not eat or drink too much carbohydrate or you will retard the gastric emptying rate, delay carbohydrate metabolism and nullify the effect you are trying to achieve.

3 Try all foods and fluids in training according to race conditions.

4 Never try any new food or drink on race day.

5 Keep use of high-fat foods to a minimum as fat takes five hours to digest. They can cause indigestion, nausea and vomiting.

♦ The refuelling diet ♦

No matter how hard you train, if you do not eat properly you will train and compete with less than adequate fuel supply. An important aspect of this is refuelling after a hard race or training. The most important nutritional considerations are the rehydration of fluids and the replenishment of glycogen stores. The sooner these are implemented after training and competition the more rapid the recovery.

Nutrition tips for refuelling

1 If you become dehydrated it may take 24 to 36 hours to become fully rehydrated. Drink fluids liberally. Do not include alcohol until rehydrated and keep coffee to a minimum. Rehydration has occurred when weight is normal and urine is 'pale and plenty'. (If you are taking a vitamin supplement the urine will be coloured.)

2 For maximum glycogen resynthesis carbohydrates are needed within the first hour after exercise. Delaying carbohydrate intake for more than two hours can mean glycogen recovery will take several days.

3 Glycogen resynthesis is greatest in the first two hours after exercise. A rate of 1–1.5 g per kg body weight per hour is recommended.

4 After the first two hours a rate of 50–100 g over two hours is sufficient, or 600 g carbohydrate over 24 hours. Recovery can then be made within 24 hours.

5 The type of carbohydrate may influence glycogen recovery. High glycaemic foods appear to result in faster glycogen resynthesis initially. Simple and complex carbohydrates in solid or liquid form can be used during the first 24 hours. From 24 to 48 hours complex carbohydrates provide better glycogen recovery.

6 Consume adequate amounts of electrolytes, especially sodium and potassium. Commercial sports recovery drinks contain added electrolytes.

7 Many endurance athletes need to train themselves to eat immediately after exercise as they often have no desire for food. Consuming an adequate carbohydrate drink is fine.

8 The refuelling diet must be part of your daily training – always include a drink and some solid food in your training bag for immediately after exercise.

9 Remember to include good quality protein in your next full meal. Protein is needed for tissue repair from training and, when you are exercising more than two hours, is needed to replace protein that has been used as energy.

The recovery diet and the training diet are regarded as the two most important aspects of an athlete's nutrition programme. Without instigating the correct dietary procedures for recovery an athlete can end up being glycogen depleted, with a resultant drop off in training, an inability to increase intensity or duration, and an increased risk of injury.

Nutrition alone will not guarantee your athletic success. By following the nutritional principles set out in this chapter, however, you can ensure that your performance is determined by skill and training, not eating habits.

Chapter 13

Endurance Training in the Future – What Can We Expect?

Endurance training will rely more and more on the detailed analysis of training and racing. More information will be gathered on an athlete's condition (physical and psychological), training volumes, training intensities, the training intensity proportions relative to training volume, total training stress, and many other specifics. This information will be analysed by coach/athlete/sports scientist in an effort to optimise the athlete's total training environment. This, in turn, will promote optimal performance.

But first must come a full understanding of the factors that contribute to the peak performance of an athlete. In order to do this a very precise training instrument will be needed. That instrument? A user-friendly log book much like that presented in this book, but the future model will be even broader in its scope and more sensitive in its measurement. The 'log book of the future' will elicit extra information on the psychological state of the athlete, on the time/distance spent at each training intensity, and on the type of training used. It will look at the 'loading index' of different types of training and the increases in training load from week to week. In short, it will be a complete training guide. The psychological inventory will pick up the stressors on an athlete, both inside and outside the sport, and will help predict overtraining situations before they occur.

♦ Training load ♦

Training volumes (distance/duration) will be combined with time/distance spent at each training intensity to provide a concise overall picture of training composition. This is because training volumes by themselves do not accurately represent 'work' done by the athlete. For instance, high-volume training done at low intensity may place a lower load on the athlete than moderate volume done at moderate intensity. Or, in terms of training load, ten minutes of intensive sprint intervals may be worth two hours of long slow distance.

By assigning each training intensity a load number or training load coefficient and multiplying it by the volume of training done at each intensity, you get a training load index number for each intensity. These index numbers are then added together to get a total training load index. This idea was originally used by Paul Kochli, who coached cycling greats Greg Lemond and Bernard Hinault. The table opposite illustrates how a weekly index is calculated.

To determine the percentage of the total training volume of each intensity, divide time/distance done at each intensity by total training volume and multiply by 100. Training load coefficients are approximated according to percentage of maximum heart rate or maximum pace. It is therefore necessary to judge for yourself how each training

Training intensity	Training volume (min)	% total training volume	Training load coefficient	Training load index
HI				
PW	0	0	1.0	0
IN	10	1.7	0.95	1.6
EX	10	1.7	0.90	1.5
SM	35	5.8	0.85	4.9
LO				
UT	0	0	0.75	0
LSD	485	80.8	0.60	48.5
AR	60	10	0.40	4.0
TOTAL	600	100		60.5

Total training volume = 600 min
Training load index = 60.5

Key: HI = high intensity; PW = power; IN = intensive sprints; EX = extensive sprints; SM = submaximal intensity; LO = low intensity; UT = up-tempo; LSD = long slow distance; AR = active recovery.

intensity feels (on a scale of 0.00 to 1.0), for example, submaximal training might be judged to require an 85 per cent effort (coefficient = 0.85).

Once athletes have worked out their training load coefficients, they can then graph training volume, training intensity proportions (percentage) and training load indices for each training intensity (*see* fig. 13.1, page 176). They can then assess increases or decreases in training load from week to week. For example, if an athlete felt the previous build-up's load was as much as they could cope with, but more speedwork was needed, the coach/ athlete could adjust the programme by incorporating more speedwork. This could be done by manipulating other variables (volume, intensity) to maintain the same training load.

Determination of training volumes at each intensity

An athlete also needs to assess how much of each training intensity they use during a build-up, i.e. how much long slow distance, submaximal training, extensive and intensive sprints they should do. There is no completely accurate way to do this the first time so it may help to set up an 'intensity bar' (*see* fig. 13.2, page 177) that equals total training volume (100 per cent). Then, using your experience (and the experience of your coach, if you have one), estimate what percentage of your training will be done at each intensity. This is difficult to do, and the assistance of a coach or an experienced athlete is very useful.

Start with the highest intensity training, for example power during speedwork, and work your way down to the lowest intensity training, for example active recovery. Work out how much each training type within each intensity contributes to total training, for

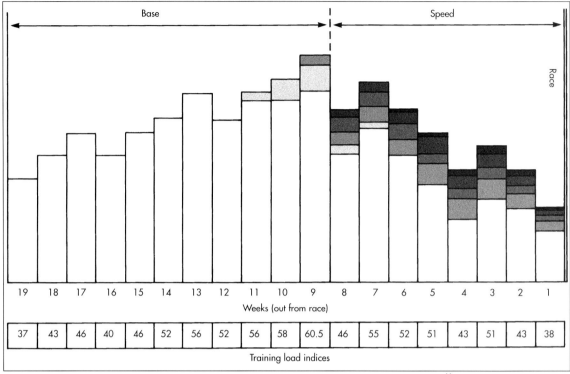

Base											Speed								Race
19	18	17	16	15	14	13	12	11	10	9	8	7	6	5	4	3	2	1	

Weeks (out from race)

37	43	46	40	46	52	56	52	56	58	60.5	46	55	52	51	43	51	43	38

Training load indices

Figure 13.1 Training volumes, training intensities and training load indices

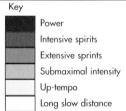

Key

Power

Intensive spirits

Extensive sprints

Submaximal intensity

Up-tempo

Long slow distance

example power may contribute 2 per cent, or it may not contribute at all. Put this first figure at the top of your 'intensity bar'. Calculate a percentage figure for each training type/intensity and fill in the bar until you have 100 per cent.

When assessing the contribution of each type of training to the programme, you need to keep in mind how much of each intensity will be needed for the race you are training for, for example a marathon runner would not do any power work as power is not an intensity needed in marathon running. (Leg speed is another issue, however, and most runners, for example, would employ this type of training at some time in their programme (*see* fig. 13.3, page 178). Once you have allocated a percentage to the speedwork, submaximal work and up-tempo work to be included in the training programme, you are left with a percentage for long slow distance training (and perhaps active recovery). You now have a percentage of total volume figure for every type of training.

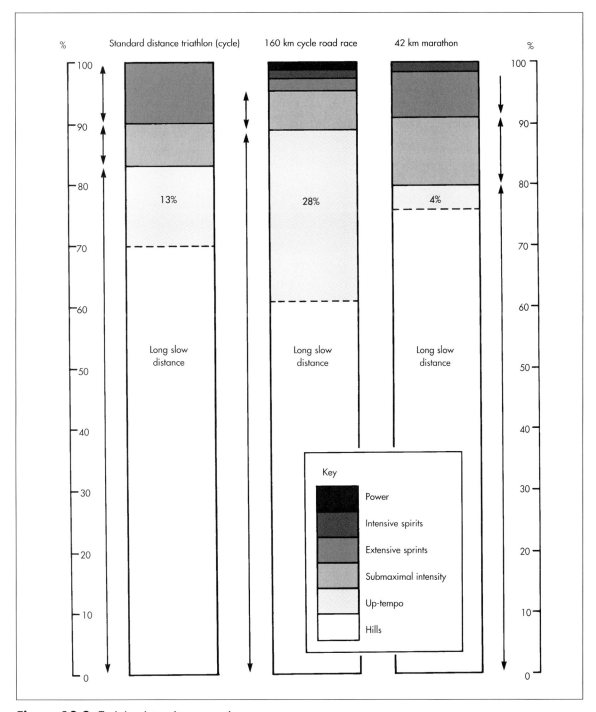

Figure 13.2 Training intensity proportions

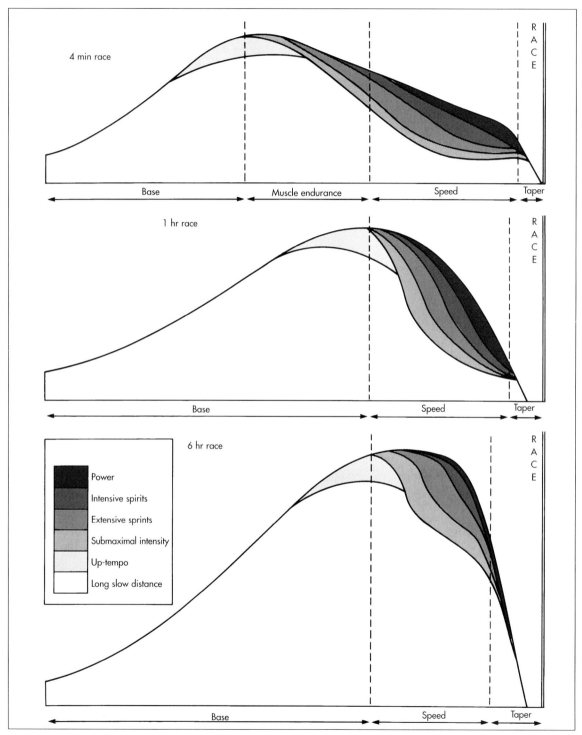

Figure 13.3 Training programmes for runners

An example follows for a cyclist training for a 160 km road race. Total training volume is 500 km per week (or 16 hr 40 min at an average of 30 kph). During speedwork the proportions of training intensities for the total training volume for the week is as follows.

Training intensity	% volume	Distance/ duration
High-intensity		
Power	0.5	2.5 km/5 min
Intensive sprint	1	5.0 km/10 min
Extensive sprint	2	10 km/20 min
Submaximal intensity		
Anaerobic threshold	9.5	47.5 km/95 min
Low-intensity		
Up-tempo	0	0 km
Long slow distance (and active recovery)	87	435 km/870 min
Total		435 km/870 min 500 km/1000 min (16 hr 40 min at 30 kph)

Of course, the intensities will not remain the same all the way through training. They start at different times and reach peak volumes at different times. How does an athlete adjust their programme to accommodate this? By using a number of 'intensity bars' at different times throughout build-up, and compiling them in the manner described above. Depending on where the athlete is at in build-up, the training intensity proportions will vary. In figure 13.4 (bottom graph, page 180) intensity bars are assessed for weeks 14, 10, 8, 6, 4 and 2 and this is shown by the change in the composition of the intensity bars. These provide continuous training intensity proportions throughout the build-up. Figure 13.4 (top graph) includes the training volumes (mileages) and mesocycles during build-up (*see* chapter 7 for how to calculate weekly mileage and mesocycles).

Once these training figures have been set up for the first time in a build-up, the log book can be used to refine the process for future build-ups. A separate graph is used to assess the more personal aspects of an athlete's response to training. These include:

- weather
- number of hours' sleep
- average training heart rate
- resting heart rate
- type of training used
- body temperature
- body weight

Also graphed are the athlete's personal assessment of:

- how they felt
- overall psychological stress level
- rating of training effectiveness
- nutrition
- general energy levels
- social, work, lifestyle and personal satisfaction and confidence levels

This means that at the end of each week the athlete/coach/sports scientist has log book information for the week plus two graphs which can be compared with previous weeks. This information is particularly useful for a post-peak analysis, when the previous training build-up can be assessed. In this case a summary graph for the entire build-up is produced. Analysis therefore occurs on a day-to-day, week-to-week, build-up-to-build-up basis. End result? Optimal training.

This systematic/analytical approach to training would also help ensure that young athletes are handled correctly and that they fulfil their potential as adults.

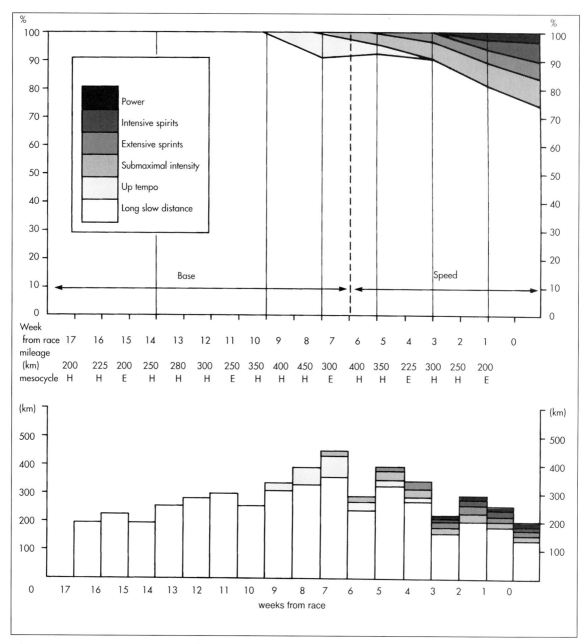

Figure 13.4 Training intensity volume assessment

♦ Re-creation – the final word ♦

If the analytical approach to training sounds too regimented, too authoritarian and too sterile, remember that an essential part of any good training programme is enjoyment. Enjoyment, of course, takes many forms – a easy jog through a forest, a gentle paddle down a river, an ocean swim on a beautiful summer's day. A good training programme, therefore, must afford you the opportunity to occasionally throw away the rule book and simply exercise. It must give you the freedom to just 'move around the planet a bit', if that's all you feel like doing. Training should be an antidote to drudgery, not a prescribed poison!

But lest we forget: enjoyment also comes under the guise of success – setting goals and achieving them; overcoming fears; exploring new boundaries; finishing with a smile, or just finishing. Yet success seldom just happens. You have almost always got to make it happen. And, yes, that can mean planning, log books, analysis, fine tuning, lateral thinking, imagination, discipline, commitment, and all that other stuff that sounds like work.

But it needn't be thought of as work. Striving can be play. Endurance training, after all, is an experiment in which you get to play both the 'guinea pig' and the 'scientist'. Enjoy both roles equally. Enjoy the physical, emotional and intellectual challenge of trying to move that body of yours further and faster. Enjoy trying to be the best athlete you can be, at whatever it is that turns you on. Enjoy being part of a personal revolution. Enjoy your personal re-creation.

Chapter 14

Specific Sample Programmes

Important note

These programmes are meant as a guide. They are designed to give you an idea of how your programme might be set up. They are not set up to be your 'perfect programme'. That is what your coach is for. He/she will be able to provide detailed specifics on a programme tailored to your individual and race requirements. Programmes are not static, they change constantly (workout to workout, day to day, week to week, month to month, year to year). They change in relation to the sport and the individual continuously and a combination of you and your coach, or an experienced athlete, will be able to keep up with the dynamics of the training process.

Explanation of sample programmes

Each section includes the following:
- weekly sample programmes for base and speed training and taper for different events
- 16-week training programmes including base, speed and taper for different events
- sport-specific training by type of intensity

Notes to sample training programmes

- Unless otherwise stated, the sample programmes are for semi-competitive to elite athletes; full-time elite athletes (elite-plus)

and novices would require adjustments to these programmes (*see* pages 105–6 for information on categories of athletes).
- The weekly programme volume/duration is the maximum for a single week (peak-mileage week) during the phase (base or speed) of training. It is not the average or standard training volume/duration.
- All the 16-week training programmes include a six-day taper.
- Bold subscript numbers in the 16-week programmes correspond to the subphases on the graph (*see* chapter 4 for more detail on subphases).
- For further information on the different types of training intensities, *see* chapter 3 and appendix 1.
- Races have not been included in the training programmes. These would need to be added with minor alterations to training volumes.
- Hydration strategies are detailed on page 167 and appendix 6.
- Race day nutrition strategies are detailed in appendix 7.

For further background on sample taining programmes *see* chapter 7.

General reminder notes for all endurance sports

Base training
Base training should mainly be carried out at a low intensity; volume or duration are more important than intensity at this stage. Racing and faster training are possible, but should be restricted to small quantities as too much speed training during this phase will cause overtraining or peaking too early. Flexibility and technique are also key areas in this phase.

Speed training
Speed training occurs four to eight weeks before peak and involves careful manipulation of all training intensities to improve race pace while retaining base fitness and without overstressing the body. Competitive phase training which follows the speed phase is a manipulation of speed training programmes.

Heart rate
If using a heart rate monitor, try to maintain target heart rate when training. If heart rate is too high, lower your training intensity. When taking your pulse manually during interval training, try to take it immediately after each interval (heart rate drops quickly).

Warming up and warming down
Always warm up and warm down for 5 to 20 minutes. The warm-up should be longer for high-intensity workouts. If you are going out for a low-intensity workout, include the warm-up and warm-down as part of the workout.

Taper and peak
A taper is a gradual reduction in training load (mileage/duration). In the last few days before a race an athlete must allow his/her body to recover from the previous intense training. Once fully recovered, they should be ready for a peak performance.

Key to sample programmes

AT	anaerobic threshold (= SM)
accels	accelerations
BRICKS	*see table note*
btwn	between
CARBO LOAD	carbohydrate loading
CONT	continuous
CONT SEA	continuous sea swim
DIST	distance
(e.g. 50% dist)	(50% of usual distance)
D/O	day off
E	easy
Flex	flexibility
H	hard
HEAT	initial race
HI	high intensity
HILLS	hill training
(e.g. 50 hills)	(50% of usual hill training)
hr	hours
INTS	intervals *see table note*
(e.g. 66% ints)	(66% of usual intervals)
IRP	Ironman race pace
km	kilometres
LO	low intensity
LONG	long workout
(e.g. 66% long)	(66% of usual workout)
m	metres
Med	medium
min	minutes
ML	medium long workout
MOD	moderate intensity
O/R	off-road
%	% of total workout per discipline per week
PLAN	plan next week's workouts
RP	race pace
R/P/C/R	ride/push/carry/ride
SANDY	training in soft/hard sand
sec	seconds
semi	race semi-final
SM	submaximal intensity
Tech	technique training
TRANS	transition training
TT	time trial
UT	up-tempo
W/UP-W/D	warm-up, warm-down
⟶	training is continuous

♦ Triathlon training ♦ programmes

Triathlons are swim/bike/run endurance time trial events. Start with two workouts per discipline per week (*see* chapter 7, section B, no. 5 semi-competitive) and progress to three to four disciplines per workout per week. This can sometimes be higher for elite triathletes. If you prefer to keep to two workouts per discipline per week, make one workout the long session and the other the speed session in the speed phase.

BASE TRAINING

Standard distance (1.5 km/40 km/10 km) base programme						
M	T	W	T	F	S	S
Swim 1.5–3 km 1 hr (27%) (LO/SM/HI)		Swim 1.5–3 km 1 hr (27%) (LO/SM/HI)		Swim* 1.5–3 km 1 hr (27%) (LO/SM/HI)	Swim 2 km 40 min (19%) (LO)(CONT)	
	Bike 30–60 km 1–2 hr (21%) (LO)		Bike 30–60 km 1–2 hr (21%) (LO)(HILLS)	DAY OFF	Bike* 20–40 km 1–1.5 hr (LO)(15%)	Bike 60–120 km 2–4 hr (LO)(43%)
Run 8–16 km 30–45 min (LO)(32%)		Run 10–20 km 45–90 min (LO)(41%)			Run 5–10 km 30–45 min (LO)(21%)	Run* 3 km 9–15 min (LO)(6%) (PLAN)

Note: * = these workouts can be removed for three workouts per discipline per week. Friday is a legs day off only. Remove the swim for a complete day off.

Ironman distance (3.8 km/180 km/42 km) base programme						
M	T	W	T	F	S	S
Swim 1.5–3.5 km 1 hr (28%) (LO/SM/HI)		Swim 1.5–3.5 km 1 hr (28%) (LO/SM/HI)		Swim* 1.5–3.5 km 1 hr (28%) (LO/SM/HI)	Swim 2 km 40 min (16%) (LO)(CONT)	
	Bike 30–60 km 1–2 hr (15%) (LO)		Bike 30–80 km 1–3 hr (24%) (LO)(HILLS)	DAY OFF	Bike* 30–60 km 1–2 hr (LO)(15%)	Bike 100–180 km 4–6 hr (LO)(46%)
Run 10–20 km 1.25–1.5 hr (LO)(25%)		Run 16–36 km 1.5–3 hr (LO)(45%)			Run 10–20 km 1.25–1.5 hr (LO)(25%)	Run* 4 km 15–20 min (LO)(5%) (PLAN)

Note: * = these workouts can be removed for three workouts per discipline per week. Friday is a legs day off only. Remove the swim for a complete day off.

SPEED TRAINING

Standard distance (1.5 km/40 km/10 km) speed programme						
M	T	W	T	F	S	S
Swim 1.5–3 km 1 hr (27%) (LO/SM/HI)		Swim 1.5–3 km 1 hr (27%) (LO/SM/HI)		Swim* 1.5–3 km 1 hr (27%) (LO/SM/HI)	Swim 2 km 40 min (19%) (LO)(CONT SEA) last 200 m (SM) ↓	
	Bike 30–60 km 1–2 hr (21%) (LO)(HILLS)		Bike 30–60 km 1–2 hr (21%) INTS 4–6 × 8 min (SM/RP) 4–1 min rest btwn (BRICKS)	DAY OFF	Bike* 20–40 km 1–1.5 hr (LO)(15%) 1st & last 10 km (SM) ↓	Bike 60–120 km 2–4 hr (LO)(43%) ↓
Run INTS 4–6 × 5 min rest btwn 4–1 min rest btwn (32%)		Run 10–20 km 45–90 min (LO)(41%)			Run 5 km (SM/RP) 3 km (LO) 2 km (SM/RP) (21%)	Run* 3 km 9–15 min (LO)(6%) (PLAN)

Note: BRICKS = 1 min (SM) bike/racing transition/1 min run (SM) × 1–4 every 2nd week; INTS = e.g. 4–6 × 5 min (SM/RP), 4–1 min rest btwn = 4–6 sets of 5 min at a submaximal or race pace intensity with 1–4 min rest between with light activity. Gradually reduce the rest period from 4 minutes down to 1 minute. * = these workouts can be removed for three workouts per discipline per week. Friday is a legs day off only. Remove the swim for a complete day off. If the number of speed sessions is too great, alter Saturday's speed training to long slow distance training.

Ironman distance (3.8 km/180 km/42 km) speed programme

M	T	W	T	F	S	S
Swim 1.5–3.5 km 1 hr (18%) (LO/SM/HI)		Swim 1.5–3.5 km 1 hr (28%) (LO/SM/HI)		Swim* 1.5–3.5 km 1 hr (28%) (LO/SM/HI)	Swim 2 km 40 min (16%) (IRP)(CONT SEA) ↓	
	Bike 30–80 km 1–3 hr (24%) (HILLS) (LO)		Bike 30–60 km 1–2 hr (15%) INTS 2–3 × 15–40 min (UT/IRP) 10–20 min rest btwn	DAY OFF	Bike* 30–60 km 1–2 hr (15%) (LO) ↓	Bike 140–180 km 4.5–6 hr (46%) 1st 80–100 km (UT/IRP) TT then 80 km (LO) ↓
Run 16–20 km 1.25–1.5 hr INTS 2–3 × 10–30 min (UT/IRP) 10–20 min rest btwn rest of run (LO)(25%)		Run 26–36 km 2–3 hr (LO)(45%)			Run 16–20 km 1.25–1.5 hr (IRP)(25%)	Run* 4 km 15–20 min (LO)(5%) (PLAN)

Note: INTS = e.g. 2–3 sets of 10–30 min of exercise at an up-tempo or Ironman race pace (UT/IRP) intensity (no faster!) with 10–20 min rest (light activity) between. * = these workouts can be removed for three workouts per discipline per week. Friday is a legs day off only. Remove the swim for a complete day off. Remove either Monday's or Thursday's or both speed workouts if the speedwork is too hard.

Race: Triathlon (sprint/Olympic)
Race date: 20 April
Training starts: 30 December

Maximum distance for the 100% week
Swim: 4 km
Bike: 100 kms
Run: 16 km

Mileage profile

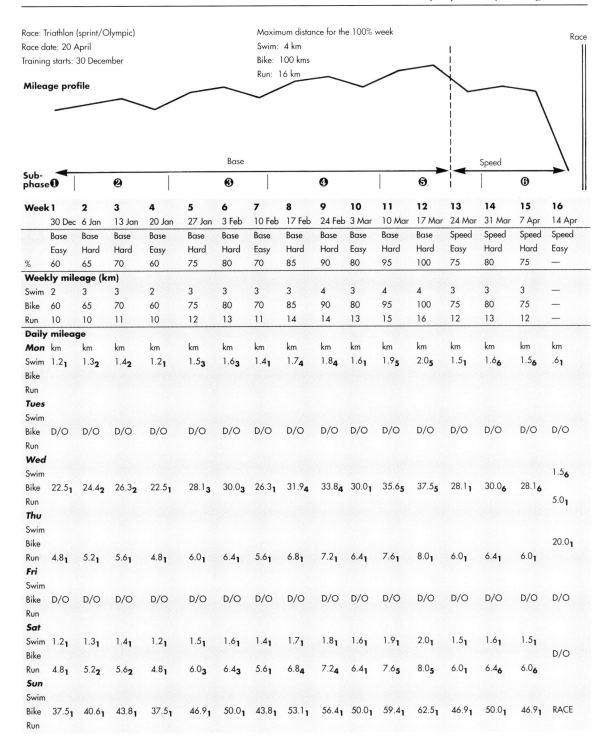

Sub-phase: ❶ ❷ ❸ ❹ ❺ ❻ — Base — Speed — Race

	1	2	3	4	5	6	7	8	9	10	11	12	13	14	15	16
Week	30 Dec	6 Jan	13 Jan	20 Jan	27 Jan	3 Feb	10 Feb	17 Feb	24 Feb	3 Mar	10 Mar	17 Mar	24 Mar	31 Mar	7 Apr	14 Apr
	Base	Base	Base	Base	Base	Base	Base	Base	Base	Base	Base	Base	Speed	Speed	Speed	Speed
	Easy	Hard	Hard	Easy	Hard	Hard	Easy	Hard	Hard	Easy	Hard	Hard	Easy	Hard	Hard	Easy
%	60	65	70	60	75	80	70	85	90	80	95	100	75	80	75	—
Weekly mileage (km)																
Swim	2	3	3	2	3	3	3	3	4	3	4	4	3	3	3	—
Bike	60	65	70	60	75	80	70	85	90	80	95	100	75	80	75	—
Run	10	10	11	10	12	13	11	14	14	13	15	16	12	13	12	—
Daily mileage																
Mon	km	km	km	km	km	km	km	km	km	km	km	km	km	km	km	km
Swim	1.2_1	1.3_2	1.4_2	1.2_1	1.5_3	1.6_3	1.4_1	1.7_4	1.8_4	1.6_1	1.9_5	2.0_5	1.5_1	1.6_6	1.5_6	$.6_1$
Bike																
Run																
Tues																
Swim																
Bike	D/O	D/O	D/O	D/O	D/O	D/O	D/O	D/O	D/O	D/O	D/O	D/O	D/O	D/O	D/O	D/O
Run																
Wed																
Swim																1.5_6
Bike	22.5_1	24.4_2	26.3_2	22.5_1	28.1_3	30.0_3	26.3_1	31.9_4	33.8_4	30.0_1	35.6_5	37.5_5	28.1_1	30.0_6	28.1_6	
Run																5.0_1
Thu																
Swim																
Bike																20.0_1
Run	4.8_1	5.2_1	5.6_1	4.8_1	6.0_1	6.4_1	5.6_1	6.8_1	7.2_1	6.4_1	7.6_1	8.0_1	6.0_1	6.4_1	6.0_1	
Fri																
Swim																
Bike	D/O	D/O	D/O	D/O	D/O	D/O	D/O	D/O	D/O	D/O	D/O	D/O	D/O	D/O	D/O	D/O
Run																
Sat																
Swim	1.2_1	1.3_1	1.4_1	1.2_1	1.5_1	1.6_1	1.4_1	1.7_1	1.8_1	1.6_1	1.9_1	2.0_1	1.5_1	1.6_1	1.5_1	
Bike																D/O
Run	4.8_1	5.2_2	5.6_2	4.8_1	6.0_3	6.4_3	5.6_1	6.8_4	7.2_4	6.4_1	7.6_5	8.0_5	6.0_1	6.4_6	6.0_6	
Sun																
Swim																
Bike	37.5_1	40.6_1	43.8_1	37.5_1	46.9_1	50.0_1	43.8_1	53.1_1	56.4_1	50.0_1	59.4_1	62.5_1	46.9_1	50.0_1	46.9_1	RACE
Run																

Race: Triathlon (sprint/Olympic)
Race date: 20 April
Training starts: 30 December

Maximum distance for the 100% week
Swim: 4 km
Bike: 180 km
Run: 25 km

Mileage profile

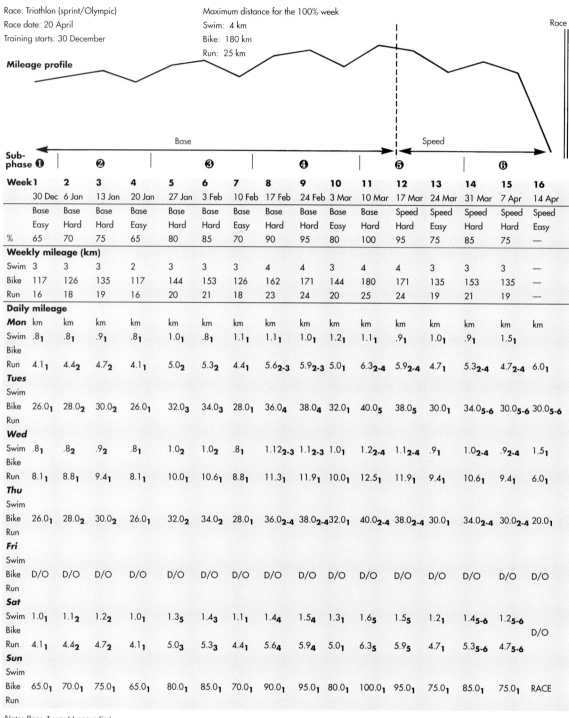

Sub-phase	❶	❷		❸		❹		❺		❻					
Week	1	2	3	4	5	6	7	8	9	10	11	12	13	14	15	16
	30 Dec	6 Jan	13 Jan	20 Jan	27 Jan	3 Feb	10 Feb	17 Feb	24 Feb	3 Mar	10 Mar	17 Mar	24 Mar	31 Mar	7 Apr	14 Apr
	Base	Base	Base	Base	Base	Base	Base	Base	Base	Base	Base	Speed	Speed	Speed	Speed	Speed
	Easy	Hard	Hard	Easy	Hard	Hard	Easy	Hard	Hard	Easy	Hard	Hard	Easy	Hard	Hard	Easy
%	65	70	75	65	80	85	70	90	95	80	100	95	75	85	75	—

Weekly mileage (km)

	1	2	3	4	5	6	7	8	9	10	11	12	13	14	15	16
Swim	3	3	3	2	3	3	3	4	4	3	4	4	3	3	3	—
Bike	117	126	135	117	144	153	126	162	171	144	180	171	135	153	135	—
Run	16	18	19	16	20	21	18	23	24	20	25	24	19	21	19	—

Daily mileage

Mon (km)

	1	2	3	4	5	6	7	8	9	10	11	12	13	14	15	16
Swim	$.8_1$	$.8_1$	$.9_1$	$.8_1$	1.0_1	$.8_1$	1.1_1	1.1_1	1.0_1	1.2_1	1.1_1	$.9_1$	1.0_1	$.9_1$	1.5_1	
Bike																
Run	4.1_1	4.4_2	4.7_2	4.1_1	5.0_2	5.3_2	4.4_1	5.6_{2-3}	5.9_{2-3}	5.0_1	6.3_{2-4}	5.9_{2-4}	4.7_1	5.3_{2-4}	4.7_{2-4}	6.0_1

Tues

	1	2	3	4	5	6	7	8	9	10	11	12	13	14	15	16
Swim																
Bike	26.0_1	28.0_2	30.0_2	26.0_1	32.0_3	34.0_3	28.0_1	36.0_4	38.0_4	32.0_1	40.0_5	38.0_5	30.0_1	34.0_{5-6}	30.0_{5-6}	30.0_{5-6}
Run																

Wed

	1	2	3	4	5	6	7	8	9	10	11	12	13	14	15	16
Swim	$.8_1$	$.8_2$	$.9_2$	$.8_1$	1.0_2	1.0_2	$.8_1$	1.1_{2-3}	1.1_{2-3}	1.0_1	1.2_{2-4}	1.1_{2-4}	$.9_1$	1.0_{2-4}	$.9_{2-4}$	1.5_1
Bike																
Run	8.1_1	8.8_1	9.4_1	8.1_1	10.0_1	10.6_1	8.8_1	11.3_1	11.9_1	10.0_1	12.5_1	11.9_1	9.4_1	10.6_1	9.4_1	6.0_1

Thu

	1	2	3	4	5	6	7	8	9	10	11	12	13	14	15	16
Swim																
Bike	26.0_1	28.0_2	30.0_2	26.0_1	32.0_2	34.0_2	28.0_1	36.0_{2-4}	38.0_{2-4}	32.0_1	40.0_{2-4}	38.0_{2-4}	30.0_1	34.0_{2-4}	30.0_{2-4}	20.0_1
Run																

Fri

	1	2	3	4	5	6	7	8	9	10	11	12	13	14	15	16
Swim																
Bike	D/O	D/O	D/O	D/O	D/O	D/O	D/O	D/O	D/O	D/O	D/O	D/O	D/O	D/O	D/O	D/O
Run																

Sat

	1	2	3	4	5	6	7	8	9	10	11	12	13	14	15	16
Swim	1.0_1	1.1_2	1.2_2	1.0_1	1.3_5	1.4_3	1.1_1	1.4_4	1.5_4	1.3_1	1.6_5	1.5_5	1.2_1	1.4_{5-6}	1.2_{5-6}	
Bike																D/O
Run	4.1_1	4.4_2	4.7_2	4.1_1	5.0_3	5.3_3	4.4_1	5.6_4	5.9_4	5.0_1	6.3_5	5.9_5	4.7_1	5.3_{5-6}	4.7_{5-6}	

Sun

	1	2	3	4	5	6	7	8	9	10	11	12	13	14	15	16
Swim																
Bike	65.0_1	70.0_1	75.0_1	65.0_1	80.0_1	85.0_1	70.0_1	90.0_1	95.0_1	80.0_1	100.0_1	95.0_1	75.0_1	85.0_1	75.0_1	RACE
Run																

Note: Base 1 would occur first.

Race: Triathlon (Olympic/Half-Ironman)
Race date: 20 April
Training starts: 30 December

Maximum distance for the 100% week
Swim: 12 km
Bike: 240 km
Run: 50 km

Race

Mileage profile

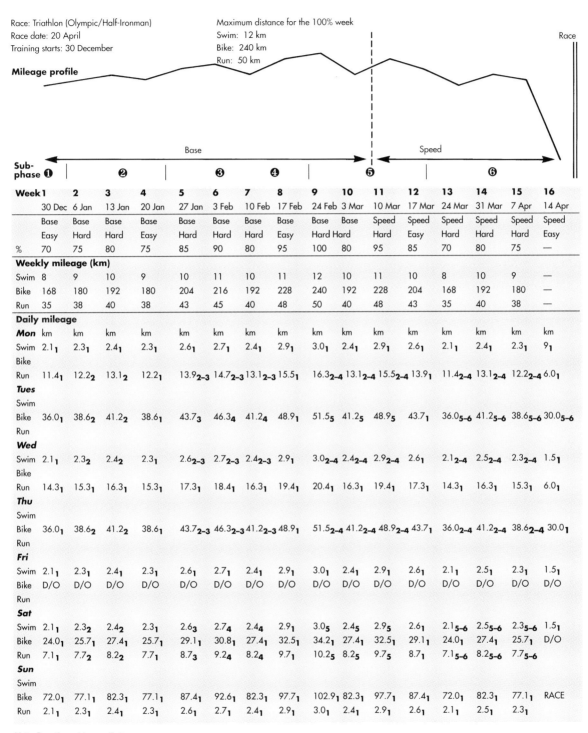

Base   Speed

Sub-phase ❶   ❷   ❸   ❹   ❺   ❻

Week	1	2	3	4	5	6	7	8	9	10	11	12	13	14	15	16
	30 Dec	6 Jan	13 Jan	20 Jan	27 Jan	3 Feb	10 Feb	17 Feb	24 Feb	3 Mar	10 Mar	17 Mar	24 Mar	31 Mar	7 Apr	14 Apr
	Base	Base	Base	Base	Base	Base	Base	Base	Base	Base	Speed	Speed	Speed	Speed	Speed	Speed
	Easy	Hard	Hard	Easy	Hard	Hard	Hard	Easy	Hard	Hard	Hard	Easy	Hard	Hard	Hard	Easy
%	70	75	80	75	85	90	80	95	100	80	95	85	70	80	75	—
Weekly mileage (km)																
Swim	8	9	10	9	10	11	10	11	12	10	11	10	8	10	9	—
Bike	168	180	192	180	204	216	192	228	240	192	228	204	168	192	180	—
Run	35	38	40	38	43	45	40	48	50	40	48	43	35	40	38	—
Daily mileage																
Mon	km	km	km	km	km	km	km	km	km	km	km	km	km	km	km	km
Swim	2.1_1	2.3_1	2.4_1	2.3_1	2.6_1	2.7_1	2.4_1	2.9_1	3.0_1	2.4_1	2.9_1	2.6_1	2.1_1	2.4_1	2.3_1	9_1
Bike																
Run	11.4_1	12.2_2	13.1_2	12.2_1	13.9_{2-3}	14.7_{2-3}	13.1_{2-3}	15.5_1	16.3_{2-4}	13.1_{2-4}	15.5_{2-4}	13.9_1	11.4_{2-4}	13.1_{2-4}	12.2_{2-4}	6.0_1
Tues																
Swim																
Bike	36.0_1	38.6_2	41.2_2	38.6_1	43.7_3	46.3_4	41.2_4	48.9_1	51.5_5	41.2_5	48.9_5	43.7_1	36.0_{5-6}	41.2_{5-6}	38.6_{5-6}	30.0_{5-6}
Run																
Wed																
Swim	2.1_1	2.3_2	2.4_2	2.3_1	2.6_{2-3}	2.7_{2-3}	2.4_{2-3}	2.9_1	3.0_{2-4}	2.4_{2-4}	2.9_{2-4}	2.6_1	2.1_{2-4}	2.5_{2-4}	2.3_{2-4}	1.5_1
Bike																
Run	14.3_1	15.3_1	16.3_1	15.3_1	17.3_1	18.4_1	16.3_1	19.4_1	20.4_1	16.3_1	19.4_1	17.3_1	14.3_1	16.3_1	15.3_1	6.0_1
Thu																
Swim																
Bike	36.0_1	38.6_2	41.2_2	38.6_1	43.7_{2-3}	46.3_{2-3}	41.2_{2-3}	48.9_1	51.5_{2-4}	41.2_{2-4}	48.9_{2-4}	43.7_1	36.0_{2-4}	41.2_{2-4}	38.6_{2-4}	30.0_1
Run																
Fri																
Swim	2.1_1	2.3_1	2.4_1	2.3_1	2.6_1	2.7_1	2.4_1	2.9_1	3.0_1	2.4_1	2.9_1	2.6_1	2.1_1	2.5_1	2.3_1	1.5_1
Bike	D/O	D/O	D/O	D/O	D/O	D/O	D/O	D/O	D/O	D/O	D/O	D/O	D/O	D/O	D/O	D/O
Run																
Sat																
Swim	2.1_1	2.3_2	2.4_2	2.3_1	2.6_3	2.7_4	2.4_4	2.9_1	3.0_5	2.4_5	2.9_5	2.6_1	2.1_{5-6}	2.5_{5-6}	2.3_{5-6}	1.5_1
Bike	24.0_1	25.7_2	27.4_2	25.7_1	29.1_1	30.8_1	27.4_1	32.5_1	34.2_1	27.4_1	32.5_1	29.1_1	24.0_1	27.4_1	25.7_1	D/O
Run	7.1_1	7.7_2	8.2_2	7.7_1	8.7_3	9.2_4	8.2_4	9.7_1	10.2_5	8.2_5	9.7_5	8.7_1	7.1_{5-6}	8.2_{5-6}	7.7_{5-6}	
Sun																
Swim																
Bike	72.0_1	77.1_1	82.3_1	77.1_1	87.4_1	92.6_1	82.3_1	97.7_1	102.9_1	82.3_1	97.7_1	87.4_1	72.0_1	82.3_1	77.1_1	RACE
Run	2.1_1	2.3_1	2.4_1	2.3_1	2.6_1	2.7_1	2.4_1	2.9_1	3.0_1	2.4_1	2.9_1	2.6_1	2.1_1	2.5_1	2.3_1	

Note: Base 1 would occur first.

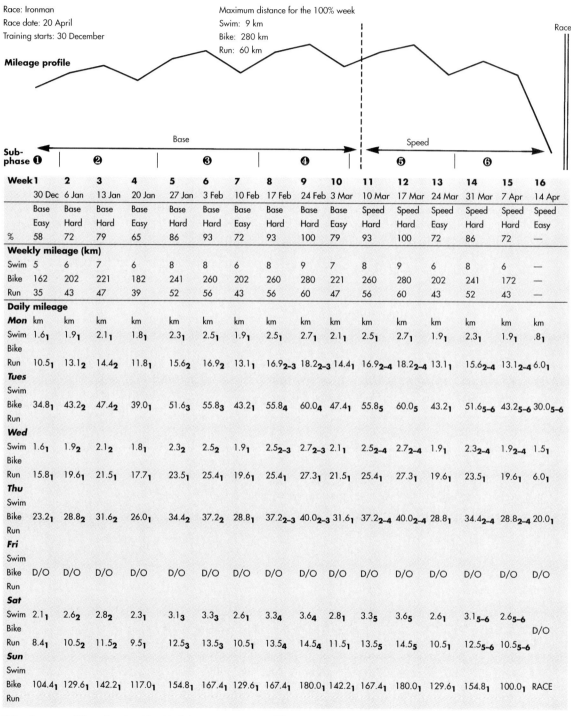

Race: Ironman
Race date: 20 April
Training starts: 30 December

Maximum distance for the 100% week
Swim: 9 km
Bike: 280 km
Run: 60 km

Mileage profile

Race

Base — Speed

Sub-phase: ❶ ❷ ❸ ❹ ❺ ❻

	Week 1	2	3	4	5	6	7	8	9	10	11	12	13	14	15	16
	30 Dec	6 Jan	13 Jan	20 Jan	27 Jan	3 Feb	10 Feb	17 Feb	24 Feb	3 Mar	10 Mar	17 Mar	24 Mar	31 Mar	7 Apr	14 Apr
	Base	Base	Base	Base	Base	Base	Base	Base	Base	Base	Speed	Speed	Speed	Speed	Speed	Speed
	Easy	Hard	Hard	Easy	Hard	Hard	Easy	Hard	Hard	Easy	Hard	Hard	Easy	Hard	Hard	Easy
%	58	72	79	65	86	93	72	93	100	79	93	100	72	86	72	—
Weekly mileage (km)																
Swim	5	6	7	6	8	8	6	8	9	7	8	9	6	8	6	—
Bike	162	202	221	182	241	260	202	260	280	221	260	280	202	241	172	—
Run	35	43	47	39	52	56	43	56	60	47	56	60	43	52	43	—

Daily mileage

Mon	km	km	km	km	km	km	km	km	km	km	km	km	km	km	km	km
Swim	1.6_1	1.9_1	2.1_1	1.8_1	2.3_1	2.5_1	1.9_1	2.5_1	2.7_1	2.1_1	2.5_1	2.7_1	1.9_1	2.3_1	1.9_1	$.8_1$
Bike																
Run	10.5_1	13.1_2	14.4_2	11.8_1	15.6_2	16.9_2	13.1_1	$16.9_{2\text{-}3}$	$18.2_{2\text{-}3}$	14.4_1	$16.9_{2\text{-}4}$	$18.2_{2\text{-}4}$	13.1_1	$15.6_{2\text{-}4}$	$13.1_{2\text{-}4}$	6.0_1
Tues																
Swim																
Bike	34.8_1	43.2_2	47.4_2	39.0_1	51.6_3	55.8_3	43.2_1	55.8_4	60.0_4	47.4_1	55.8_5	60.0_5	43.2_1	$51.6_{5\text{-}6}$	$43.2_{5\text{-}6}$	$30.0_{5\text{-}6}$
Run																
Wed																
Swim	1.6_1	1.9_2	2.1_2	1.8_1	2.3_2	2.5_2	1.9_1	$2.5_{2\text{-}3}$	$2.7_{2\text{-}3}$	2.1_1	$2.5_{2\text{-}4}$	$2.7_{2\text{-}4}$	1.9_1	$2.3_{2\text{-}4}$	$1.9_{2\text{-}4}$	1.5_1
Bike																
Run	15.8_1	19.6_2	21.5_1	17.7_1	23.5_1	25.4_1	19.6_1	25.4_1	27.3_1	21.5_1	25.4_1	27.3_1	19.6_1	23.5_1	19.6_1	6.0_1
Thu																
Swim																
Bike	23.2_1	28.8_2	31.6_2	26.0_1	34.4_2	37.2_2	28.8_1	$37.2_{2\text{-}3}$	$40.0_{2\text{-}3}$	31.6_1	$37.2_{2\text{-}4}$	$40.0_{2\text{-}4}$	28.8_1	$34.4_{2\text{-}4}$	$28.8_{2\text{-}4}$	20.0_1
Run																
Fri																
Swim																
Bike	D/O	D/O	D/O	D/O	D/O	D/O	D/O	D/O	D/O	D/O	D/O	D/O	D/O	D/O	D/O	D/O
Run																
Sat																
Swim	2.1_1	2.6_2	2.8_2	2.3_1	3.1_3	3.3_3	2.6_1	3.3_4	3.6_4	2.8_1	3.3_5	3.6_5	2.6_1	$3.1_{5\text{-}6}$	$2.6_{5\text{-}6}$	
Bike																D/O
Run	8.4_1	10.5_2	11.5_2	9.5_1	12.5_3	13.5_3	10.5_1	13.5_4	14.5_4	11.5_1	13.5_5	14.5_5	10.5_1	$12.5_{5\text{-}6}$	$10.5_{5\text{-}6}$	
Sun																
Swim																
Bike	104.4_1	129.6_1	142.2_1	117.0_1	154.8_1	167.4_1	129.6_1	167.4_1	180.0_1	142.2_1	167.4_1	180.0_1	129.6_1	154.8_1	100.0_1	RACE
Run																

Note: mileages would be set based on this guide. In Ironman training more 180 km bike rides may be done. Base 1 would occur first.

Race: Ironman
Race date: 20 April
Training starts: 30 December

Mileage profile

Maximum distance for the 100% week
Swim: 12 km
Bike: 360 km
Run: 75 km

Race

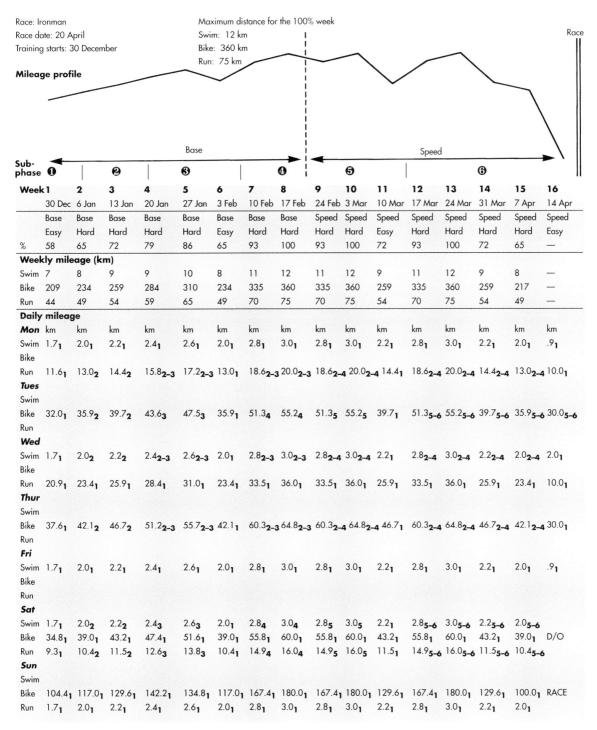

Sub-phase	❶		❷		❸		❹		❺		❻					
Week	1	2	3	4	5	6	7	8	9	10	11	12	13	14	15	16
	30 Dec	6 Jan	13 Jan	20 Jan	27 Jan	3 Feb	10 Feb	17 Feb	24 Feb	3 Mar	10 Mar	17 Mar	24 Mar	31 Mar	7 Apr	14 Apr
	Base	Base	Base	Base	Base	Base	Base	Base	Speed	Speed	Speed	Speed	Speed	Speed	Speed	Speed
	Easy	Hard	Hard	Hard	Hard	Easy	Hard	Hard	Hard	Hard	Easy	Hard	Hard	Hard	Hard	Easy
%	58	65	72	79	86	65	93	100	93	100	72	93	100	72	65	—
Weekly mileage (km)																
Swim	7	8	9	9	10	8	11	12	11	12	9	11	12	9	8	—
Bike	209	234	259	284	310	234	335	360	335	360	259	335	360	259	217	—
Run	44	49	54	59	65	49	70	75	70	75	54	70	75	54	49	—
Daily mileage																
Mon	km	km	km	km	km	km	km	km	km	km	km	km	km	km	km	km
Swim	1.7_1	2.0_1	2.2_1	2.4_1	2.6_1	2.0_1	2.8_1	3.0_1	2.8_1	3.0_1	2.2_1	2.8_1	3.0_1	2.2_1	2.0_1	$.9_1$
Bike																
Run	11.6_1	13.0_2	14.4_2	15.8_{2-3}	17.2_{2-3}	13.0_1	18.6_{2-3}	20.0_{2-3}	18.6_{2-4}	20.0_{2-4}	14.4_1	18.6_{2-4}	20.0_{2-4}	14.4_{2-4}	13.0_{2-4}	10.0_1
Tues																
Swim																
Bike	32.0_1	35.9_2	39.7_2	43.6_3	47.5_3	35.9_1	51.3_4	55.2_4	51.3_5	55.2_5	39.7_1	51.3_{5-6}	55.2_{5-6}	39.7_{5-6}	35.9_{5-6}	30.0_{5-6}
Run																
Wed																
Swim	1.7_1	2.0_2	2.2_2	2.4_{2-3}	2.6_{2-3}	2.0_1	2.8_{2-3}	3.0_{2-3}	2.8_{2-4}	3.0_{2-4}	2.2_1	2.8_{2-4}	3.0_{2-4}	2.2_{2-4}	2.0_{2-4}	2.0_1
Bike																
Run	20.9_1	23.4_1	25.9_1	28.4_1	31.0_1	23.4_1	33.5_1	36.0_1	33.5_1	36.0_1	25.9_1	33.5_1	36.0_1	25.9_1	23.4_1	10.0_1
Thur																
Swim																
Bike	37.6_1	42.1_2	46.7_2	51.2_{2-3}	55.7_{2-3}	42.1_1	60.3_{2-3}	64.8_{2-3}	60.3_{2-4}	64.8_{2-4}	46.7_1	60.3_{2-4}	64.8_{2-4}	46.7_{2-4}	42.1_{2-4}	30.0_1
Run																
Fri																
Swim	1.7_1	2.0_1	2.2_1	2.4_1	2.6_1	2.0_1	2.8_1	3.0_1	2.8_1	3.0_1	2.2_1	2.8_1	3.0_1	2.2_1	2.0_1	$.9_1$
Bike																
Run																
Sat																
Swim	1.7_1	2.0_2	2.2_2	2.4_3	2.6_3	2.0_1	2.8_4	3.0_4	2.8_5	3.0_5	2.2_1	2.8_{5-6}	3.0_{5-6}	2.2_{5-6}	2.0_{5-6}	
Bike	34.8_1	39.0_1	43.2_1	47.4_1	51.6_1	39.0_1	55.8_1	60.0_1	55.8_1	60.0_1	43.2_1	55.8_1	60.0_1	43.2_1	39.0_1	D/O
Run	9.3_1	10.4_2	11.5_2	12.6_3	13.8_3	10.4_1	14.9_4	16.0_4	14.9_5	16.0_5	11.5_1	14.9_{5-6}	16.0_{5-6}	11.5_{5-6}	10.4_{5-6}	
Sun																
Swim																
Bike	104.4_1	117.0_1	129.6_1	142.2_1	134.8_1	117.0_1	167.4_1	180.0_1	167.4_1	180.0_1	129.6_1	167.4_1	180.0_1	129.6_1	100.0_1	RACE
Run	1.7_1	2.0_1	2.2_1	2.4_1	2.6_1	2.0_1	2.8_1	3.0_1	2.8_1	3.0_1	2.2_1	2.8_1	3.0_1	2.2_1	2.0_1	

Base ← → Speed

Note: mileages would be set based on this guide. In Ironman training more 180 km bike rides may be done. Base 1 would occur first.

TAPER AND PEAK

Standard distance low-priority taper (and following week resuming normal training)

Week 1

M	T	W	T	F	S	S
Swim		Swim		Swim (50% DIST)	DAY OFF	R
	Bike (HILLS)		Bike (50% INTS)			A
						C
Run (INTS)		Run (66% LONG)		Run (E)		E

Week 2

M	T	W	T	F	S	S
DAY OFF		Swim		Swim		Swim
	Bike (E)		Bike (HILLS)		Bike (E)	Bike (LONG)
		Run (LONG)		DAY OFF	Run (E)	Run (E)

Note: Friday is a legs day off. Remove the swim for a complete day off.

Standard distance high-priority taper

M	T	W	T	F	S	S
Swim		Swim		DAY OFF	DAY OFF	R
	Bike (BRICKS) (E)		Bike (E) (TRANS)			A
						C
Run (50% INTS)	Run (E)	Run (E)	CARBO LOAD ⟶			E W/UP–W/D

Ironman distance taper

Week 1

M	T	W	T	F	S	S
Swim		Swim		Swim	Swim	
	Bike (HILLS)		Bike (IRP)	DAY OFF		Bike (60% DIST) (IRP TT)
Run (E)		Run (70% DIST)			Run (IRP)	Run (E)

Week 2

M	T	W	T	F	S	S
Swim (E)		Swim (E)		DAY OFF	DAY OFF	I R O N M A N
	Bike (E)		TRANS (E)			
Run (E)		Run (30% DIST)				
			CARBO LOAD	────────────────────▶		GENTLE W/UP

Note: Friday is a legs day off. Remove the swim for a complete day off.

SPORT-SPECIFIC TRAINING USED FOR TRIATHLON

Type (intensity)	When initiated	Effect	Example	Race use
Power	—	—	—	—
Intensive sprints	—	—	—	—
Extensive sprints	—	—	—	—
Submaximal	Speed phase	Improves max steady state race pace	4–6 × 6–8 min 4–1 min rest btwn or 20–30 min TT	standard, sprint, Half-Iron
Up-tempo	Late base, early speed, speed	Transition from base to speedwork or long dist race pace – Ironman speedwork recovery rate	1–2 × 10–30 min rest 10–20 min btwn	standard, sprint, Half-Iron, Ironman
Long slow distance	Base/speed	Improves ability to do mileage, builds training tolerance and improves recovery rate	Continuous	All
Active recovery	Base/speed	Assists recovery (only if needed)	Continuous	All

Proportions:
1 Base – 100% long slow distance and active recovery; some speedwork may be used.
2 Speed – approx. 85–90% long slow distance and active recovery; approx. 10–15% up-tempo and submaximal intensity.

Changes in triathlon

Since the first edition of this book, many new triathlon events have emerged. Very short swim/bike/run races are now raced with up to three races on the same day. The order of disciplines has also changed. In many triathlons, drafting is now used in the cycle stage, making swimming and running training more important than cycle training if you don't have the necessary cycle racing skills. To cover all these variables would create too many diverse programmes, so I advise the following:

simulate race conditions and intensities. If the races are shorter and repeated in the same day, adjust your training to suit. Do higher intensity training (extensive and intensive sprints) and a little more speedwork, balanced by less volume. Simulate multiple races in your workouts (e.g. S/B/R/S/B/R). As far as drafting is concerned, reduce your cycling volumes by about 20–30 per cent, and increase running and swimming volumes by 10–20 per cent. Learn how to draft in the swim; learn the skills and tactics of cycle racing in a bunch, and learn how to run like hell!

Multiple coaches

For multiple discipline sports such as triathlon, having more than one coach can be very useful (particularly if each is a specialist in one of the disciplines). One problem, though, is coordinating the input of each coach into a structured and balanced programme. Often, each coach will emphasise his or her sport too much. This can lead to overtraining.

Try to set up your coaching so that the training for each discipline is complementary in terms of phasing, volume and intensity each week. Ensure each coach has the same goal!

Racing tips for triathlons

Ironman athletes are often regarded as the intellectuals of triathlon because the Ironman is as much a measure of an athlete's training and racing administration as it is a measure of athletic ability. Here are a few things to look out for.

Tidal patterns
Work out whether the tide is coming in or going out and if it is going to determine the best place to be on the start line for the swim. Being at the wrong end of the start line may mean you get pushed off course by the tide or that you have to swim against it slightly. Either way, it will be extra work you don't need! So, do your homework and use the tide to your advantage if at all possible.

Wind on the course
This has nothing to do with diet! In both the New Zealand and the Hawaii Ironman there is generally a tail wind over the first 40 km of the bike. Less experienced athletes often don't know this and they worry that they have started too fast or 'overstretched' themselves

and, consequently, slow down. They then turn around and 'grind' back into wind. This may result in a less than optimal bike time. Sponge more often when running with the wind as there is less evaporation and you tend to overheat more.

Fluid and energy replacement
Make sure you know what your fluid and energy requirements will be for the entire race. Devise a schedule and stick to it. Poor drinking/eating practices can destroy six months of excellent training no matter how well prepared you are physically. This cannot be emphasised enough for the Ironman – fluid and food must be consumed at the right time. For instance, when you come out of the water you will be slightly dehydrated after not taking on fluid for about an hour – swallowing sea water doesn't count! Rectify this as soon as you get on the bike.

Pace judgement
Pace judgement is critical in the Ironman. In the 1988 Hawaii Ironman the racing heart rates of many athletes were monitored. It was found the heart rates of the elite competitors fluctuated by 10 bpm or less for the entire journey. The heart rates of the lesser athletes, however, fluctuated a great deal more. The key to optimal performance is to maintain a steady pace (and HR) throughout the race.

Urinating during competition
Why do you never see top triathletes urinating? Think about it!

♦ Duathlon training ♦ programmes

Duathlons are run/bike or run/bike/run endurance time trial events. The duathlon (run 5 km/bike 20 km/run 5 km) weekly and 16-week programmes are based on chapter 7, no. 15 semi-competitive. The duathlon (run 10 km/bike 60 km/run 10 km) weekly and 16-week programmes are based on chapter 7, no. 19 elite.

BASE TRAINING

			Duathlon (run 5 km/bike 20 km/run 5 km) base programme			
M	T	W	T	F	S	S
Run 10 km 1 hr (26.3%) (LO)	Bike 40 km 1.5hr (25%) (LO)	Run 18 km 1.5 hr (47.4%) (LO)	Bike 40 km 1.5 hr (25%) (LO)	DAY OFF	Bike 20 km 45 min (12.5%) (LO) Run 8 km 50 min (21%) (LO)	Bike 60 km 2 hr (37.5%) (LO) (PLAN) Run 2 km 10 min (5.3%) (LO)

		Duathlon (run 10 km/bike 60 km/run 10 km) base programme				
M	T	W	T	F	S	S
Run 15 km 1.25 hr) (21.7%) (LO)	Bike 60 km 2 hr (18.7%) (LO) (HILLS)	Bike 30 km 1 hr (9.5%) (LO) (EASY) Run 25 km 2.25 hr (36.2%) (LO)	Bike 50 km 1.6 hr (15.6%) (LO) Run 6 km 40 min (8.7%) (LO)	DAY OFF	Bike 60 km 2 hr (18.7%) (LO) Run 20 km 1.5 hr) (29%) (LO) (HILLS)	Bike 120 km 4 hr (37.5%) (LO) Run 3 km 15 min (4.4%) (LO) (PLAN)

SPEED TRAINING

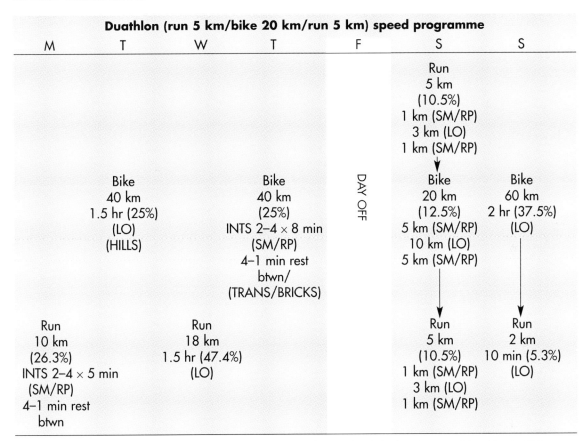

Duathlon (run 5 km/bike 20 km/run 5 km) speed programme

M	T	W	T	F	S	S
					Run 5 km (10.5%) 1 km (SM/RP) 3 km (LO) 1 km (SM/RP) ↓	
	Bike 40 km 1.5 hr (25%) (LO) (HILLS)		Bike 40 km (25%) INTS 2–4 × 8 min (SM/RP) 4–1 min rest btwn/ (TRANS/BRICKS)	DAY OFF	Bike 20 km (12.5%) 5 km (SM/RP) 10 km (LO) 5 km (SM/RP) ↓	Bike 60 km 2 hr (37.5%) (LO) ↓
Run 10 km (26.3%) INTS 2–4 × 5 min (SM/RP) 4–1 min rest btwn		Run 18 km 1.5 hr (47.4%) (LO)			Run 5 km (10.5%) 1 km (SM/RP) 3 km (LO) 1 km (SM/RP)	Run 2 km 10 min (5.3%) (LO)

Note: (TRANS/BRICKS) = transition training and bricks (1 min SM bike/racing transition/1 min SM run × 1–4 every 2nd week); INTS = e.g. 2–4 × 5 min (SM/RP) 4–1 min rest btwn = 2–4 repetitions of 5 minute intervals at submaximal or race pace intensity with light activity between. Rest periods progress from 4 minutes down to 1 minute. Remove Saturday's speed workout if speedwork is too much.

Duathlon (run 10 km/bike 60 km/run 10 km) speed programme

M	T	W	T	F	S	S
					Run 10 km (14.5%) 3 km (SM/RP) 4 km (LO) 3 km (SM/RP) ↓	
	Bike 60 km 2 hr (18.7%) (LO) (HILLS)	Bike 30 km 1 hr (9.5%) (LO)	Bike 50 km 1.6 hr (15.6%) INTS 4–6 × 8 min (SM/RP) 4–1 min rest btwn	DAY OFF	Bike 60 km 2 hr (18.7%) 5–10 km (SM/RP) 40–50 km (LO) 5–10 km (SM/RP) ↓	Bike 120 km 4 hr (37.5%) ↓
Run 15 km 1.25 hr (21.7%) INTS 4–6 × 5 min 4–1 min rest btwn		Run 25 km 2.25 hr (36.2%) (LO)	Run 6 km 40 min (8.7%) (LO)		Run 10 km 1.5 hr (14.5%) 3 km (SM/RP) 4 km (LO) 3 km (SM/RP)	Run 3 km (4.4%) (LO)

Note: (TRANS/BRICKS) = transition training and bricks (1 min SM bike/racing transition/1 min SM run × 1–4 every 2nd week); INTS = e.g. 2–4 × 5 min (SM/RP) 4–1 min rest btwn = 2–4 repetitions of 5 minute intervals at submaximal or race pace intensity with light activity between. Rest periods progress from 4 minutes down to 1 minute. Remove Saturday's speed workout if speedwork is too much.

Race: Duathlon 4 km/20/ km/4 km
Race date: 20 April
Training starts: 30 December

Maximum distance for the 100% week
Run: 38 km
Bike: 160 km

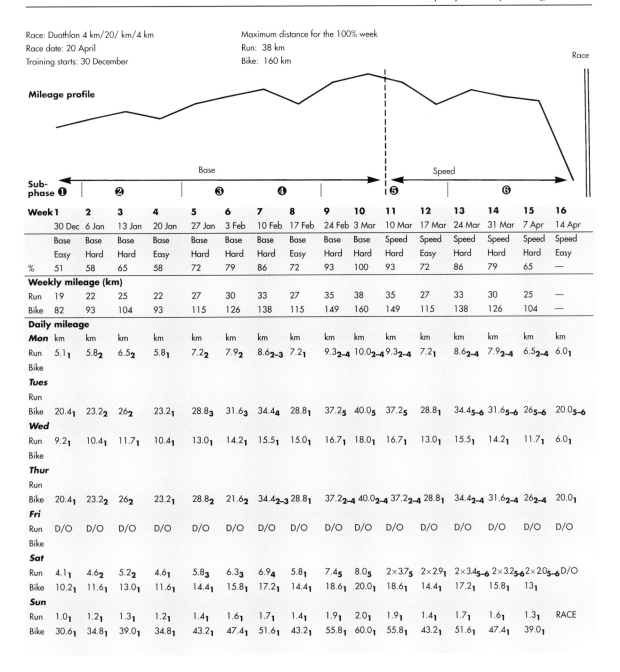

Mileage profile

Sub-phase	❶	❷		❸	❹		❺		❻		
				Base				Speed			

Week	1	2	3	4	5	6	7	8	9	10	11	12	13	14	15	16
	30 Dec	6 Jan	13 Jan	20 Jan	27 Jan	3 Feb	10 Feb	17 Feb	24 Feb	3 Mar	10 Mar	17 Mar	24 Mar	31 Mar	7 Apr	14 Apr
	Base	Base	Base	Base	Base	Base	Base	Base	Base	Base	Speed	Speed	Speed	Speed	Speed	Speed
	Easy	Hard	Hard	Easy	Hard	Hard	Hard	Easy	Hard	Hard	Hard	Easy	Hard	Hard	Hard	Easy
%	51	58	65	58	72	79	86	72	93	100	93	72	86	79	65	—
Weekly mileage (km)																
Run	19	22	25	22	27	30	33	27	35	38	35	27	33	30	25	—
Bike	82	93	104	93	115	126	138	115	149	160	149	115	138	126	104	—
Daily mileage																
Mon	km	km	km	km	km	km	km	km	km	km	km	km	km	km	km	km
Run	5.1_1	5.8_2	6.5_2	5.8_1	7.2_2	7.9_2	8.6_{2-3}	7.2_1	9.3_{2-4}	10.0_{2-4}	9.3_{2-4}	7.2_1	8.6_{2-4}	7.9_{2-4}	6.5_{2-4}	6.0_1
Bike																
Tues																
Run																
Bike	20.4_1	23.2_2	26_2	23.2_1	28.8_3	31.6_3	34.4_4	28.8_1	37.2_5	40.0_5	37.2_5	28.8_1	34.4_{5-6}	31.6_{5-6}	26_{5-6}	20.0_{5-6}
Wed																
Run	9.2_1	10.4_1	11.7_1	10.4_1	13.0_1	14.2_1	15.5_1	15.0_1	16.7_1	18.0_1	16.7_1	13.0_1	15.5_1	14.2_1	11.7_1	6.0_1
Bike																
Thur																
Run																
Bike	20.4_1	23.2_2	26_2	23.2_1	28.8_2	21.6_2	34.4_{2-3}	28.8_1	37.2_{2-4}	40.0_{2-4}	37.2_{2-4}	28.8_1	34.4_{2-4}	31.6_{2-4}	26_{2-4}	20.0_1
Fri																
Run	D/O	D/O	D/O	D/O	D/O	D/O	D/O	D/O	D/O	D/O	D/O	D/O	D/O	D/O	D/O	D/O
Bike																
Sat																
Run	4.1_1	4.6_2	5.2_2	4.6_1	5.8_3	6.3_3	6.9_4	5.8_1	7.4_5	8.0_5	$2\times3.7_5$	$2\times2.9_1$	$2\times3.4_{5-6}$	$2\times3.2_{5-6}$	$2\times2.0_{5-6}$	D/O
Bike	10.2_1	11.6_1	13.0_1	11.6_1	14.4_1	15.8_1	17.2_1	14.4_1	18.6_1	20.0_1	18.6_1	14.4_1	17.2_1	15.8_1	13_1	
Sun																
Run	1.0_1	1.2_1	1.3_1	1.2_1	1.4_1	1.6_1	1.7_1	1.4_1	1.9_1	2.0_1	1.9_1	1.4_1	1.7_1	1.6_1	1.3_1	RACE
Bike	30.6_1	34.8_1	39.0_1	34.8_1	43.2_1	47.4_1	51.6_1	43.2_1	55.8_1	60.0_1	55.8_1	43.2_1	51.6_1	47.4_1	39.0_1	

Race: Duathlon 10 km/60 km/10 km
Race date: 20 April
Training starts: 30 December

Maximum distance for the 100% week
Run: 69 km
Bike: 320 km

Race

Mileage profile

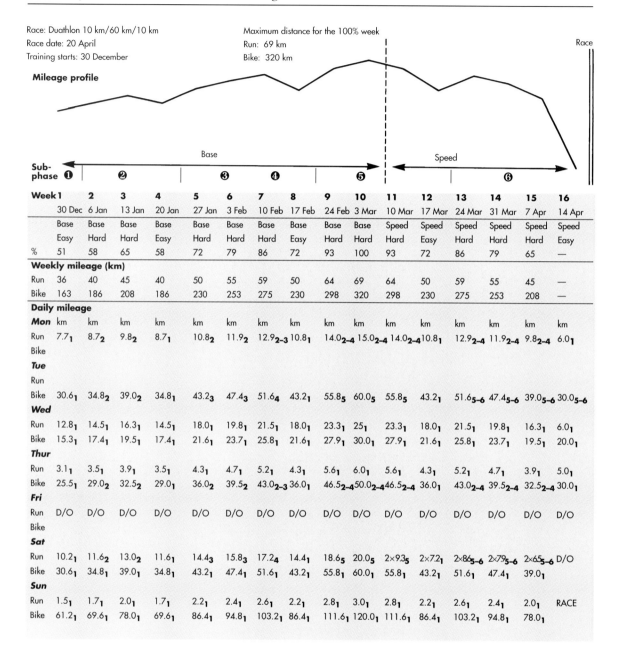

Sub-phase ❶ ❷ ❸ ❹ ❺ ❻ — Base / Speed

Week	1	2	3	4	5	6	7	8	9	10	11	12	13	14	15	16
	30 Dec	6 Jan	13 Jan	20 Jan	27 Jan	3 Feb	10 Feb	17 Feb	24 Feb	3 Mar	10 Mar	17 Mar	24 Mar	31 Mar	7 Apr	14 Apr
	Base Easy	Base Hard	Base Hard	Base Easy	Base Hard	Base Hard	Base Hard	Base Easy	Base Hard	Base Hard	Speed Hard	Speed Easy	Speed Hard	Speed Hard	Speed Hard	Speed Easy
%	51	58	65	58	72	79	86	72	93	100	93	72	86	79	65	—
Weekly mileage (km)																
Run	36	40	45	40	50	55	59	50	64	69	64	50	59	55	45	—
Bike	163	186	208	186	230	253	275	230	298	320	298	230	275	253	208	—
Daily mileage																
Mon	km	km	km	km	km	km	km	km	km	km	km	km	km	km	km	km
Run	7.7_1	8.7_2	9.8_2	8.7_1	10.8_2	11.9_2	12.9_{2-3}	10.8_1	14.0_{2-4}	15.0_{2-4}	14.0_{2-4}	10.8_1	12.9_{2-4}	11.9_{2-4}	9.8_{2-4}	6.0_1
Bike																
Tue																
Run																
Bike	30.6_1	34.8_2	39.0_2	34.8_1	43.2_3	47.4_3	51.6_4	43.2_1	55.8_5	60.0_5	55.8_5	43.2_1	51.6_{5-6}	47.4_{5-6}	39.0_{5-6}	30.0_{5-6}
Wed																
Run	12.8_1	14.5_1	16.3_1	14.5_1	18.0_1	19.8_1	21.5_1	18.0_1	23.3_1	25_1	23.3_1	18.0_1	21.5_1	19.8_1	16.3_1	6.0_1
Bike	15.3_1	17.4_1	19.5_1	17.4_1	21.6_1	23.7_1	25.8_1	21.6_1	27.9_1	30.0_1	27.9_1	21.6_1	25.8_1	23.7_1	19.5_1	20.0_1
Thur																
Run	3.1_1	3.5_1	3.9_1	3.5_1	4.3_1	4.7_1	5.2_1	4.3_1	5.6_1	6.0_1	5.6_1	4.3_1	5.2_1	4.7_1	3.9_1	5.0_1
Bike	25.5_1	29.0_2	32.5_2	29.0_1	36.0_2	39.5_2	43.0_{2-3}	36.0_1	46.5_{2-4}	50.0_{2-4}	46.5_{2-4}	36.0_1	43.0_{2-4}	39.5_{2-4}	32.5_{2-4}	30.0_1
Fri																
Run	D/O	D/O	D/O	D/O	D/O	D/O	D/O	D/O	D/O	D/O	D/O	D/O	D/O	D/O	D/O	D/O
Bike																
Sat																
Run	10.2_1	11.6_2	13.0_2	11.6_1	14.4_3	15.8_3	17.2_4	14.4_1	18.6_5	20.0_5	$2{\times}9.3_5$	$2{\times}7.2_1$	$2{\times}8.6_{5-6}$	$2{\times}7.9_{5-6}$	$2{\times}6.5_{5-6}$	D/O
Bike	30.6_1	34.8_1	39.0_1	34.8_1	43.2_1	47.4_1	51.6_1	43.2_1	55.8_1	60.0_1	55.8_1	43.2_1	51.6_1	47.4_1	39.0_1	
Sun																
Run	1.5_1	1.7_1	2.0_1	1.7_1	2.2_1	2.4_1	2.6_1	2.2_1	2.8_1	3.0_1	2.8_1	2.2_1	2.6_1	2.4_1	2.0_1	RACE
Bike	61.2_1	69.6_1	78.0_1	69.6_1	86.4_1	94.8_1	103.2_1	86.4_1	111.6_1	120.0_1	111.6_1	86.4_1	103.2_1	94.8_1	78.0_1	

TAPER AND PEAK

Duathlon low-priority taper

Week 1

M	T	W	T	F	S	S
	Bike (50% HILLS)	Bike* (E)	Bike (50% INTS)	Bike (E)	DAY OFF	R A C E
Run (INTS)		Run (66% LONG)		Run (E) (BRICKS)		W/UP–W/D

Week 2

M	T	W	T	F	S	S
DAY OFF	Bike (E)	Bike* (E) Run (LONG)	Bike (HILLS) Run (E)	DAY OFF	Run (E) Bike (E) Run (E)	Bike (LONG) Run (E)

Duathlon high-priority taper

M	T	W	T	F	S	S
	Bike (E)	Bike* (E)	Bike (E)	DAY OFF	DAY OFF	R A C E
Run (50% INTS		Run (BRICKS) (E)	Run (BRICKS) (E)			

Note: * = this workout can be dropped; BRICKS = 5 km bike (LO)/race transition/1 km run (LO).

SPORT-SPECIFIC TRAINING USED FOR DUATHLONS

Type (intensity)	When initiated	Effect	Example	Race use
Power	—	—	—	—
Intensive sprints	—	—	—	—
Extensive sprints	—	—	—	—
Submaximal	Speed phase	Improves max steady state race pace	4–6 × 6–8 min 4–1 min rest btwn or 20–30 min TT	Duathlon
Up-tempo	Late base, early speed,	Transition from base to speedwork	1–2 × 10–30 min rest 10–20 min btwn	Duathlon long dist duathlon (4 hrs +)
Long slow distance	Base/speed	Improves ability to do mileage, builds training tolerance and improves recovery rate	Continuous	All
Active recovery	Base/speed	Assists recovery (only if needed)	Continuous	All

Proportions:
1 Base – 100% long slow distance and active recovery; some speedwork may be used.
2 Speed – approx. 85–90% long slow distance and active recovery; approx. 10–15% up-tempo and submaximal intensity.

♦ Multisport training ♦ programmes

These programmes are designed for multi-sport events such as New Zealand's Coast to Coast and Mountains to Sea races.

Coast to Coast is a one- and two-day multisport (cycling, running and kayaking) race that spans the width of the South Island. Day 1 consists of 2.8 km run/58 km cycle/26 km mountain run; day 2 involves a 15 km cycle/67 km kayak/70 km cycle. The Longest Day race combines the two-day event to form a gruelling one-day race. The weekly and 16-week programmes are based on chapter 7, no. 21 elite.

Mountains to Sea is a three-day multisport (kayak/bike/run) event held in the central North Island of New Zealand. Day 1 involves a 23 km run, a 61 km cycle and a 35 km kayak; day 2 is a tough 87 km paddle, and day 3 is a 30 km run followed by a 54 km cycle. The weekly and 16-week programmes are based on chapter 7, no. 24 elite.

Do as many kayaks as possible in white-water river conditions close to the conditions you will race in. Time (min) is used for off-road running and for kayaking as it is difficult to measure kilometres in both cases.

BASE TRAINING

Coast to Coast race base programme						
M	T	W	T	F	S	S
Run 3 hr (51.4%) (LONG) (O/R) (LO)		Run 1.5 hr (25.7%) (LO)	Run* 20 min (5.7%) (LO) (SANDY)	DAY OFF	Run 1 hr (17.2%) (LO) (O/R)	
Bike* 30–40 km 1–1.5 hr (17%) (LO)	Bike 60 km 2 hr (24%) (LO)		Bike 80–100 km 3–4 hr (42%) (LO)(LONG)		Bike 30–40 km 1–1.5 hr (17%) (LO)(HILLS)	
	Kayak 1 hr (12.5%) (LO)	Kayak 2 hr (25%) (LO)			Kayak* 1 hr (12.5%) (LO)	Kayak 4 hr (50%) (LO)

*Note: * = these workouts can be removed for a three-discipline per workout per week programme.*

			Mountains to Sea race base programme				
M	T	W	T	F	S	S	
Run 3 hr (43%) (LONG) (O/R) (LO)		Run 1.5 hr (21.4%) (LO)	Run* 40 min–1 hr (14.2%) (LO)	DAY OFF	Run 1–2 hr (21.4%) (O/R) (LO)		
Bike* 30–40 km 1–1.5 hr (21%) (LO)	Bike 40 km 1.5 hr (21%) (LO)		Bike 60–80 km 2–3 hr (42%) (LO)(LONG)		Bike 20–30 km 0.6–1 hr (16%) (LO)(HILLS)		
	Kayak 1 hr (11%) (LO)	Kayak 2 hr (22%) (LO)			Kayak* 1 hr (11%) (LO)	Kayak 5 hr (56%) (LO)	

Note: Include a lot of downhill (long descents) running as your legs will have to be very used to this; * = these workouts can be removed for a three-discipline per workout per week programme.

SPEED TRAINING

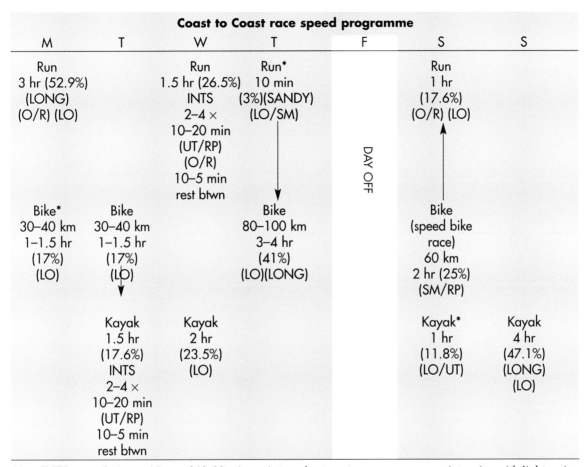

M	T	W	T	F	S	S
Coast to Coast race speed programme						
Run 3 hr (52.9%) (LONG) (O/R) (LO)		Run 1.5 hr (26.5%) INTS 2–4 × 10–20 min (UT/RP) (O/R) 10–5 min rest btwn	Run* 10 min (3%)(SANDY) (LO/SM)	DAY OFF	Run 1 hr (17.6%) (O/R) (LO)	
Bike* 30–40 km 1–1.5 hr (17%) (LO)	Bike 30–40 km 1–1.5 hr (17%) (LO)		Bike 80–100 km 3–4 hr (41%) (LO)(LONG)		Bike (speed bike race) 60 km 2 hr (25%) (SM/RP)	
	Kayak 1.5 hr (17.6%) INTS 2–4 × 10–20 min (UT/RP) 10–5 min rest btwn	Kayak 2 hr (23.5%) (LO)			Kayak* 1 hr (11.8%) (LO/UT)	Kayak 4 hr (47.1%) (LONG) (LO)

Note: INTS = e.g. 2–4 repetitions of 10–20 minute intervals at up-tempo or race pace intensity with light activity between. Rest periods progress from 10 minutes down to 5 minutes; * = workouts that can be dropped.

Mountain to Sea race speed programme

M	T	W	T	F	S	S
Run 3 hr (45%) (LONG) (O/R) (LO)		Run 1.5 hr (22.5%) (SPEED) 2–4 × 10–20 min (UT/RP) (O/R) 10–5 min rest btwn 1.5 hr (22.5%)	Run* 40 min (10%) (LO)	DAY OFF	Run 1.5 hr (22.5%) (O/R) (LO)	
Bike* 30–40 km 1–1.5 hr (21%) (LO)	Bike 30 km 1 hr (16%) (LO)		Bike 60 km 2 hr (42%) (LONG) (LO)		Bike 40 km 1.5 hr (21%) (SPEED) 2–4 × 10–20 min (UT/RP) 10–5 min rest btwn	
	Kayak 1.5 hr (15.8%) (SPEED) 2–4 × 10–20 min (UT/RP) 10–5 min rest btwn	Kayak 2 hr (15.8%) (LO)			Kayak* 1 hr (10.6%) (LO/UT)	Kayak 5 hr (52.6%) (LONG) (LO)

Note: INTS = e.g. 2–4 repetitions of 10–20 minute intervals at up-tempo or race pace intensity with light activity between. Rest periods progress from 10 minutes down to 5 minutes; * = workouts that can be dropped.

Race: Coast to Coast
Day 1: 2.8 km run/58 km cycle/26 km mountain run
Day 2: 15 km cycle/67 km kayak/70 km cycle
Race date: 20 April
Training starts: 30 December

Maximum distance for the 100% week
Cycle: 240 km
Run: 350 min
Kayak: 480 min

Race

Mileage profile

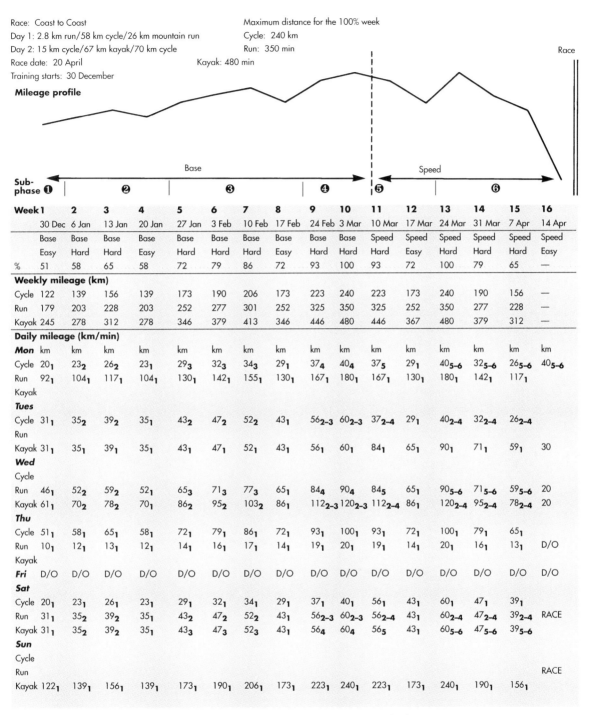

Sub-phase	❶		❷		❸			❹			❺			❻		
	Base										Speed					
Week	1	2	3	4	5	6	7	8	9	10	11	12	13	14	15	16
	30 Dec	6 Jan	13 Jan	20 Jan	27 Jan	3 Feb	10 Feb	17 Feb	24 Feb	3 Mar	10 Mar	17 Mar	24 Mar	31 Mar	7 Apr	14 Apr
	Base	Base	Base	Base	Base	Base	Base	Base	Base	Base	Speed	Speed	Speed	Speed	Speed	Speed
	Easy	Hard	Hard	Easy	Hard	Hard	Hard	Easy	Hard	Hard	Hard	Easy	Hard	Hard	Hard	Easy
%	51	58	65	58	72	79	86	72	93	100	93	72	100	79	65	—
Weekly mileage (km)																
Cycle	122	139	156	139	173	190	206	173	223	240	223	173	240	190	156	—
Run	179	203	228	203	252	277	301	252	325	350	325	252	350	277	228	—
Kayak	245	278	312	278	346	379	413	346	446	480	446	367	480	379	312	—
Daily mileage (km/min)																
Mon	km	km	km	km	km	km	km	km	km	km	km	km	km	km	km	km
Cycle	20_1	23_2	26_2	23_1	29_3	32_3	34_3	29_1	37_4	40_4	37_5	29_1	$40_{5\text{-}6}$	$32_{5\text{-}6}$	$26_{5\text{-}6}$	$40_{5\text{-}6}$
Run	92_1	104_1	117_1	104_1	130_1	142_1	155_1	130_1	167_1	180_1	167_1	130_1	180_1	142_1	117_1	
Kayak																
Tues																
Cycle	31_1	35_2	39_2	35_1	43_2	47_2	52_2	43_1	$56_{2\text{-}3}$	$60_{2\text{-}3}$	$37_{2\text{-}4}$	29_1	$40_{2\text{-}4}$	$32_{2\text{-}4}$	$26_{2\text{-}4}$	
Run																
Kayak	31_1	35_1	39_1	35_1	43_1	47_1	52_1	43_1	56_1	60_1	84_1	65_1	90_1	71_1	59_1	30
Wed																
Cycle																
Run	46_1	52_2	59_2	52_1	65_3	71_3	77_3	65_1	84_4	90_4	84_5	65_1	$90_{5\text{-}6}$	$71_{5\text{-}6}$	$59_{5\text{-}6}$	20
Kayak	61_1	70_2	78_2	70_1	86_2	95_2	103_2	86_1	$112_{2\text{-}3}$	$120_{2\text{-}3}$	$112_{2\text{-}4}$	86_1	$120_{2\text{-}4}$	$95_{2\text{-}4}$	$78_{2\text{-}4}$	20
Thu																
Cycle	51_1	58_1	65_1	58_1	72_1	79_1	86_1	72_1	93_1	100_1	93_1	72_1	100_1	79_1	65_1	D/O
Run	10_1	12_1	13_1	12_1	14_1	16_1	17_1	14_1	19_1	20_1	19_1	14_1	20_1	16_1	13_1	D/O
Kayak																
Fri	D/O	D/O	D/O	D/O	D/O	D/O	D/O	D/O	D/O	D/O	D/O	D/O	D/O	D/O	D/O	D/O
Sat																
Cycle	20_1	23_1	26_1	23_1	29_1	32_1	34_1	29_1	37_1	40_1	56_1	43_1	60_1	47_1	39_1	
Run	31_1	35_2	39_2	35_1	43_2	47_2	52_2	43_1	$56_{2\text{-}3}$	$60_{2\text{-}3}$	$56_{2\text{-}4}$	43_1	$60_{2\text{-}4}$	$47_{2\text{-}4}$	$39_{2\text{-}4}$	RACE
Kayak	31_1	35_2	39_2	35_1	43_3	47_3	52_3	43_1	56_4	60_4	56_5	43_1	$60_{5\text{-}6}$	$47_{5\text{-}6}$	$39_{5\text{-}6}$	
Sun																
Cycle																
Run																RACE
Kayak	122_1	139_1	156_1	139_1	173_1	190_1	206_1	173_1	223_1	240_1	223_1	173_1	240_1	190_1	156_1	

Note: Base 1 would occur first. Cycle volumes are displayed in kilometres; kayak and running volumes are in minutes.

Race: Mountains to Sea
Day 1: 23 km run/61 km cycle/35 km kayak
Day 2: 87 km kayak
Day 3: 30 km run/54 km cycle
Race date: 20 April
Training starts: 30 December

Mileage profile

Maximum distance for the 100% week
Cycle: 190 km
Run: 420 min
Kayak: 540 min

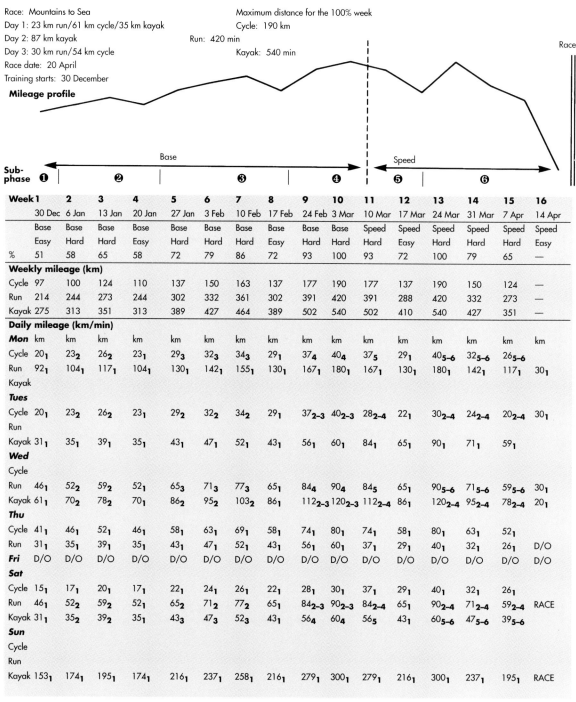

Sub-phase ❶ ❷ ❸ ❹ ❺ ❻ — Base phase (weeks 1–10), Speed phase (weeks 11–16)

Week	1	2	3	4	5	6	7	8	9	10	11	12	13	14	15	16
	30 Dec	6 Jan	13 Jan	20 Jan	27 Jan	3 Feb	10 Feb	17 Feb	24 Feb	3 Mar	10 Mar	17 Mar	24 Mar	31 Mar	7 Apr	14 Apr
	Base	Base	Base	Base	Base	Base	Base	Base	Base	Base	Speed	Speed	Speed	Speed	Speed	Speed
	Easy	Hard	Hard	Easy	Hard	Hard	Hard	Easy	Hard	Hard	Hard	Easy	Hard	Hard	Hard	Easy
%	51	58	65	58	72	79	86	72	93	100	93	72	100	79	65	—
Weekly mileage (km)																
Cycle	97	100	124	110	137	150	163	137	177	190	177	137	190	150	124	—
Run	214	244	273	244	302	332	361	302	391	420	391	288	420	332	273	—
Kayak	275	313	351	313	389	427	464	389	502	540	502	410	540	427	351	—

Daily mileage (km/min)

	1	2	3	4	5	6	7	8	9	10	11	12	13	14	15	16
Mon km	km	km	km	km	km	km	km	km	km	km	km	km	km	km	km
Cycle	20_1	23_2	26_2	23_1	29_3	32_3	34_3	29_1	37_4	40_4	37_5	29_1	$40_{5\text{-}6}$	$32_{5\text{-}6}$	$26_{5\text{-}6}$	
Run	92_1	104_1	117_1	104_1	130_1	142_1	155_1	130_1	167_1	180_1	167_1	130_1	180_1	142_1	117_1	30_1
Kayak																
Tues																
Cycle	20_1	23_2	26_2	23_1	29_2	32_2	34_2	29_1	$37_{2\text{-}3}$	$40_{2\text{-}3}$	$28_{2\text{-}4}$	22_1	$30_{2\text{-}4}$	$24_{2\text{-}4}$	$20_{2\text{-}4}$	30_1
Run																
Kayak	31_1	35_1	39_1	35_1	43_1	47_1	52_1	43_1	56_1	60_1	84_1	65_1	90_1	71_1	59_1	
Wed																
Cycle																
Run	46_1	52_2	59_2	52_1	65_3	71_3	77_3	65_1	84_4	90_4	84_5	65_1	$90_{5\text{-}6}$	$71_{5\text{-}6}$	$59_{5\text{-}6}$	30_1
Kayak	61_1	70_2	78_2	70_1	86_2	95_2	103_2	86_1	$112_{2\text{-}3}$	$120_{2\text{-}3}$	$112_{2\text{-}4}$	86_1	$120_{2\text{-}4}$	$95_{2\text{-}4}$	$78_{2\text{-}4}$	20_1
Thu																
Cycle	41_1	46_1	52_1	46_1	58_1	63_1	69_1	58_1	74_1	80_1	74_1	58_1	80_1	63_1	52_1	
Run	31_1	35_1	39_1	35_1	43_1	47_1	52_1	43_1	56_1	60_1	37_1	29_1	40_1	32_1	26_1	D/O
Fri	D/O	D/O	D/O	D/O	D/O	D/O	D/O	D/O	D/O	D/O	D/O	D/O	D/O	D/O	D/O	D/O
Sat																
Cycle	15_1	17_1	20_1	17_1	22_1	24_1	26_1	22_1	28_1	30_1	37_1	29_1	40_1	32_1	26_1	
Run	46_1	52_2	59_2	52_1	65_2	71_2	77_2	65_1	$84_{2\text{-}3}$	$90_{2\text{-}3}$	$84_{2\text{-}4}$	65_1	$90_{2\text{-}4}$	$71_{2\text{-}4}$	$59_{2\text{-}4}$	RACE
Kayak	31_1	35_2	39_2	35_1	43_3	47_3	52_3	43_1	56_4	60_4	56_5	43_1	$60_{5\text{-}6}$	$47_{5\text{-}6}$	$39_{5\text{-}6}$	
Sun																
Cycle																
Run																
Kayak	153_1	174_1	195_1	174_1	216_1	237_1	258_1	216_1	279_1	300_1	279_1	216_1	300_1	237_1	195_1	RACE

Note: Base 1 would occur first. Cycle volumes are displayed in kilometres; kayak and running volumes are in minutes.

TAPER AND PEAK

Multisport taper

Week 1

M	T	W	T	F	S	S
Run (50% DIST) Bike (E)	Bike (E) Kayak (INTS)	Run (INTS) Kayak (E)	Run (E) Bike (50% DIST)	DAY OFF	Run (E) Bike (E) Kayak (E)	Kayak (50% DIST)

Week 2

M	T	W	T	F	S	S	M
Run (E) Bike (E)	TRANS (E)	Run (E) Kayak (E) CARBO LOAD	DAY OFF	DAY OFF	RACE	RACE	RACE

ADDITIONAL SPEED TRAINING

During the speed phase, do several race format simulations (up-tempo weeks) on a weekend. This means getting the body used to racing over several days. For example:

Coast to Coast
    Sat: Run, bike, run;
    Sun: Bike, kayak, bike. If you are doing the one day event, do all on the same day.

Mountain to Sea
    Sat: Run, cycle, kayak;
    Sun: Kayak;
    Mon: Run, cycle

It is not necessary to do full distances in your simulation.

Up-tempo weeks, Coast to Coast

Week 1

M	T	W	T	F	S	S
Run (66% DIST) Bike (E)	Bike (E) Kayak (INTS)	Run (INTS) Kayak (E)	Run (E) Bike (50% DIST)	DAY OFF	Run (UT) Bike (UT) Run (UT)	Run (UT) Kayak (UT) Bike (UT)

Week 2

M	T	W	T	F	S	S
DAY OFF	Bike (E) Kayak (E)	Run (E) Kayak (E)	Run (E) Bike (66% DIST)	DAY OFF	Run (E) Bike (INTS) Kayak (E)	Kayak (LONG)

Up-tempo weeks, Mountain to Sea

Week 1

M	T	W	T	F	S	S
Run (66% DIST) Bike (E)	Bike (E) Kayak (INTS)	Run (INTS) Kayak (E)	Run (E) Bike (50% DIST)	DAY OFF	Run (UT) Bike (UT) Kayak (UT)	Kayak (UT)

Week 2

M	T	W	T	F	S	S
Run (UT) Bike (UT)	DAY OFF	Run (E) Kayak (E)	Run (E) Bike (66% DIST)	DAY OFF	Run (E) Bike (INTS) Kayak (E)	Kayak (LONG)

SPORT-SPECIFIC TRAINING USED FOR MULTISPORT EVENTS

Type (intensity)	When initiated	Effect	Example	Race use
Power	—	—	—	—
Intensive sprints	—	—	—	—
Extensive sprints	Late speed phase	Improves extended sprint	4–6 × 1–3 m rest to recovery bike race, initial run	Coast to Coast bike ride initial run
Submaximal	Speed phase	Improves max steady state race pace	4–6 × 6–8 m 4–1 min rest btwn or 20–30 min TT.	All (small amount if in 4 hr+ races)
Up-tempo	Late base, early speed	Transition from base to speedwork	1–2 × 10–30 min rest 10–20 min btwn	All
Long slow distance	Base/speed	Improves ability to do mileage, builds training tolerance and improves recovery rate	Continuous	All
Active recovery	Base/speed	Assists recovery (only if needed)	Continuous	All

Proportions:
1 Base – 100% long slow distance and active recovery; some speedwork may be used.
2 Speed – approx. 85–90% long slow distance and active recovery; approx. 10–15% up-tempo and submaximal intensity.

♦ Rowing training ♦ programmes

BASE TRAINING

Start with minimal (between one and three) weekly workouts and progress to four to six workouts per week. Base 1 and Base 2 are each split into two parts to allow a gradual increase in workouts and rowing from land-based training to 'on the water' training.

Off-season rowing programme (2000-metre distance); sculling one to three times per week

	Training type	Training intensity	% of total week	Hard/easy day
Base 1A				
Mon	Row Tech	LO	31.5%	H
	Strength (gradual build-up) + Flex			
Tue	Day off			E
Wed	Strength (gradual build-up) + Flex			H
Thur	Row Tech (land training after)	LO	31.5%	H
Fri	Day off			E
Sat	Long row Tech	LO	37%	H
Sun	Day off			E
Base 1B				
Mon	Day off			E
Tues	Strength + Ergometer + Flex	LO	14%	H
Wed	Med row Tech	LO	22%	E
Thurs	Strength + Ergometer + Flex	LO	14%	H
Fri	Day off			E
Sat	Long row Tech + Flex	LO	25%	H
Sun	Long row Tech + Flex	LO	25%	H
Base 2A				
Mon	Row tech + Flex	LO	15%	E
Tues	Row Mod/Tech + muscle endurance (gym) + Flex	LO	15%	H
Wed	Row Tech + Flex	LO	15%	E
Thurs	Row Mod/Tech + muscle endurance (gym) + Flex	LO	15%	H
Fri	Day off			
Sat	Long row Tech + Flex	LO	23%	H
Sun	Row Mod/Tech + muscle endurance (gym) + Flex	LO	17%	H
Base 2B				
Mon	Row Tech + Flex	LO	12%	E
Tues	Row med/long + Flex (some up-tempo if no race Sat/Sun)	LO/SM	17%	H
Wed	Row Tech + Flex	LO	12%	E
Thurs	Row med/long + Flex	LO	17%	H
Fri	Day off			E
Sat	Long row or early season race + Flex	LO/SM/HI	23%	H
Sun	Long row Tech + Flex	LO	19%	H

SPEED TRAINING

Rowing (2000-metre distance) speed programme

	Training type	Training intensity	% of total week	Hard/easy day
Mon	Row Tech + Flex Aim: recovery, Tech	LO	13%	E
Tues	Intervals 4–7 × 1 min Rest 2 min–30 sec btwn Then 2–6 × 2 min + 2–4 × 4–5 min 2 min–30 sec rest btwn Aim: increase AT + Flex	LO/SM/HI	18%	H
Wed	Intervals 1–2 × 250–500 m, 2–4 × 250–1000 m, Rest to recovery. Between race pace, race rating + Flex. Aim: race pace	LO/SM/HI	16%	H
Thur	Row Tech (starts) + Flex Aim: Tech, starts	Mainly LO	16%	E
Fri	Day off			E
Sat	Race + Flex Aim: race pace	LO/SM/HI	18%	H
Sun	Long row Tech + Flex	LO	22%	H

Race: Rowing coxed 4 (2000 m)
Race date: 20 April
Training starts: 30 December

Maximum hours for the 100% week
Row: 5 hr 50 min

Race

Mileage profile

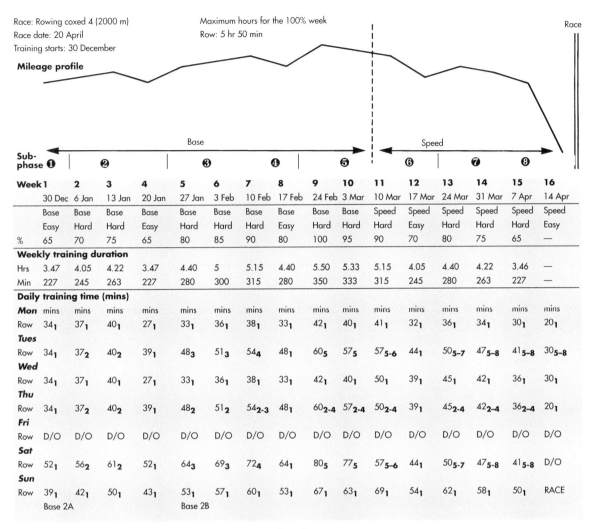

Sub-phase	❶		❷		❸		❹		❺		❻		❼		❽	

Base (phases ❶–❺) — Speed (phases ❻–❽)

Week	1	2	3	4	5	6	7	8	9	10	11	12	13	14	15	16
	30 Dec	6 Jan	13 Jan	20 Jan	27 Jan	3 Feb	10 Feb	17 Feb	24 Feb	3 Mar	10 Mar	17 Mar	24 Mar	31 Mar	7 Apr	14 Apr
	Base	Base	Base	Base	Base	Base	Base	Base	Base	Base	Speed	Speed	Speed	Speed	Speed	Speed
	Easy	Hard	Hard	Easy	Hard	Hard	Hard	Easy	Hard	Hard	Hard	Easy	Hard	Hard	Hard	Easy
%	65	70	75	65	80	85	90	80	100	95	90	70	80	75	65	—
Weekly training duration																
Hrs	3.47	4.05	4.22	3.47	4.40	5	5.15	4.40	5.50	5.33	5.15	4.05	4.40	4.22	3.46	—
Min	227	245	263	227	280	300	315	280	350	333	315	245	280	263	227	—
Daily training time (mins)																
Mon	mins	mins	mins	mins	mins	mins	mins	mins	mins	mins	mins	mins	mins	mins	mins	mins
Row	34_1	37_1	40_1	27_1	33_1	36_1	38_1	33_1	42_1	40_1	41_1	32_1	36_1	34_1	30_1	20_1
Tues																
Row	34_1	37_2	40_2	39_1	48_3	51_3	54_4	48_1	60_5	57_5	57_{5-6}	44_1	50_{5-7}	47_{5-8}	41_{5-8}	30_{5-8}
Wed																
Row	34_1	37_1	40_1	27_1	33_1	36_1	38_1	33_1	42_1	40_1	50_1	39_1	45_1	42_1	36_1	30_1
Thu																
Row	34_1	37_2	40_2	39_1	48_2	51_2	54_{2-3}	48_1	60_{2-4}	57_{2-4}	50_{2-4}	39_1	45_{2-4}	42_{2-4}	36_{2-4}	20_1
Fri																
Row	D/O	D/O	D/O	D/O	D/O	D/O	D/O	D/O	D/O	D/O	D/O	D/O	D/O	D/O	D/O	D/O
Sat																
Row	52_1	56_2	61_2	52_1	64_3	69_3	72_4	64_1	80_5	77_5	57_{5-6}	44_1	50_{5-7}	47_{5-8}	41_{5-8}	D/O
Sun																
Row	39_1	42_1	50_1	43_1	53_1	57_1	60_1	53_1	67_1	63_1	69_1	54_1	62_1	58_1	50_1	RACE
	Base 2A				Base 2B											

Note: times given are actual rowing times, not training times Base 1A and Base 1B would occur first.

Race: Rowing coxed 4 (2000 m)
Race date: 20 April
Training starts: 30 December

Maximum distance for the 100% week
Row: 100 km

Race

Mileage profile

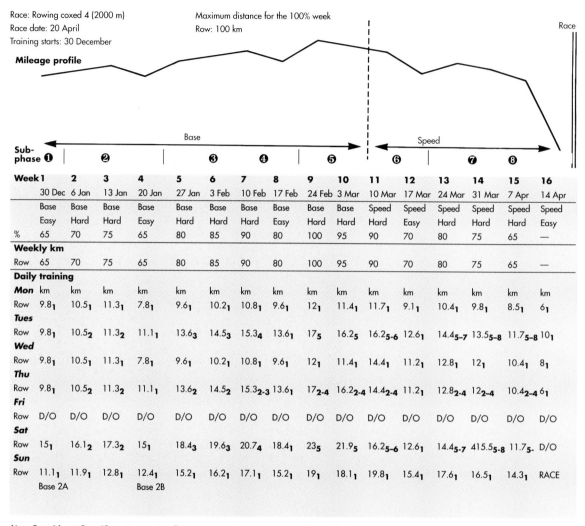

Sub-phase: ❶ ❷ ❸ ❹ ❺ | ❻ ❼ ❽ — Base (phases ❶–❺) / Speed (phases ❻–❽)

	1	2	3	4	5	6	7	8	9	10	11	12	13	14	15	16
Week	1	2	3	4	5	6	7	8	9	10	11	12	13	14	15	16
	30 Dec	6 Jan	13 Jan	20 Jan	27 Jan	3 Feb	10 Feb	17 Feb	24 Feb	3 Mar	10 Mar	17 Mar	24 Mar	31 Mar	7 Apr	14 Apr
	Base	Base	Base	Base	Base	Base	Base	Base	Base	Base	Speed	Speed	Speed	Speed	Speed	Speed
	Easy	Hard	Hard	Easy	Hard	Hard	Hard	Easy	Hard	Hard	Hard	Easy	Hard	Hard	Hard	Easy
%	65	70	75	65	80	85	90	80	100	95	90	70	80	75	65	—
Weekly km																
Row	65	70	75	65	80	85	90	80	100	95	90	70	80	75	65	—
Daily training																
Mon km	km	km	km	km	km	km	km	km	km	km	km	km	km	km	km	km
Row	9.8_1	10.5_1	11.3_1	7.8_1	9.6_1	10.2_1	10.8_1	9.6_1	12_1	11.4_1	11.7_1	9.1_1	10.4_1	9.8_1	8.5_1	6_1
Tues Row	9.8_1	10.5_2	11.3_2	11.1_1	13.6_3	14.5_3	15.3_4	13.6_1	17_5	16.2_5	16.2_{5-6}	12.6_1	14.4_{5-7}	13.5_{5-8}	11.7_{5-8}	10_1
Wed Row	9.8_1	10.5_1	11.3_1	7.8_1	9.6_1	10.2_1	10.8_1	9.6_1	12_1	11.4_1	14.4_1	11.2_1	12.8_1	12_1	10.4_1	8_1
Thu Row	9.8_1	10.5_2	11.3_2	11.1_1	13.6_2	14.5_2	15.3_{2-3}	13.6_1	17_{2-4}	16.2_{2-4}	14.4_{2-4}	11.2_1	12.8_{2-4}	12_{2-4}	10.4_{2-4}	6_1
Fri Row	D/O	D/O	D/O	D/O	D/O	D/O	D/O	D/O	D/O	D/O	D/O	D/O	D/O	D/O	D/O	D/O
Sat Row	15_1	16.1_2	17.3_2	15_1	18.4_3	19.6_3	20.7_4	18.4_1	23_5	21.9_5	16.2_{5-6}	12.6_1	14.4_{5-7}	415.5_{5-8}	11.7_{5-}	D/O
Sun Row	11.1_1	11.9_1	12.8_1	12.4_1	15.2_1	16.2_1	17.1_1	15.2_1	19_1	18.1_1	19.8_1	15.4_1	17.6_1	16.5_1	14.3_1	RACE
	Base 2A			Base 2B												

Note: Base 1A and Base 1B would occur first. This programme is based on chapter 7, no. 45 elite.

TAPER AND PEAK

Rowing (2000-metre distance) low-priority taper (and following training week)

Week 1

M	T	W	T	F	S	S
Tech	66% INTS	50% INTS	Tech	DAY OFF	RACE	50% LONG or D/O
E	H	H	E		H	H/E

Week 2

M	T	W	T	F	S	S
Tech	Tech or 66% INTS	Tech or INTS	Tech	DAY OFF	LONG	LONG
E	H/E	H/E	E		H	H
	(E if racing next Sat)					

Rowing (2000-metre distance) high-priority taper

Week 1

M	T	W	T	F	S	S
Tech	INTS	66% INTS	Tech starts	Tech	DAY OFF	DAY OFF
E	H	H	E	E		

Week 2

M	T	W	T	F	S	S
2 × race (HEAT)	1 × race (Heat)	2 × race (SEMI)	DAY OFF	race (FINAL)	race (FINAL)	DAY OFF
	CARBO LOAD					
Recovery very important						

217

SPORT-SPECIFIC TRAINING USED FOR ROWING

Type (intensity)	When initiated	Effect	Example
Power	Late speed phase	Faster, more powerful stroke	Starts, rest to recovery
Intensive sprints	Late speed phase	Improves starts and finishes	Extended start, 20–30 strokes
Extensive sprints	Speed phase	Improves extended starts and finishes	4–6×1–3 m rest to recovery
Submaximal	Early speed phase	Improves max steady state race pace	4–6×6–8 m 4–1 min rest btwn
Up-tempo	Late base, early speed	Transition from base to speedwork	20–40 min pieces, rest to recovery btwn
Long slow distance	Base/speed	Improves ability to do mileage, builds training tolerance and improves recovery rate	Continuous
Active	Base/speed	Assists recovery	Continuous

Proportions:
1 Base – 100% long slow distance and active recovery; some speedwork may be used.
2 Speed – approx. 85–90% long slow distance and active recovery; approx. 10–15% submaximal intensity and higher intensities. Training to allow peak performance in the rowing race.

Training notes for rowing

Land-based training for rowing

Starting with full 'on the water' rowing training at the beginning of the season may not be effective in terms of the overall programme. Too much rowing may negatively affect rowing technique as you are likely to tire quickly early in the season and lose form. Therefore, the aim might be to start with a lot of land training and limited rowing training which, at this point in the season, will emphasise technique. (Land training should always follow rowing training so as not to affect technique.)

The technique work at this time is important as technique established in the early part of the season sets the technical rowing ability for the remainder of the season. With a lot of early season land training and limited rowing training you will gain cardiovascular and muscular benefit without causing a deterioration in rowing technique. The rowing training itself, which is technical in early season, will enhance rowing performance later on. This also fits in quite well with the philosophy of doing base training first.

As you become fitter, more 'on the water' training occurs, with a gradual reduction in land-based training. Finally, towards the end of base most, if not all, training is done 'on the water'. This allows a gradual progression to full rowing training without sacrificing technique.

Technique vs duration and intensity

In all sports with a technical component the ability to perform the given task required by the sport in a precise manner is crucial. Technique should not be sacrificed through tiredness or too much intensity or duration. It is commonly accepted that technique begins to deteriorate as you tire. Therefore, intensity/duration training must be carried out with minimum effect on technique. Strategies for this are:

1 Technique in target sport training followed by 'like sport' training: Technique is performed in the target or specific sport first, followed by extra training in the 'like sport' to boost muscular and cardiovascular fitness without compromising the technique in the target sport. Start with minimal target sport training and mostly 'like sport' training, progressing as you become fitter and better able to maintain technique for longer, to almost all target sport training and minimal 'like sport' training.

Always train in the target sport first, concentrating on technique while still 'fresh', then follow this with 'like sport' training. 'Like sports' useful for rowing training are a rowing ergometer and rowing-specific land-based gym exercises.

2 Split workouts: Training workouts are split up over a day, instead of doing one single long workout where technique may be affected by fatigue in the later stages. The athlete splits training into shorter workouts in the morning and evening, with a recovery period in between. This allows the athlete to be 'fresher' during training, so that correct technique can be maintained.

Rowing in small boats at the beginning of the season

Using smaller boats at the beginning of the season (e.g. race in a coxless four but train in a pair) can be a very good way of improving technique – rowing the smaller boats is obviously a lot less forgiving on bad rowing technique. Later in the season the key is to begin to train the full crew in the type of boat (e.g. coxless four) in which they will race. At this point the coach can begin to mould the crew together to row as one unit.

◆ Road cycling training ◆ programmes

BASE TRAINING

Start base training with a minimal number of workouts (between one and three per week), and progress up to full workouts (five to ten a week).

Road cycling base programme (160 km)

		Training intensity	% of weekly mileage	Hard/easy
Base 1 (total distance for week 210–385 km)				
Mon	Day off			E
Tues	2–3 weeks easy, gradually introduce hills	LO	21.5%	H
Wed	Day off			E
Thurs	Easy Spin/Tech (45–90 km);	LO	21.5%	H
Fri	Day off			E
Sat	Easy medium distance (50–80 km); gym training if needed	LO	18.5%	H
Sun	Long cycle (70–135)	LO	32.5%	H
Base 2 (total distance for week 350–700 km)				
Mon	Easy cycle (40–80 km)	LO	9%	E
Tues	Hills (60–120 km)	LO	17%	H
Wed	Easy cycle (40–80 km)	LO	9%	E
Thurs	Hills (60–120 km)	LO	17%	H
Fri	Day off			E
Sat	Up-tempo, medium distance or early season race (50–100 km)	LO/SM/HI	14%	H
Sun	Long cycle (100–200 km)	LO	28%	H

SPEED TRAINING

Road cycling speed programme (160 km)

		Training intensity	% of weekly mileage	Hard/easy
Speed (total distance for week 595–630 km)				
Mon	Easy/Hills (50–55 km)	LO	9%	E
Tues	Time trial or intervals 4–6 × 6–8 min (SM) (110–120 km); rest 4–1 mins between. All terrain. Later add motorpacing for leg speed. Start long up-tempo ints then increase intensity to SM. Short ints to long ints. Can finish with some up-tempo continuous training	LO/SM	17%	H
Wed	Easy ride, finish with sprints 2–10 × 1–2 min (HI). Random recovery (110–120 km). Progress to shorter rest periods. Last weeks = power + power climbs	LO/HI	17%	H
Thurs	Easy cycle; finish with spinning sprints downhill (50–55 km)	LO	9%	E
Fri	Day off			E
Sat	Race or up-tempo. Long intervals. If race long w/up 30 min; w/down 30 min (90–95 km)	LO/SM/HI	14%	H
Sun	Long cycle (180–190 km)	LO	28%	H

Race: Cycle (40 km) Maximum distance for the 100% week
Race date: 20 April   Cycle: 160 km
Training starts: 30 December

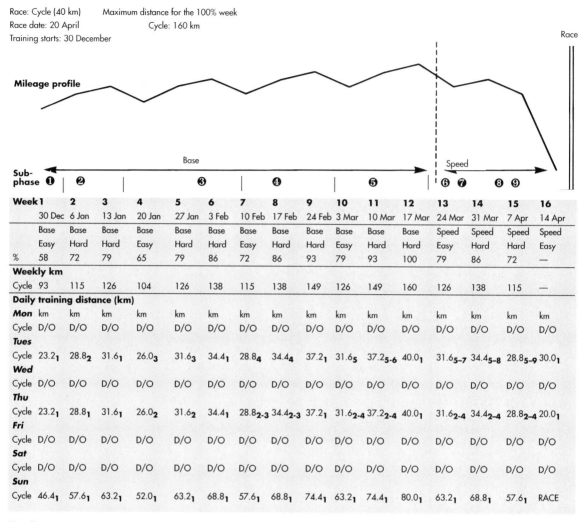

Mileage profile

Base — Speed — Race

Sub-phase	❶	❷			❸		❹		❺		❻ ❼	❽ ❾

Week	1	2	3	4	5	6	7	8	9	10	11	12	13	14	15	16
	30 Dec	6 Jan	13 Jan	20 Jan	27 Jan	3 Feb	10 Feb	17 Feb	24 Feb	3 Mar	10 Mar	17 Mar	24 Mar	31 Mar	7 Apr	14 Apr
	Base	Base	Base	Base	Base	Base	Base	Base	Base	Base	Base	Base	Speed	Speed	Speed	Speed
	Easy	Hard	Hard	Easy	Hard	Hard	Easy	Hard	Hard	Easy	Hard	Hard	Easy	Hard	Hard	Easy
%	58	72	79	65	79	86	72	86	93	79	93	100	79	86	72	—
Weekly km																
Cycle	93	115	126	104	126	138	115	138	149	126	149	160	126	138	115	—

Daily training distance (km)

	Week 1	2	3	4	5	6	7	8	9	10	11	12	13	14	15	16
Mon km	km	km	km	km	km	km	km	km	km	km	km	km	km	km	km
Cycle	D/O	D/O	D/O	D/O	D/O	D/O	D/O	D/O	D/O	D/O	D/O	D/O	D/O	D/O	D/O	D/O
Tues																
Cycle	23.2_1	28.8_2	31.6_1	26.0_3	31.6_3	34.4_1	28.8_4	34.4_4	37.2_1	31.6_5	$37.2_{5\text{-}6}$	40.0_1	$31.6_{5\text{-}7}$	$34.4_{5\text{-}8}$	$28.8_{5\text{-}9}$	30.0_1
Wed																
Cycle	D/O	D/O	D/O	D/O	D/O	D/O	D/O	D/O	D/O	D/O	D/O	D/O	D/O	D/O	D/O	D/O
Thu																
Cycle	23.2_1	28.8_1	31.6_1	26.0_2	31.6_2	34.4_1	$28.8_{2\text{-}3}$	$34.4_{2\text{-}3}$	37.2_1	$31.6_{2\text{-}4}$	$37.2_{2\text{-}4}$	40.0_1	$31.6_{2\text{-}4}$	$34.4_{2\text{-}4}$	$28.8_{2\text{-}4}$	20.0_1
Fri																
Cycle	D/O	D/O	D/O	D/O	D/O	D/O	D/O	D/O	D/O	D/O	D/O	D/O	D/O	D/O	D/O	D/O
Sat																
Cycle	D/O	D/O	D/O	D/O	D/O	D/O	D/O	D/O	D/O	D/O	D/O	D/O	D/O	D/O	D/O	D/O
Sun																
Cycle	46.4_1	57.6_1	63.2_1	52.0_1	63.2_1	68.8_1	57.6_1	68.8_1	74.4_1	63.2_1	74.4_1	80.0_1	63.2_1	68.8_1	57.6_1	RACE

Note: This programme is based on chapter 7, no. 26 novice.

Race: Cycle (80 km)
Race date: 20 April
Training starts: 30 December

Maximum distance for the 100% week
Cycle: 350 km

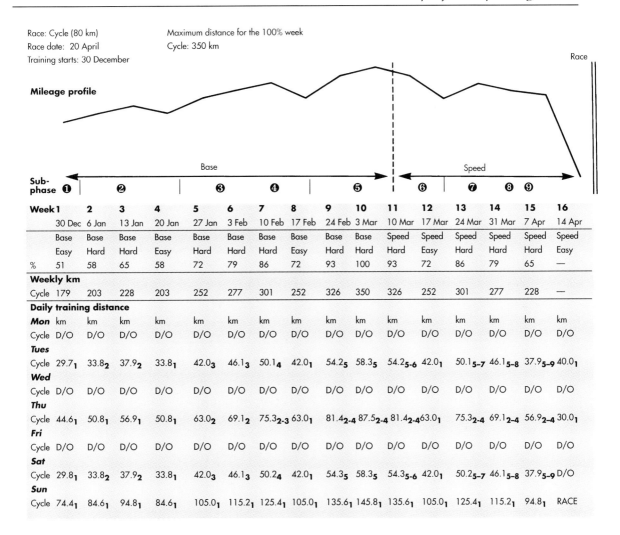

Mileage profile

	Base									Speed						Race
Sub-phase	❶	❷		❸	❹			❺		❻	❼		❽	❾		
Week	1	2	3	4	5	6	7	8	9	10	11	12	13	14	15	16
	30 Dec	6 Jan	13 Jan	20 Jan	27 Jan	3 Feb	10 Feb	17 Feb	24 Feb	3 Mar	10 Mar	17 Mar	24 Mar	31 Mar	7 Apr	14 Apr
	Base	Base	Base	Base	Base	Base	Base	Base	Base	Base	Speed	Speed	Speed	Speed	Speed	Speed
	Easy	Hard	Hard	Easy	Hard	Hard	Hard	Easy	Hard	Hard	Hard	Easy	Hard	Hard	Hard	Easy
%	51	58	65	58	72	79	86	72	93	100	93	72	86	79	65	—
Weekly km																
Cycle	179	203	228	203	252	277	301	252	326	350	326	252	301	277	228	—

Daily training distance

	1	2	3	4	5	6	7	8	9	10	11	12	13	14	15	16
Mon km																
Cycle	D/O	D/O	D/O	D/O	D/O	D/O	D/O	D/O	D/O	D/O	D/O	D/O	D/O	D/O	D/O	D/O
Tues																
Cycle	29.7_1	33.8_2	37.9_2	33.8_1	42.0_3	46.1_3	50.1_4	42.0_1	54.2_5	58.3_5	54.2_{5-6}	42.0_1	50.1_{5-7}	46.1_{5-8}	37.9_{5-9}	40.0_1
Wed																
Cycle	D/O	D/O	D/O	D/O	D/O	D/O	D/O	D/O	D/O	D/O	D/O	D/O	D/O	D/O	D/O	D/O
Thu																
Cycle	44.6_1	50.8_1	56.9_1	50.8_1	63.0_2	69.1_2	75.3_{2-3}	63.0_1	81.4_{2-4}	87.5_{2-4}	81.4_{2-4}	63.0_1	75.3_{2-4}	69.1_{2-4}	56.9_{2-4}	30.0_1
Fri																
Cycle	D/O	D/O	D/O	D/O	D/O	D/O	D/O	D/O	D/O	D/O	D/O	D/O	D/O	D/O	D/O	D/O
Sat																
Cycle	29.8_1	33.8_2	37.9_2	33.8_1	42.0_3	46.1_3	50.2_4	42.0_1	54.3_5	58.3_5	54.3_{5-6}	42.0_1	50.2_{5-7}	46.1_{5-8}	37.9_{5-9}	D/O
Sun																
Cycle	74.4_1	84.6_1	94.8_1	84.6_1	105.0_1	115.2_1	125.4_1	105.0_1	135.6_1	145.8_1	135.6_1	105.0_1	125.4_1	115.2_1	94.8_1	RACE

Race: Cycle (80 km)
Race date: 20 April
Training starts: 30 December

Maximum distance for the 100% week
Cycle: 400 km

Mileage profile

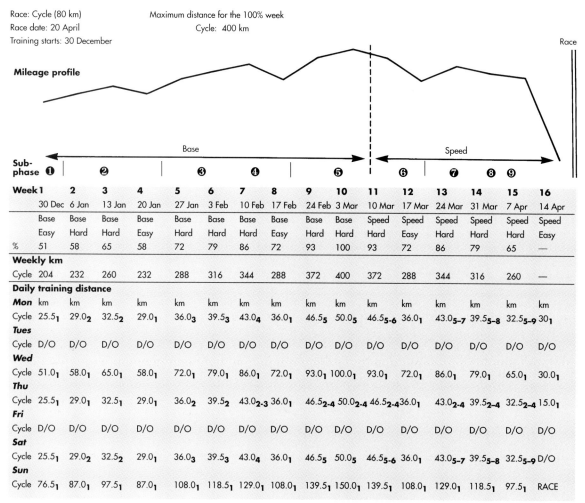

Sub-phase	❶		❷		❸		❹		❺		❻		❼	❽	❾	
Week	1	2	3	4	5	6	7	8	9	10	11	12	13	14	15	16
	30 Dec	6 Jan	13 Jan	20 Jan	27 Jan	3 Feb	10 Feb	17 Feb	24 Feb	3 Mar	10 Mar	17 Mar	24 Mar	31 Mar	7 Apr	14 Apr
	Base	Base	Base	Base	Base	Base	Base	Base	Base	Base	Speed	Speed	Speed	Speed	Speed	Speed
	Easy	Hard	Hard	Easy	Hard	Hard	Hard	Easy	Hard	Hard	Hard	Easy	Hard	Hard	Hard	Easy
%	51	58	65	58	72	79	86	72	93	100	93	72	86	79	65	—
Weekly km																
Cycle	204	232	260	232	288	316	344	288	372	400	372	288	344	316	260	—
Daily training distance																
Mon km	km	km	km	km	km	km	km	km	km	km	km	km	km	km	km
Cycle	25.5_1	29.0_2	32.5_2	29.0_1	36.0_3	39.5_3	43.0_4	36.0_1	46.5_5	50.0_5	46.5_{5-6}	36.0_1	43.0_{5-7}	39.5_{5-8}	32.5_{5-9}	30_1
Tues																
Cycle	D/O	D/O	D/O	D/O	D/O	D/O	D/O	D/O	D/O	D/O	D/O	D/O	D/O	D/O	D/O	D/O
Wed																
Cycle	51.0_1	58.0_1	65.0_1	58.0_1	72.0_1	79.0_1	86.0_1	72.0_1	93.0_1	100.0_1	93.0_1	72.0_1	86.0_1	79.0_1	65.0_1	30.0_1
Thu																
Cycle	25.5_1	29.0_1	32.5_1	29.0_1	36.0_2	39.5_2	43.0_{2-3}	36.0_1	46.5_{2-4}	50.0_{2-4}	46.5_{2-4}	36.0_1	43.0_{2-4}	39.5_{2-4}	32.5_{2-4}	15.0_1
Fri																
Cycle	D/O	D/O	D/O	D/O	D/O	D/O	D/O	D/O	D/O	D/O	D/O	D/O	D/O	D/O	D/O	D/O
Sat																
Cycle	25.5_1	29.0_2	32.5_2	29.0_1	36.0_3	39.5_3	43.0_4	36.0_1	46.5_5	50.0_5	46.5_{5-6}	36.0_1	43.0_{5-7}	39.5_{5-8}	32.5_{5-9}	D/O
Sun																
Cycle	76.5_1	87.0_1	97.5_1	87.0_1	108.0_1	118.5_1	129.0_1	108.0_1	139.5_1	150.0_1	139.5_1	108.0_1	129.0_1	118.5_1	97.5_1	RACE

Note: Base 1 would occur first.

Race: Cycle (100 km)
Race date: 20 April
Training starts: 30 December

Maximum distance for the 100% week
Cycle: 500 km

Mileage profile

Race

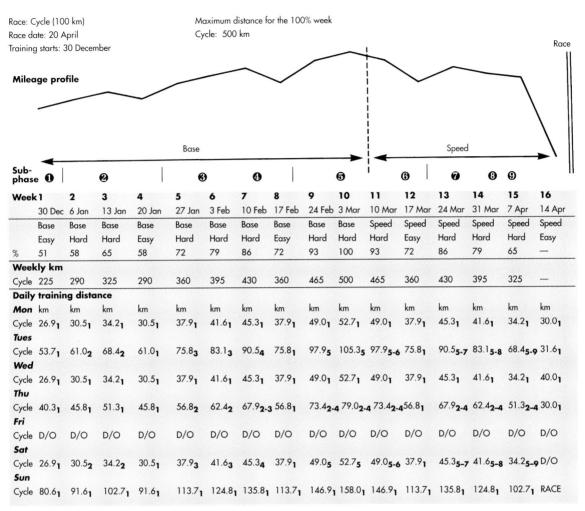

Base ⟷ Speed

Sub-phase: ❶ ❷ ❸ ❹ ❺ ❻ ❼ ❽ ❾

Week	Date	Phase	Type	%	Weekly km (Cycle)	Mon	Tues	Wed	Thu	Fri	Sat	Sun
1	30 Dec	Base	Easy	51	225	26.9_1	53.7_1	26.9_1	40.3_1	D/O	26.9_1	80.6_1
2	6 Jan	Base	Hard	58	290	30.5_1	61.0_2	30.5_1	45.8_1	D/O	30.5_2	91.6_1
3	13 Jan	Base	Hard	65	325	34.2_1	68.4_2	34.2_1	51.3_1	D/O	34.2_2	102.7_1
4	20 Jan	Base	Easy	58	290	30.5_1	61.0_1	30.5_1	45.8_1	D/O	30.5_1	91.6_1
5	27 Jan	Base	Hard	72	360	37.9_1	75.8_3	37.9_1	56.8_2	D/O	37.9_3	113.7_1
6	3 Feb	Base	Hard	79	395	41.6_1	83.1_3	41.6_1	62.4_2	D/O	41.6_3	124.8_1
7	10 Feb	Base	Hard	86	430	45.3_1	90.5_4	45.3_1	67.9_{2-3}	D/O	45.3_4	135.8_1
8	17 Feb	Base	Easy	72	360	37.9_1	75.8_1	37.9_1	56.8_1	D/O	37.9_1	113.7_1
9	24 Feb	Base	Hard	93	465	49.0_1	97.9_5	49.0_1	73.4_{2-4}	D/O	49.0_5	146.9_1
10	3 Mar	Base	Hard	100	500	52.7_1	105.3_5	52.7_1	79.0_{2-4}	D/O	52.7_5	158.0_1
11	10 Mar	Speed	Hard	93	465	49.0_1	97.9_{5-6}	49.0_1	73.4_{2-4}	D/O	49.0_{5-6}	146.9_1
12	17 Mar	Speed	Easy	72	360	37.9_1	75.8_1	37.9_1	56.8_1	D/O	37.9_1	113.7_1
13	24 Mar	Speed	Hard	86	430	45.3_1	90.5_{5-7}	45.3_1	67.9_{2-4}	D/O	45.3_{5-7}	135.8_1
14	31 Mar	Speed	Hard	79	395	41.6_1	83.1_{5-8}	41.6_1	62.4_{2-4}	D/O	41.6_{5-8}	124.8_1
15	7 Apr	Speed	Hard	65	325	34.2_1	68.4_{5-9}	34.2_1	51.3_{2-4}	D/O	34.2_{5-9}	102.7_1
16	14 Apr	Speed	Easy	—	—	30.0_1	31.6_1	40.0_1	30.0_1	D/O	D/O	RACE

Note: Base 1 would occur first.

Race: Cycle (160 km)
Race date: 20 April
Training starts: 30 December

Maximum distance for the 100% week
Cycle: 600 km

Mileage profile

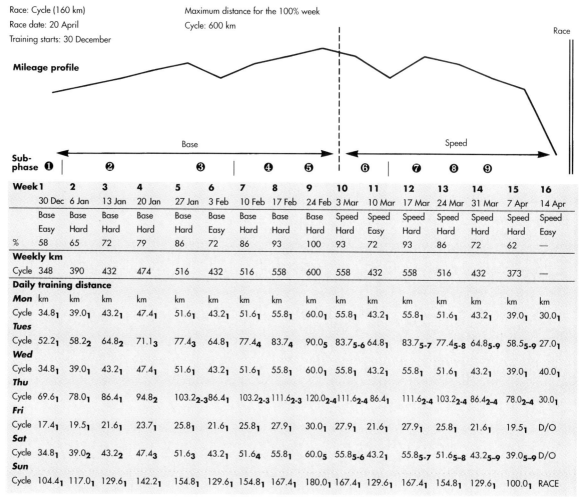

Sub-phase	❶		❷		❸		❹	❺		❻		❼	❽	❾		Race
Week	1	2	3	4	5	6	7	8	9	10	11	12	13	14	15	16
	30 Dec	6 Jan	13 Jan	20 Jan	27 Jan	3 Feb	10 Feb	17 Feb	24 Feb	3 Mar	10 Mar	17 Mar	24 Mar	31 Mar	7 Apr	14 Apr
	Base	Base	Base	Base	Base	Base	Base	Base	Base	Speed	Speed	Speed	Speed	Speed	Speed	Speed
	Easy	Hard	Hard	Hard	Hard	Easy	Hard	Hard	Hard	Hard	Easy	Hard	Hard	Hard	Hard	Easy
%	58	65	72	79	86	72	86	93	100	93	72	93	86	72	62	—
Weekly km																
Cycle	348	390	432	474	516	432	516	558	600	558	432	558	516	432	373	—
Daily training distance																
Mon km	km	km	km	km	km	km	km	km	km	km	km	km	km	km	km	km
Cycle	34.8_1	39.0_1	43.2_1	47.4_1	51.6_1	43.2_1	51.6_1	55.8_1	60.0_1	55.8_1	43.2_1	55.8_1	51.6_1	43.2_1	39.0_1	30.0_1
Tues Cycle	52.2_1	58.2_2	64.8_2	71.1_3	77.4_3	64.8_1	77.4_4	83.7_4	90.0_5	83.7_{5-6}	64.8_1	83.7_{5-7}	77.4_{5-8}	64.8_{5-9}	58.5_{5-9}	27.0_1
Wed Cycle	34.8_1	39.0_1	43.2_1	47.4_1	51.6_1	43.2_1	51.6_1	55.8_1	60.0_1	55.8_1	43.2_1	55.8_1	51.6_1	43.2_1	39.0_1	40.0_1
Thu Cycle	69.6_1	78.0_1	86.4_1	94.8_2	103.2_{2-3}	86.4_1	103.2_{2-3}	111.6_{2-3}	120.0_{2-4}	111.6_{2-4}	86.4_1	111.6_{2-4}	103.2_{2-4}	86.4_{2-4}	78.0_{2-4}	30.0_1
Fri Cycle	17.4_1	19.5_1	21.6_1	23.7_1	25.8_1	21.6_1	25.8_1	27.9_1	30.0_1	27.9_1	21.6_1	27.9_1	25.8_1	21.6_1	19.5_1	D/O
Sat Cycle	34.8_1	39.0_2	43.2_2	47.4_3	51.6_3	43.2_1	51.6_4	55.8_1	60.0_5	55.8_{5-6}	43.2_1	55.8_{5-7}	51.6_{5-8}	43.2_{5-9}	39.0_{5-9}	D/O
Sun Cycle	104.4_1	117.0_1	129.6_1	142.2_1	154.8_1	129.6_1	154.8_1	167.4_1	180.0_1	167.4_1	129.6_1	167.4_1	154.8_1	129.6_1	100.0_1	RACE

Note: Base 1 would occur first.

226

Race: Tour (700 km)
Race date: 20 April
Training starts: 30 December

Maximum distance for the 100% week
Cycle: 800 km

Race

Mileage profile

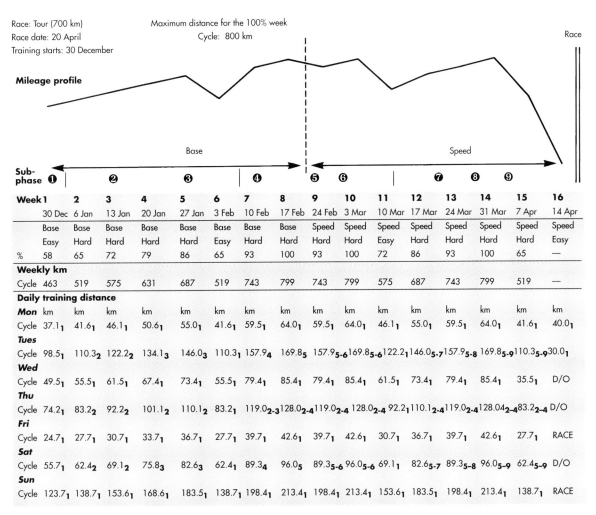

Base   Speed

Sub-phase ❶ ❷ ❸ ❹ ❺ ❻ ❼ ❽ ❾

	Week 1	2	3	4	5	6	7	8	9	10	11	12	13	14	15	16
	30 Dec	6 Jan	13 Jan	20 Jan	27 Jan	3 Feb	10 Feb	17 Feb	24 Feb	3 Mar	10 Mar	17 Mar	24 Mar	31 Mar	7 Apr	14 Apr
	Base	Base	Base	Base	Base	Base	Base	Base	Speed	Speed	Speed	Speed	Speed	Speed	Speed	Speed
	Easy	Hard	Hard	Hard	Hard	Easy	Hard	Hard	Hard	Hard	Easy	Hard	Hard	Hard	Hard	Easy
%	58	65	72	79	86	65	93	100	93	100	72	86	93	100	65	—
Weekly km																
Cycle	463	519	575	631	687	519	743	799	743	799	575	687	743	799	519	—
Daily training distance																
Mon km	km	km	km	km	km	km	km	km	km	km	km	km	km	km	km
Cycle	37.1_1	41.6_1	46.1_1	50.6_1	55.0_1	41.6_1	59.5_1	64.0_1	59.5_1	64.0_1	46.1_1	55.0_1	59.5_1	64.0_1	41.6_1	40.0_1
Tues																
Cycle	98.5_1	110.3_2	122.2_2	134.1_3	146.0_3	110.3_1	157.9_4	169.8_5	$157.9_{5\text{-}6}$	$169.8_{5\text{-}6}$	122.2_1	$146.0_{5\text{-}7}$	$157.9_{5\text{-}8}$	$169.8_{5\text{-}9}$	$110.3_{5\text{-}9}$	30.0_1
Wed																
Cycle	49.5_1	55.5_1	61.5_1	67.4_1	73.4_1	55.5_1	79.4_1	85.4_1	79.4_1	85.4_1	61.5_1	73.4_1	79.4_1	85.4_1	35.5_1	D/O
Thu																
Cycle	74.2_1	83.2_2	92.2_2	101.1_2	110.1_2	83.2_1	$119.0_{2\text{-}3}$	$128.0_{2\text{-}4}$	$119.0_{2\text{-}4}$	$128.0_{2\text{-}4}$	92.2_1	$110.1_{2\text{-}4}$	$119.0_{2\text{-}4}$	$128.04_{2\text{-}4}$	$83.2_{2\text{-}4}$	D/O
Fri																
Cycle	24.7_1	27.7_1	30.7_1	33.7_1	36.7_1	27.7_1	39.7_1	42.6_1	39.7_1	42.6_1	30.7_1	36.7_1	39.7_1	42.6_1	27.7_1	RACE
Sat																
Cycle	55.7_1	62.4_2	69.1_2	75.8_3	82.6_3	62.4_1	89.3_4	96.0_5	$89.3_{5\text{-}6}$	$96.0_{5\text{-}6}$	69.1_1	$82.6_{5\text{-}7}$	$89.3_{5\text{-}8}$	$96.0_{5\text{-}9}$	$62.4_{5\text{-}9}$	D/O
Sun																
Cycle	123.7_1	138.7_1	153.6_1	168.6_1	183.5_1	138.7_1	198.4_1	213.4_1	198.4_1	213.4_1	153.6_1	183.5_1	198.4_1	213.4_1	138.7_1	RACE

Note: Base 1 would occur first.

227

TAPER AND PEAK

Single-day road races/criterium – low-priority taper (and following training week)

Week 1

M	T	W	T	F	S	S
HILLS	INTS	50% INTS	EASY	DAY OFF	RACE	DAY OFF or easy ride
E	H	H	E		H	E

Week 2

M	T	W	T	F	S	S
EASY (NO HILLS)	HILLS	INTS	EASY	DAY OFF	LONG	LONG
E	E	H	E		H	H

Single-day road races/criterium – high-priority taper

M	T	W	T	F	S	S
EASY	50% INTS	EASY	DAY OFF or easy	DAY OFF or easy	RACE	DAY OFF or easy
E	E	H	E	E	H	E

Tour – high-priority taper

Week 1

M	T	W	T	F	S	S
HILLS	RACE	50% INTS	EASY	DAY OFF	HILLS	LONG (33% DIST)
E	H	H	E		E	H

Week 2

M	T	W	T	F	S	S
50% INTS	EASY	DAY OFF or easy	DAY OFF or easy	TOUR PROLOGUE	TOUR	TOUR
E	E	E	E	H	H	H

Note: Do tour simulations in training where you train/race three to four long days in a row. Do this between one and three times before you race.

SPORT-SPECIFIC TRAINING USED IN ROAD CYCLING

Type (intensity)	When initiated	Effect	Example
Power	Late speed phase	Improves jump accels	4–6 × 10–15 sec rest to recovery
Intensive sprints	Late speed phase	Improves full sprint phase	6–10 × 30 sec–1 min rest to recovery or short rest < 1 min
Extensive sprints	Speed phase	Improves long sprint bridging gaps	4–6 × 1–3 min rest to recovery or 1–2 min btwn
Submaximal	Speed phase	Improves max steady state pace in TTs peloton and breaks	4–6 × 6–8 min 4–1 min rest btwn or 20–30 min TT
Up-tempo	Late base, early speed	Transition from base to speedwork	1–2 × 5–10 km rest 5 km btwn
Long slow distance	Base/speed	Improves ability to do mileage, builds training tolerance and improves recovery rate	Continuous
Active recovery	Base/speed	Assists recovery	Continuous

Proportions:
1 Base – 100% long slow distance and active recovery; some speedwork may be used.
2 Speed – approx. 85–90% long slow distance and active recovery; approx. 10–15% submaximal intensity and higher intensities.

Training notes for road cycling

Spinning, cadence and gear selection in base training

A lot of cyclists tend to start their build-up by pushing big gears at a slow cadence, for example 65–80 rpm. This can cause stress on the knees and injuries may occur. It is more beneficial to start in a very easy gear, such as 42×18, and maintain a high rpm, for example 85–95 rpm. This is an optimal time trial cadence for triathletes; 90–110 is good for cyclists and mountain bikers. These cadences will help prevent injury, and improve fitness, pedalling fluidity and technique. Bigger gears will be used later in the season when the body can tolerate the load.

Spinning is also very important for a number of other reasons. For instance, it allows you to sprint quickly if another cyclist trys to 'jump'. In a big gear at low rpm it is harder to respond quickly to a 'jump' as the big gear would need to be 'wound up'. At high rpm, however, the response can be much quicker and the acceleration needed to match the 'jump' can also be achieved rapidly. Spinning in a smaller gear initially also means you can change to a bigger gear as you build up speed following the 'jump'.

Spinning is also good for conserving strength. Pushing big gears is much harder work than pushing the equivalent loads at higher rpms. If you push too high a gear, you may find that towards the end of the race you have tired legs. You may as a result be dropped on a hill or lose the sprint despite being fit enough to stay with the bunch right up to the final 200–300 metres.

In triathlons, particularly the Ironman, the big gear pushers often tire and slow in the second half of the bike and on the run. Spinning is one of the best ways of improving cycling performance.

Possible gearing in pre-season

Base 1 (6 weeks)

2 weeks: $42 \times 18+$ (only). This limits leg fatigue, helps prevent injury, increases fitness and improves pedalling technique.

2 weeks: $42 \times 16+$ (only).

2 weeks: Open gears but still use planned cadence; that is, cadence must remain at 85–95 rpm for triathletes and 90–110 rpm for cyclists.

Base 2 and Speed

Open gears, maintain optimal cadence in all rides.

Note: In Base 2 and speed phases, limit easy rides to smaller gears to aid recovery; all easy rides $42 \times 16+$ only.

Cycle tours vs single-day cycle races

The major training emphasis for tours is mileage. If you are going to be racing 500 km in four days, or 900 km in a week, you need to be able to do this in training. Peak-mileage weeks for tours are very different to those for single-day races. For tours, the peak mileages are much higher and they are maintained approximately up until the last four weeks before the race. (Some cyclists use another tour as a warm-up.) For single-day racing peak mileages are smaller and occur further away from race day (four to eight weeks) as more speedwork is required between base and peak. Too many single-day cyclists maintain mileage too close to the race. This leaves them too slow (not enough speedwork) and fatigued (too much too close).

Approximate timing of peak mileage

Long tours (more than a week): two to four weeks before peak race; short tours (less than a week): three to four weeks before peak race; 160 km race: four to six weeks before peak race; 40–80 km: six to eight weeks before peak race.

◆ Mountain biking ◆ training programmes

All rides not specified 'off road' are on the road; time is used as it is difficult to determine distance off road.

BASE TRAINING

Mountain biking base programme

	Training type	Training intensity	% of weekly mileage	Hard/easy
Base 1				
Mon	Day off			E
Tues	2–3 weeks easy, gradually introduce hills; 1–1.5 hrs	LO	23%	H
Wed	Day off			E
Thurs	Easy Spin 1–1.5 hrs	LO	23%	H
Fri	Day off			E
Sat	Tech ride off road 1–1.5 hrs	LO	23%	H
Sun	Long ride off or on road 1–1.5 hrs	LO	31%	H
Base 2 (total km = 84)				
Mon	Easy ride Tech off road 1–2 hrs)	LO	12.5%	E
Tues	Ride 2–3 hrs	LO	18.8%	H
Wed	Ride 1–2 hrs Tech off road	LO	12.5%	E
Thurs	Ride 2–3 hrs hills	LO	18.8%	H
Fri	Day off			E
Sat	Ride Tech off road 2 hrs	LO	12.4%	H
Sun	Long ride off or on road 3–4 hrs	LO	25%	H

SPEED TRAINING

Mountain biking speed programme

	Training type	Training intensity	% of weekly mileage	Hard/easy
Mon	Easy ride Tech off road 1–2 hrs	LO	15.4%	E
Tues	INTS (2)*; (SM) = 80% (HI) = 20%; off road undulating	SM/HI	15.4%	H
Wed	INTS (1)* hilly uphill R/P/C/R; progress to off road (SM)	SM	15.4%	H
Thurs	Ride easy	LO	7.8%	E
Fri	Day off			E
Sat	Race or med dist ride	LO/SM	15.4%	H/E
Sun	Long ride off road	LO	30.8%	H

Intervals (1) on Wednesday: uphill R/P/C/R (SM) hilly

First two to four weeks: ride 4–6 mins at SM uphill followed by a racing dismount to either run pushing or carrying your mountain bike for 1–2 min. This is followed by a racing mount to ride a further 4–6 min at SM uphill. Do this two to four times. Rest with 10–20 min easy pedalling between.

Second two to four weeks: off road rides, time trials and long intervals (6–8 min); do this two to four times at SM.

Intervals (2) on Tuesday: 80% SM and 20% HI

80% (SM) = 2–6 reps of 4–8 min at SM. Rest for 8–10 min between;
20% (HI) = 2–4 reps of 2–3 min at HI. Variable rest periods; rest to recovery to less that 30 sec rest.

Move Wednesday's speedwork to Thursday if you are not racing or find two speed workouts in a row too much. Alternatively, remove Wednesday's speedwork altogether and have a day off or an easy day.

Refer to 'Road cycling', page 228, for taper programmes.

Race: Mountain bike
Race date 15 Jan

Maximum time for the 100% week
Mountain bike: 10.5 hrs (630 mins)

Race

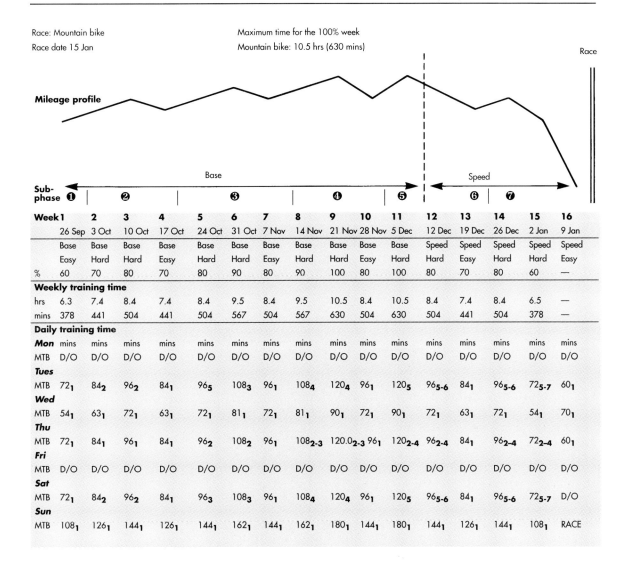

Mileage profile

Base — Speed

Sub-phase	❶	❷		❸		❹	❺	❻	❼

Week	1	2	3	4	5	6	7	8	9	10	11	12	13	14	15	16
	26 Sep	3 Oct	10 Oct	17 Oct	24 Oct	31 Oct	7 Nov	14 Nov	21 Nov	28 Nov	5 Dec	12 Dec	19 Dec	26 Dec	2 Jan	9 Jan
	Base	Base	Base	Base	Base	Base	Base	Base	Base	Base	Base	Speed	Speed	Speed	Speed	Speed
	Easy	Hard	Hard	Easy	Hard	Hard	Easy	Hard	Hard	Easy	Hard	Hard	Easy	Hard	Hard	Easy
%	60	70	80	70	80	90	80	90	100	80	100	80	70	80	60	—

Weekly training time

	1	2	3	4	5	6	7	8	9	10	11	12	13	14	15	16
hrs	6.3	7.4	8.4	7.4	8.4	9.5	8.4	9.5	10.5	8.4	10.5	8.4	7.4	8.4	6.5	—
mins	378	441	504	441	504	567	504	567	630	504	630	504	441	504	378	—

Daily training time

	1	2	3	4	5	6	7	8	9	10	11	12	13	14	15	16
Mon	mins	mins	mins	mins	mins	mins	mins	mins	mins	mins	mins	mins	mins	mins	mins	mins
MTB	D/O	D/O	D/O	D/O	D/O	D/O	D/O	D/O	D/O	D/O	D/O	D/O	D/O	D/O	D/O	D/O
Tues																
MTB	72_1	84_2	96_2	84_1	96_5	108_3	96_1	108_4	120_4	96_1	120_5	$96_{5\text{-}6}$	84_1	$96_{5\text{-}6}$	$72_{5\text{-}7}$	60_1
Wed																
MTB	54_1	63_1	72_1	63_1	72_1	81_1	72_1	81_1	90_1	72_1	90_1	72_1	63_1	72_1	54_1	70_1
Thu																
MTB	72_1	84_1	96_1	84_1	96_2	108_2	96_1	$108_{2\text{-}3}$	$120.0_{2\text{-}3}$	96_1	$120_{2\text{-}4}$	$96_{2\text{-}4}$	84_1	$96_{2\text{-}4}$	$72_{2\text{-}4}$	60_1
Fri																
MTB	D/O	D/O	D/O	D/O	D/O	D/O	D/O	D/O	D/O	D/O	D/O	D/O	D/O	D/O	D/O	D/O
Sat																
MTB	72_1	84_2	96_2	84_1	96_3	108_3	96_1	108_4	120_4	96_1	120_5	$96_{5\text{-}6}$	84_1	$96_{5\text{-}6}$	$72_{5\text{-}7}$	D/O
Sun																
MTB	108_1	126_1	144_1	126_1	144_1	162_1	144_1	162_1	180_1	144_1	180_1	144_1	126_1	144_1	108_1	RACE

Race: Mountain bike (2.5 hrs advanced   )
Race date: 15 Jan

Maximum time for 100% week
Mountain bike: 16 hrs (960 mins)

Race

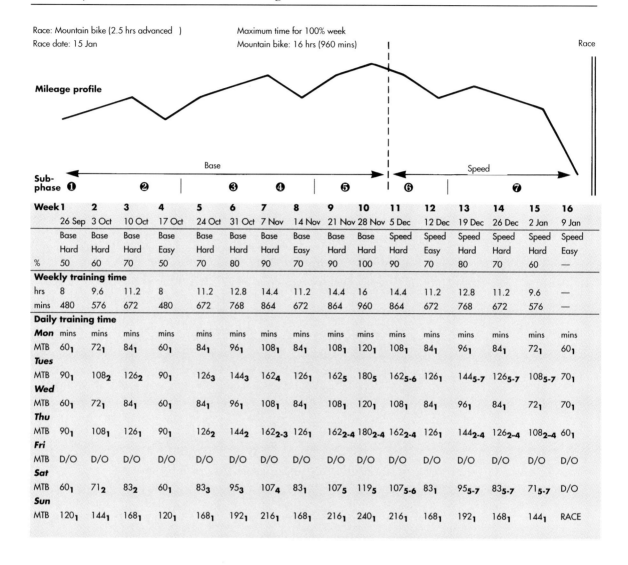

Mileage profile

Base | Speed

Sub-phase: ❶ ❷ | ❸ ❹ | ❺ | ❻ | ❼

Week	1	2	3	4	5	6	7	8	9	10	11	12	13	14	15	16
	26 Sep	3 Oct	10 Oct	17 Oct	24 Oct	31 Oct	7 Nov	14 Nov	21 Nov	28 Nov	5 Dec	12 Dec	19 Dec	26 Dec	2 Jan	9 Jan
	Base	Base	Base	Base	Base	Base	Base	Base	Base	Base	Speed	Speed	Speed	Speed	Speed	Speed
	Hard	Hard	Hard	Easy	Hard	Hard	Hard	Easy	Hard	Hard	Hard	Easy	Hard	Hard	Hard	Easy
%	50	60	70	50	70	80	90	70	90	100	90	70	80	70	60	—
Weekly training time																
hrs	8	9.6	11.2	8	11.2	12.8	14.4	11.2	14.4	16	14.4	11.2	12.8	11.2	9.6	—
mins	480	576	672	480	672	768	864	672	864	960	864	672	768	672	576	—
Daily training time																
Mon	mins	mins	mins	mins	mins	mins	mins	mins	mins	mins	mins	mins	mins	mins	mins	mins
MTB	60_1	72_1	84_1	60_1	84_1	96_1	108_1	84_1	108_1	120_1	108_1	84_1	96_1	84_1	72_1	60_1
Tues																
MTB	90_1	108_2	126_2	90_1	126_3	144_3	162_4	126_1	162_5	180_5	$162_{5\text{-}6}$	126_1	$144_{5\text{-}7}$	$126_{5\text{-}7}$	$108_{5\text{-}7}$	70_1
Wed																
MTB	60_1	72_1	84_1	60_1	84_1	96_1	108_1	84_1	108_1	120_1	108_1	84_1	96_1	84_1	72_1	70_1
Thu																
MTB	90_1	108_1	126_1	90_1	126_2	144_2	$162_{2\text{-}3}$	126_1	$162_{2\text{-}4}$	$180_{2\text{-}4}$	$162_{2\text{-}4}$	126_1	$144_{2\text{-}4}$	$126_{2\text{-}4}$	$108_{2\text{-}4}$	60_1
Fri																
MTB	D/O	D/O	D/O	D/O	D/O	D/O	D/O	D/O	D/O	D/O	D/O	D/O	D/O	D/O	D/O	D/O
Sat																
MTB	60_1	71_2	83_2	60_1	83_3	95_3	107_4	83_1	107_5	119_5	$107_{5\text{-}6}$	83_1	$95_{5\text{-}7}$	$83_{5\text{-}7}$	$71_{5\text{-}7}$	D/O
Sun																
MTB	120_1	144_1	168_1	120_1	168_1	192_1	216_1	168_1	216_1	240_1	216_1	168_1	192_1	168_1	144_1	RACE

SPORT-SPECIFIC TRAINING USED IN MOUNTAIN BIKING

Type (intensity)	When initiated	Effect	Example
Power	—	—	—
Intensive sprints	—	—	—
Extensive sprints	Speed phase	Improves short hill climbs and starts	4–6 × 1–3 min rest to recovery or 1–2 min btwn
Submaximal	Speed phase	Improves max steady state pace for racing	4–6 × 6–8 min 4–1 min rest btwn or 20–30 min TT
Up-tempo	Late base, early speed	Transition from base to speedwork	1–2 × 5–10 km rest 5 km btwn
Long slow distance	Base/speed	Improves ability to do mileage builds training tolerance and improves recovery rate	Continuous
Active recovery	Base/speed	Assists recovery	Continuous
Spinning (cadence) (*see* page 230)			

♦ Distance running ♦ training programmes

BASE TRAINING

Start with two workouts per discipline per week and progress up to three to four workouts per week.

10 km distance running base programme

	Training type	Training intensity	% of weekly mileage	Hard/easy
Base 1 (total km = 37)				
Mon	Day off			E
Tues	Easy run 4–6 km (hilly) (20–30 min)	LO	16.2%	H
Wed	Day off			E
Thurs	Run 5–10 km (30–50 min)	LO	27%	H
Fri	Day off			E
Sat	Run 4–6 km (20–30 min)	LO	16.2%	H
Sun	Long run 10–15 km (50 min–1 hr 15 min)	LO	40.6%	H
Base 2 (total km = 70)				
Mon	Easy run 4–6 km (20–30 min)	LO	8.6%	E
Tues	Med run 8–12 km (hilly) (40–60 min)	LO	17%	H
Wed	Easy run 5–10 km (30–50 min)	LO	8.6%	E
Thurs	Med long run 10–16 km (50 min–1 hr 20 min)	LO	22.8%	H
Fri	Day off			E
Sat	Easy run 4–6 km	LO	8.6%	H
Sun	Long run 10–20 km (50 min–1 hr 20 min)	LO	29%	H

Marathon distance running base programme

	Training type	Training intensity	% of total week	Hard/easy
Base 1 (total km = 47)				
Mon	Day off			E
Tues	Run 4–6 km (20–30 min)	LO	12.8%	H
Wed	Day off			E
Thurs	Run 5–10 km (50 min–1 hr 15 min)	LO	31.9%	H
Fri	Day off			E
Sat	Run 4–6 km (20–30 min)	LO	12.8%	H
Sun	Run 10–20 km (50 min–1 hr 15 min)	LO	42.5%	H
Base 2 (total km = 84)				
Mon	Easy run 4–6 km (20–30 min)	LO	7.1%	E
Tues	Med 6–12 km (30–60 min)	LO	14.3%	H
Wed	Easy run 4–6 km (20–30 min)	LO	7.1%	E
Thurs	Med long 15–20 km (1 hr 15 min–1 hr 40 min)	LO	23.8%	H
Fri	Day off			E
Sat	Easy run 5–10 km (25–50 min)	LO	11.9%	H
Sun	Long run 30 km (2.5 hr)	LO	35.8%	H

SPEED TRAINING

10 km distance running speed programme

	Training type	Training intensity	% of total week	Hard/easy
Speed: (total km = 64)				
Mon	Easy run 6 km (30 min)	LO	9.4%	E
Tues	INTS or TT 10 km (50 min)	LO/SM/UT	15.6%	H
Wed	Easy 6 km (30 min)	LO	9.4%	E
Thurs	Med long 16 km (1 hr 20 min)	LO/UT	25%	H
Fri	Day off			E
Sat	INTS 4–6 × 6–8 min 6 km (30 min)	SM	9.4%	H
Sun	Long run 20 km (1 hr 40 min)	LO	31.2%	H

Marathon distance running speed programme

	Training type	Training intensity	% of total week	Hard/easy
Speed: (total km = 78)				
Mon	Easy run 6 km (30 min)	LO	7.7%	E
Tues	INTS 4–6 × 6–8 min (SM) 4–1 min rest btwn = 10 km (50 min)	LO/SM	12.8%	H
Wed	Easy run 6 km (30 min)	LO	7.7%	E
Thurs	Med long 20 km (1 hr 40 min)	LO/UT	25.6%	H
Fri	Day off			E
Sat	INTS 2–4 × 10–15 min (RP); rest 10–2 min btwn = 12 km (60 min)	LO/RP	7.7%	H
Sun	Long 30 km (2.5 hrs)	LO	38.5%	H

BASIC HALF-MARATHON PROGRAMMES

Base 1: (30 km)

M	T	W	T	F	S	S
DAY OFF	R (H) 6 km	DAY OFF	R (M/L) 8 km	DAY OFF	R E 6 km	R (LONG) 10 km

Base 2: (76 km)

M	T	W	T	F	S	S
R (E) 4–6 km	R (H) 8–14 km	R (E) 4–6 km	R (ML) 15–18 km	DAY OFF	R E 4–6 km	R (LONG) 21–26 km

Speed: (69 km)

M	T	W	T	F	S	S
R (E) 4–5 km	R (SPEED) 6–10 km	R (E) 4–5 km	R (ML) 15–18 km	DAY OFF	R (SPEED) 4–5 km	R (LONG) 21–26 km

Race: Marathon
Race date: 20 April
Training starts: 30 December

Maximum distance for the 100% week
Run: 84 km

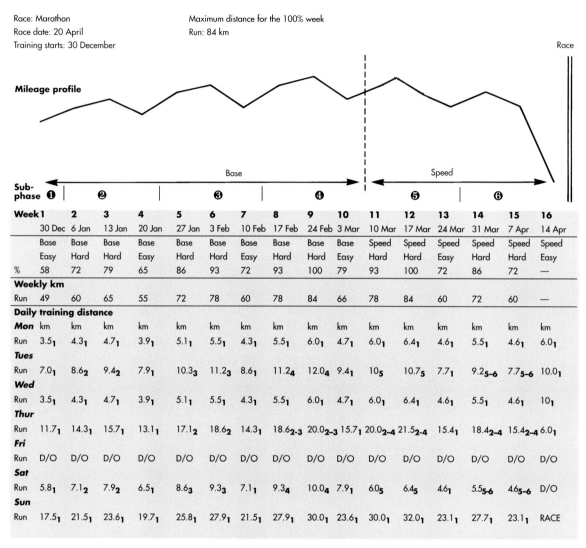

Mileage profile

Base — Speed

Sub-phase: ❶ ❷ ❸ ❹ ❺ ❻

Week	1	2	3	4	5	6	7	8	9	10	11	12	13	14	15	16
	30 Dec	6 Jan	13 Jan	20 Jan	27 Jan	3 Feb	10 Feb	17 Feb	24 Feb	3 Mar	10 Mar	17 Mar	24 Mar	31 Mar	7 Apr	14 Apr
	Base	Base	Base	Base	Base	Base	Base	Base	Base	Base	Speed	Speed	Speed	Speed	Speed	Speed
	Easy	Hard	Hard	Easy	Hard	Hard	Easy	Hard	Hard	Easy	Hard	Hard	Easy	Hard	Hard	Easy
%	58	72	79	65	86	93	72	93	100	79	93	100	72	86	72	—
Weekly km																
Run	49	60	65	55	72	78	60	78	84	66	78	84	60	72	60	—

Daily training distance

	Week 1	2	3	4	5	6	7	8	9	10	11	12	13	14	15	16
Mon Run	3.5_1	4.3_1	4.7_1	3.9_1	5.1_1	5.5_1	4.3_1	5.5_1	6.0_1	4.7_1	6.0_1	6.4_1	4.6_1	5.5_1	4.6_1	6.0_1
Tues Run	7.0_1	8.6_2	9.4_2	7.9_1	10.3_3	11.2_3	8.6_1	11.2_4	12.0_4	9.4_1	10_5	10.7_5	7.7_1	$9.2_{5\text{-}6}$	$7.7_{5\text{-}6}$	10.0_1
Wed Run	3.5_1	4.3_1	4.7_1	3.9_1	5.1_1	5.5_1	4.3_1	5.5_1	6.0_1	4.7_1	6.0_1	6.4_1	4.6_1	5.5_1	4.6_1	10_1
Thur Run	11.7_1	14.3_1	15.7_1	13.1_1	17.1_2	18.6_2	14.3_1	$18.6_{2\text{-}3}$	$20.0_{2\text{-}3}$	15.7_1	$20.0_{2\text{-}4}$	$21.5_{2\text{-}4}$	15.4_1	$18.4_{2\text{-}4}$	$15.4_{2\text{-}4}$	6.0_1
Fri Run	D/O	D/O	D/O	D/O	D/O	D/O	D/O	D/O	D/O	D/O	D/O	D/O	D/O	D/O	D/O	D/O
Sat Run	5.8_1	7.1_2	7.9_2	6.5_1	8.6_3	9.3_3	7.1_1	9.3_4	10.0_4	7.9_1	6.0_5	6.4_5	4.6_1	$5.5_{5\text{-}6}$	$4.6_{5\text{-}6}$	D/O
Sun Run	17.5_1	21.5_1	23.6_1	19.7_1	25.8_1	27.9_1	21.5_1	27.9_1	30.0_1	23.6_1	30.0_1	32.0_1	23.1_1	27.7_1	23.1_1	RACE

Note: Base 1 would occur first

Race: 10 km
Race date: 20 April
Training starts: 30 December

Maximum distance for the 100% week
Run: 70 km

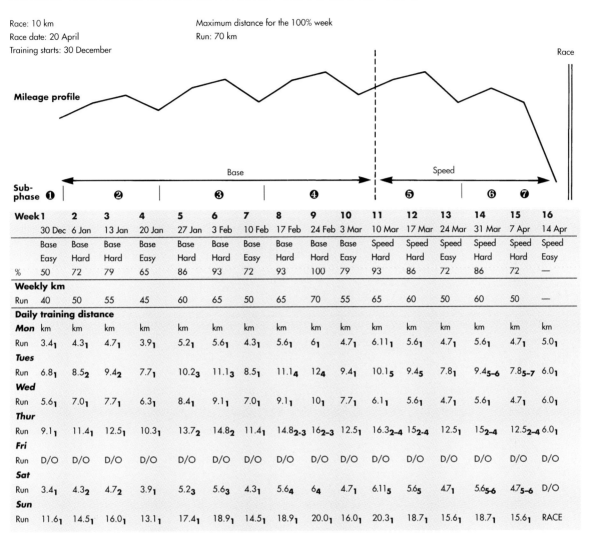

Mileage profile

Base Speed Race

Sub-phase	❶	❷		❸		❹		❺		❻	❼	
Week	1	2	3	4	5	6	7	8	9	10	11	12	13	14	15	16
	30 Dec	6 Jan	13 Jan	20 Jan	27 Jan	3 Feb	10 Feb	17 Feb	24 Feb	3 Mar	10 Mar	17 Mar	24 Mar	31 Mar	7 Apr	14 Apr
	Base	Base	Base	Base	Base	Base	Base	Base	Base	Base	Speed	Speed	Speed	Speed	Speed	Speed
	Easy	Hard	Hard	Easy	Hard	Hard	Easy	Hard	Hard	Easy	Hard	Hard	Easy	Hard	Hard	Easy
%	50	72	79	65	86	93	72	93	100	79	93	86	72	86	72	—

Weekly km

Run	40	50	55	45	60	65	50	65	70	55	65	60	50	60	50	—

Daily training distance

Mon	km	km	km	km	km	km	km	km	km	km	km	km	km	km	km	km
Run	3.4_1	4.3_1	4.7_1	3.9_1	5.2_1	5.6_1	4.3_1	5.6_1	6_1	4.7_1	6.11_1	5.6_1	4.7_1	5.6_1	4.7_1	5.0_1
Tues																
Run	6.8_1	8.5_2	9.4_2	7.7_1	10.2_3	11.1_3	8.5_1	11.1_4	12_4	9.4_1	10.1_5	9.4_5	7.8_1	9.4_{5-6}	7.8_{5-7}	6.0_1
Wed																
Run	5.6_1	7.0_1	7.7_1	6.3_1	8.4_1	9.1_1	7.0_1	9.1_1	10_1	7.7_1	6.1_1	5.6_1	4.7_1	5.6_1	4.7_1	6.0_1
Thur																
Run	9.1_1	11.4_1	12.5_1	10.3_1	13.7_2	14.8_2	11.4_1	14.8_{2-3}	16_{2-3}	12.5_1	16.3_{2-4}	15_{2-4}	12.5_1	15_{2-4}	12.5_{2-4}	6.0_1
Fri																
Run	D/O	D/O	D/O	D/O	D/O	D/O	D/O	D/O	D/O	D/O	D/O	D/O	D/O	D/O	D/O	D/O
Sat																
Run	3.4_1	4.3_2	4.7_2	3.9_1	5.2_3	5.6_3	4.3_1	5.6_4	6_4	4.7_1	6.11_5	5.6_5	4.7_1	5.6_{5-6}	4.7_{5-6}	D/O
Sun																
Run	11.6_1	14.5_1	16.0_1	13.1_1	17.4_1	18.9_1	14.5_1	18.9_1	20.0_1	16.0_1	20.3_1	18.7_1	15.6_1	18.7_1	15.6_1	RACE

Note: Base 1 would occur first

Race: Half-marathon
Race date: 20 April
Training starts: 30 December

Maximum distance for the 100% week
Run: 53 km

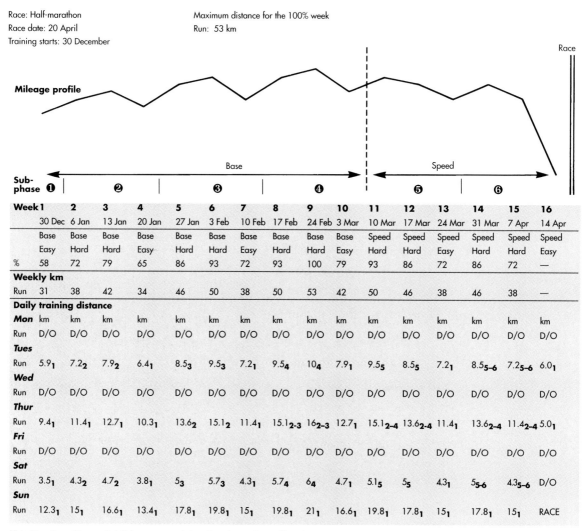

Mileage profile

Sub-phase: Base (❶ ❷ ❸ ❹) — Speed (❺ ❻) — Race

Week	1	2	3	4	5	6	7	8	9	10	11	12	13	14	15	16
	30 Dec	6 Jan	13 Jan	20 Jan	27 Jan	3 Feb	10 Feb	17 Feb	24 Feb	3 Mar	10 Mar	17 Mar	24 Mar	31 Mar	7 Apr	14 Apr
	Base	Base	Base	Base	Base	Base	Base	Base	Base	Base	Speed	Speed	Speed	Speed	Speed	Speed
	Easy	Hard	Hard	Easy	Hard	Hard	Easy	Hard	Hard	Easy	Hard	Hard	Easy	Hard	Hard	Easy
%	58	72	79	65	86	93	72	93	100	79	93	86	72	86	72	—
Weekly km																
Run	31	38	42	34	46	50	38	50	53	42	50	46	38	46	38	—
Daily training distance																
Mon	km	km	km	km	km	km	km	km	km	km	km	km	km	km	km	km
Run	D/O	D/O	D/O	D/O	D/O	D/O	D/O	D/O	D/O	D/O	D/O	D/O	D/O	D/O	D/O	D/O
Tues																
Run	5.9_1	7.2_2	7.9_2	6.4_1	8.5_3	9.5_3	7.2_1	9.5_4	10_4	7.9_1	9.5_5	8.5_5	7.2_1	8.5_{5-6}	7.2_{5-6}	6.0_1
Wed																
Run	D/O	D/O	D/O	D/O	D/O	D/O	D/O	D/O	D/O	D/O	D/O	D/O	D/O	D/O	D/O	D/O
Thur																
Run	9.4_1	11.4_1	12.7_1	10.3_1	13.6_2	15.1_2	11.4_1	15.1_{2-3}	16_{2-3}	12.7_1	15.1_{2-4}	13.6_{2-4}	11.4_1	13.6_{2-4}	11.4_{2-4}	5.0_1
Fri																
Run	D/O	D/O	D/O	D/O	D/O	D/O	D/O	D/O	D/O	D/O	D/O	D/O	D/O	D/O	D/O	D/O
Sat																
Run	3.5_1	4.3_2	4.7_2	3.8_1	5_3	5.7_3	4.3_1	5.7_4	6_4	4.7_1	5.1_5	5_5	4.3_1	5_{5-6}	4.3_{5-6}	D/O
Sun																
Run	12.3_1	15_1	16.6_1	13.4_1	17.8_1	19.8_1	15_1	19.8_1	21_1	16.6_1	19.8_1	17.8_1	15_1	17.8_1	15_1	RACE

Note: Base 1 would occur first. This programme is based on chapter 7, no. 51 novice.

TAPER AND PEAK

Short distance low-priority race taper programme

Week 1

M	T	W	T	F	S	S
E	INTS	E	ML	E	DAY OFF	RACE

Week 2

M	T	W	T	F	S	S
DAY OFF	E	E	ML	DAY OFF	INTS	LONG

High-priority race (10 km or marathon) taper programme

Week 1

M	T	W	T	F	S	S
E	INTS	E	66% DIST	DAY OFF	50% INTS	50% INTS

Week 2

M	T	W	T	F	S	S
E	25% INTS	E	20% DIST CARBO LOAD ⟶	DAY OFF	DAY OFF	RACE

SPORT-SPECIFIC TRAINING USED FOR RUNNING 10 KM AND MARATHON

Type (intensity)	When initiated	Effect	Example
Power	—	—	—
Intensive sprints	—	—	—
Extensive sprints	Speed phase	Ability to employ race strategy, 'Leg speed'	2–3 × 1–3 min rest to recovery
Submaximal	Speed phase	Improves max steady state race pace	4–6 × 6–8 min 4–1 min rest btwn or 20–30 min TT
Up-tempo	Late base, early speed	Transition from base to speedwork	1–2 × 5–10 km rest 5 km btwn
Long slow distance	Base/speed	Improves ability to do mileage, builds training tolerance and improves recovery rate	Continuous
Active recovery	Base/speed	Assists recovery	Continuous

Appendix 1

Karvonen Formula Calculations

$$HR^{max} - HR^{rest} \times (\% \text{ exercise intensity}) + HR^{rest}$$

HR^{max} = maximum heart rate
HR^{rest} = resting pulse
% exercise intensity (see below)
Your maximum heart rate: .... (either by physical test or 220 – age)
Your resting heart rate: .... (in bed lying down on waking)

Fill in the spaces in the calculations below, using the Karvonen formula, to work out your training ranges for each intensity. Accurate training heart rate ranges are impossible to obtain; these percentages are designed only to give you an approximate level as a guide for your training. For more detail on the Karvonen formula, the different types of intensities and the types of training for each intensity, refer back to chapter 3.

High intensity (HI) – anaerobic = 95–100%

(a)   (.......... – ....) × 95% + ... = ...

(b)   (.......... – ....) × 100% + ... = ...

Your HI training range is (a) – (b) = ... – ....

Submaximal intensity (SM) –
maximum steady state pace/anaerobic threshold = 85–95%

(a)   (.......... – ....) × 85% + ... = ...

(b)   (.......... – ....) × 95% + ... = ...

Your SM training range is (a) – (b) = ... – ....

Low intensity (LO) – aerobic = 60–85%

Up-tempo = 75–85%

(a)   (.......... – ....) × 75% + ... = ...

(b)   (.......... – ....) × 85% + ... = ...

Your up-tempo training range is (a) – (b) = ... – ....

Long slow distance = 60–75%

(a)   (.......... – ....) × 60% + ... = ...

(b)   (.......... – ....) × 75% + ... = ...

Your long slow distance training range is (a) – (b) = ... – ....

Active recovery = less than 60%

(a)   (.......... – ....) × 60% + ... = ...

Your active recovery training range is less than (a) = less than ....

Basic VO$_2$max Test

Here is a very basic running test to determine VO$_2$max. It is not the ideal test as it is not specific and not 100% accurate, but it doesn't require $100,000 worth of testing equipment and you don't have to be Einstein to calculate it.

Modified Margaria et al. run test formula

You need to record the distance you run and the time in which you complete it. The test must be done at the fastest pace you can hold for the full duration of the test (i.e. race pace).

If you do this test:

1 Do not test over a distance less than 3000 m or more than 10,000 m.

2 Do a good warm-up and be very careful. Cyclists, rowers and other non-running athletes who aren't used to running could get injured.

3 If you are at all worried about doing the test, consult a doctor before doing it. Doing the test if you are not prepared can be dangerous.

4 Make sure you are well rested prior to the test.

$$VO_2max \ (ml/kg/min) = \frac{m + (30 \times t)}{5 \ (t + 1)}$$

where m = distance in metres; t = time in minutes

For example, 3000 metres run in 12 minutes: (seconds must be expressed in decimal form, for instance, 30 sec = 0.5 min)

$$
\begin{aligned}
VO_2max \ &= \frac{3000 + (30 \times 12)}{5 \ (12 + 1)} \\
&= \frac{(3000 + 360)}{5 \times 13} \\
&= \frac{3360}{65} \\
&= 51.7 \ ml/kg/min
\end{aligned}
$$

Appendix 3

Basic Anaerobic Threshold Tests

Why test anaerobic threshold?

- To determine optimal training intensities to improve performance
- To check performance and physical condition

What is anaerobic threshold?

This is the zone where the body moves from being predominantly in the aerobic (continuous) training system to being predominantly in the anaerobic (sprinting) training system. The anaerobic system is where the body produces more lactic acid (an exercise by-product) than it is able to eliminate. An athlete cannot remain in this system for very long (no more than two to four minutes). This is where the muscles do not have time to process oxygen and so switch to an energy production that does not include oxygen. Anaerobic threshold is therefore your maximum steady state pace, or the fastest pace you can hold without sprinting or going into oxygen debt for periods over four minutes or, more accurately, around one hour. Training in this zone allows you to improve your fastest endurance pace, leading to a faster race pace. It is very useful for your training to know where this zone is.

Running test

First, a basic way of predicting anaerobic threshold during a running test. It is not the most accurate in the world, but it is still a useful guide. This test was developed in 1989 by Dr Art Weltman at the University of Virginia.

The test involves a 3200 m time trial run and can be used to determine the percentage of your maximum you can sustain in a race. It is not specific for non-runners but can provide a very loose guide to training. Time is measured in minutes, e.g. 30 sec = 0.5 min.

> For men:
> $VO_2 = 122.0 - (5.310 \times \text{time for 3200-m run})$

> For women:
> $VO_2 = (-1.120 \times \text{time for 3200-m run}) + 61.57$
> (Note the negative in this equation.)

For example, a 40-year-old male with a 3200 m time of 14 min

$$VO_2\text{max} = 122 - (5.31 \times 14)$$
$$= 122 - (74.34)$$
$$= 47.66$$

Divide your result (47.66) by your VO_2max (56) and multiply by 100 to reach a percentage figure:

$$(47.66 \div 56) \times 100 = 85\%$$

Therefore anaerobic threshold is at 85% of VO₂max. *See* 'Basic VO₂max Test', appendix 2 to get your VO₂max.

Anaerobic threshold test – Conconi Test

This test is very strenuous! Get medical clearance if you are unsure about your ability to cope with it, particularly if you are over the age of 35.

One of the more notable experts in developing techniques for testing anaerobic threshold was an Italian physician and physiologist named Francesco Conconi. He developed a method for determining anaerobic threshold without needing to take blood samples. This was achieved by monitoring the athlete's heart rate as he or she steadily increased exercise effort. Conconi and his test became very famous when it was used successfully to train a cyclist named Francesco Moser to break the World One-Hour Cycling record.

Why use the Conconi Test?
The advantage of the Conconi Test is that it is very simple, does not require a lot of expensive testing equipment and, with the help of a couple of assistants, you can conduct it yourself.

For runners (including run discipline in triathlon)
You will need:
- an accurate heart rate monitor;
- two helpers, one equipped with a stopwatch and the other with a bike set up with a bike computer that measures kph – the bike can be optional;
- a 200 m indoor track (or 400 m outdoor track but test in windless conditions).

The test
Measure and mark a section of track 50 m in length (for 400 m track mark two 50 m sections 200 m apart).

After a good warm-up (at least 20 min) start the test running with the cyclist at a very comfortable pace. Run behind or beside the bike around the track (preferably beside bike on outside). The cyclist must maintain an even speed throughout each lap. The cyclist is there to control the runner's pace and speed exactly, using a cycle computer. After each 200 m lap the cyclist must increase the pace for the runner by 0.5 kph (if testing without a cyclist, increase running speed by 5 seconds per kilometre).

The second helper will be timing the final 50 m of each 200 m section so your actual running speed can be determined and to double check the cycle computer. Each time you pass the end of the marked 50 m call out your heart rate. Your assistant will record the heart rate next to the time for that 50 m section (there are monitors available that will record this so you don't have call out heart rates). Continue until you feel that you have passed your anaerobic threshold (once heart rate is no longer increasing as fast as running speed, breathing frequency dramatically increases and you find it difficult or impossible to increase your pace further).

For cyclists/mountain bikers (including cycle discipline in triathlon)
You will need:
- accurate heart rate monitor;
- an assistant to record heart rates/speeds;
- a bike computer that measures speed and cadence;
- a velodrome (choose a windless day) or a stationary cycle trainer.

The test

Warm up for ten to twenty minutes. Each lap should be between 300 and 450 m. If you use a windtrainer, use an appropriate time interval (30–50 sec between speed increases). You can change gears if you are an experienced cyclist (cadence must remain constant though); if you are not experienced you should start in a moderately large gear and not gear change during the test. Ride in your racing position and maintain constant pace during each lap. Increase your speed by 1 or 2 kph for each lap (use the same increase each lap.) Keep increasing the speed until your legs are too tired to continue. At the end of each lap call out your heart rate so that it can be recorded by your assistant.

Note: triathletes need to test both running and cycling anaerobic threshold as the heart rates and speeds recorded may be vastly different. Tests should be conducted on sepa-

rate days with enough time to recover fully in between. These protocols can be adapted for kayaking, swimming and rowing but practicalities make tests more difficult to conduct.

How to calculate anaerobic threshold

Calculate your speed (running or cycling) per section of lap (refer to 'Useful Calculations', appendix 8). On a graph plot your recorded heart rates on the vertical axis and your speed on the horizontal axis. If your test has gone as planned, your graph should show an evenly sloping line until the point where your heart rate was unable to increase at the same rate as speed – your heart rate plateau (*see* fig. 3.1A). These zones on the graph just before and just after where the sloping line deflects are the top and bottom heart rates for your anaerobic threshold zone (preferably a five to ten beat range). You can record your test results and plot them on the graph provided at the end of this appendix.

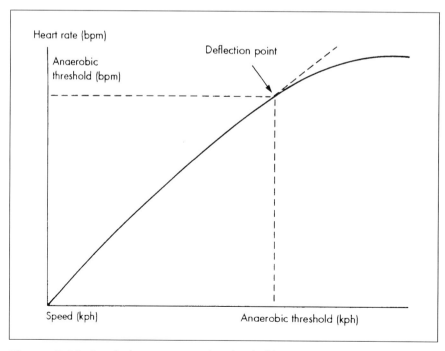

Figure 3.1A Graph showing anaerobic threshold test (Conconi), with heart rate vs speed

How often do you need to test?

Test every two to eight weeks towards the end of an easy week in your mesocycles. Rest for 18 to 24 hours before the test to freshen up. Test every two weeks in the speed phase and every eight weeks in the base phase. Figure 3.2A shows how your anaerobic threshold can change.

This test is useful but a lot of controversy does surround it (there is even controversy over whether anaerobic threshold exists at all). With extensive research being carried out in this area, exercise physiologists will produce further advances. In the meantime, this test is easy to conduct, inexpensive and relatively accurate.

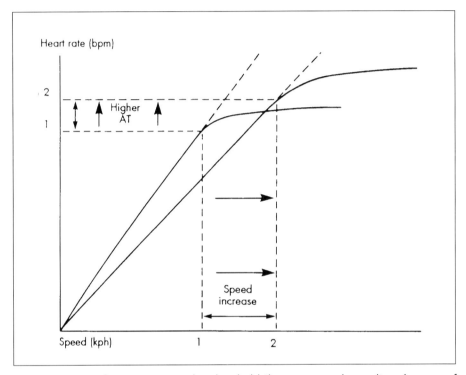

Figure 3.2A Change in anaerobic threshold (heart rate and speed) at the start of speedwork (1) and after peak (2)

Anaerobic Threshold Conconi Test Record Sheet

Name:

Date:

Lap:	Heart rate	Time (sec/50 m)	Speed (kph)
1	....	....	....
2	....	....	....
3	....	....	....
4	....	....	....
5	....	....	....
6	....	....	....
7	....	....	....
8	....	....	....
9	....	....	....
10	....	....	....
11	....	....	....
12	....	....	....
13	....	....	....
14	....	....	....
15	....	....	....
16	....	....	....
17	....	....	....
18	....	....	....
19	....	....	....
20	....	....	....

Anaerobic Threshold Conconi Test Graph

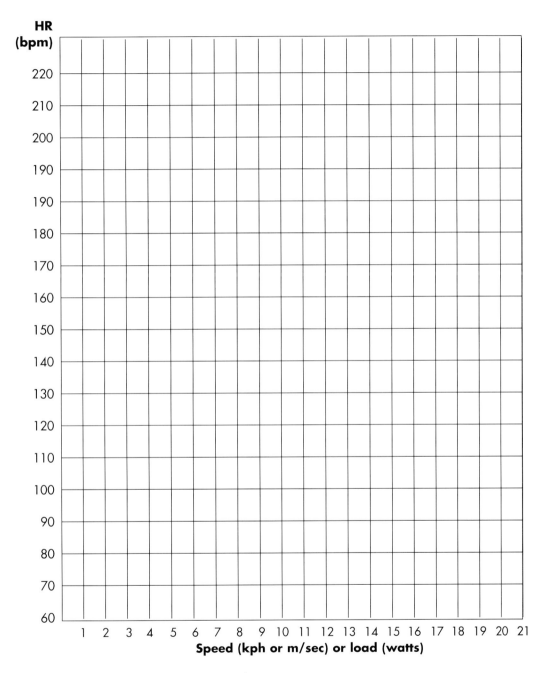

Test duration: ....

Basic Exercise Economy Test

This basic Exercise Economy Test is used to measure increases in fitness and performance. It determines whether speed increases over a set distance at a set heart rate. This is effective in monitoring performance/fitness improvements and can be conducted every two to eight weeks (preferably every six to eight weeks). You must ensure that you are totally fresh for the test – being tired will greatly affect the test and make it invalid.

Heart rate settings

Fill in below the target heart rates that you have determined for each of the specified intensities.

		Example
Anaerobic threshold	....	170
Up-tempo	....	160
Long slow distance	....	145

Test procedure

Warm up at active recovery heart rate for five to ten minutes. If performing more than one test in a row (that is, more than one intensity) start the first test at long slow distance, followed by the up-tempo test and then the anaerobic threshold test. Walk for ten minutes between each test. The tests should be conducted at the end of an easy week with at least 24 hours rest beforehand. You must maintain the same test protocol each time (if you test three intensities, you must test them each time).

Running test
Distance = 2 km
Write in your set heart rate and record the time taken to complete the 2 km. Next determine the min/km pace using the calculation below. Test conditions must be as close to identical as possible (no wind, same test venue).

AT HR ..... Time to complete ..... min/km pace .....
UT HR ..... Time to complete ..... min/km pace .....
LSD HR..... Time to complete ..... min/km pace .....

min/km pace calculation: time (min/km) ÷ 2 km = min/km pace

Cycling test
Distance = 5 km
Write in your set heart rate and record the time taken to complete the 5 km. Next determine the kph pace using the calculation below. Test conditions must be as close to identical as possible (no wind, same test venue).

AT HR ..... Time to complete ..... kph pace .....
UT HR ..... Time to complete ..... kph pace .....
LSD HR..... Time to complete ..... kph pace .....

kph pace calculation: km ÷ time (min) × 60 = kph pace

Variation in exercise economy

The aim now is to measure whether your exercise economy has improved. If your time is faster (speed faster) than previous tests for exactly the same heart rate, your exercise economy has improved. Write your previous pace (speed) and current pace into the spaces below. Use the following calculation to determine the percentage difference in pace.

(Current pace ÷ previous pace × 100) − 100 = % difference

For example:

(30 kph ÷ 28 kph × 100) − 100 = 7.1% increase

	Previous pace	Current pace	% difference
Sport...			
AT	....	....	....
UT	....	....	....
LSD	....	....	....
Sport...			
AT	....	....	....
UT	....	....	....
LSD	....	....	....

Appendix 5

Orthostatic Heart Rate Test and Time Trial Test

Measuring training recovery: orthostatic heart rate test

The orthostatic heart rate test is a measure of overtiredness and is determined by calculating the difference between the standing heart rate and the resting heart rate: a 5 to 10 beat difference is usual, 15 to 20 beats indicates overtiredness.

1 Calculate resting heart rate

Heart rate is taken in bed lying down upon waking. If you use an alarm, you must lie quietly for several minutes before taking your pulse. Try to take it lying in the same position every morning and note that a need to urinate may raise your heart rate slightly. Take this over a full minute.

HR^{rest} = ...

2 Calculate standing heart rate

Taken as soon as you stand up out of bed.

$HR^{standing}$ = ...

3 Calculate the difference in heart rate

$HR^{diff} = HR^{standing} - HR^{rest}$

HR^{diff} = ...

Note: differences between standing and resting heart rates may vary more than stated; if this is the case, use averages.

Time trial test

A time trial test is conducted around a short circuit where cumulative distance, time, speed and heart rate are recorded. For reference on how to conduct the test, *see* page 131.

Time Trial

Lap	Cumulative distance	Cumulative time	Speed for lap	Heart rate
1	....	....	....	....
2	....	....	....	....
3	....	....	....	....
4	....	....	....	....
5	....	....	....	....
6	....	....	....	....
7	....	....	....	....
8	....	....	....	....
9	....	....	....	....
10	....	....	....	....

Speed calculations:

1 Distance (km) – time (min) × 60 = speed (kph)
2 Distance (metres) – time (sec) = speed (m/sec)
3 Time (min) – distance (km) = speed (min/km)

For example, during test for laps:

Total cumulative time ÷ previous lap cumulative time = time

Total cumulative distance – previous lap cumulative distance = distance

Appendix 6

Fluid Balance Test

Test procedure

Exercise for 30 min or one hour at moderate intensity in moderate conditions without eating or drinking. Weigh yourself immediately before and after the exercise test without clothes (some fluid lost during exercise will be absorbed into your clothes). Weigh yourself on electronic scales so you have accuracy to within 0.1 kg. Every 0.1 kg = 100 ml of water lost. For example:

pre-test weight   = 70 kg
post-test weight = 69.5 kg; 500 ml fluid
                              required per hour
post-test weight = 68 kg; 2000 ml fluid
                              required per hour.

Most adult males require 600 to 1000 ml of water per hour in moderate conditions.

Variables that affect fluid consumption
1 Intensity: as intensity increases so do fluid requirements
2 Temperature: temperature increases fluid requirements
3 Altitude: altitude can also raise fluid requirements initially

If any of these variables is noticeably above normal, fluid consumption would need to be increased by up to 35 per cent. Your drinking frequency may also need to increase from every fifteen minutes to every ten minutes.

Test results

Temp (°C)	Humidity	HR	Pre Wght
....	....	....	....
Pst Wght	Diff	Fld Rqmt	% Diff
....	....	....	....

Key: Temp (°C) = temperature; HR = heart rate; Pre Wght = pre-exercise weight; Pst Wght = post-exercise weight; Diff = difference between pre- and post-exercise weights; Fld Rqmt = fluid requirement calculated; % Diff = percentage difference between pre- and post-exercise weights – therefore % fluid loss.

Required fluid intake:
Per hour   ....

Per half hour   ....

Per 15 min   ....

Per 10 min   ....

Use a cycle water bottle (clear plastic so you can see the fluid inside) and mark off your required drinking quantities for either ten or fifteen minute drinking schedules.

Calculations:

1 Diff: Pre Wght (kg) – Pst Wght (kg) = Diff (kg)

2 Fld Rqmt: Diff (kg) × 1000 = Fld Rqmt (ml)

3 Fld Rqmt per min: Fld Rqmt ÷ No. of min of test

4 Actual fluid Rqmt: Fld Rqmt per min × No. min (e.g. race duration)

5 % Diff: Pre Wght ÷ Pst Wght × 100–100 = % Diff

Research has shown that athletes must drink a minimum of 50 per cent of fluid lost during exercise to minimise the effects of dehydration. The maximum you should drink is 65 per cent. For example, if 1 kg is lost during exercise:

- minimum of 500 ml should be drunk
- maximum of 650 ml should be drunk

Appendix 7

Nutritional Calculations

Aim: To establish correct fluid and carbohydrate intake during racing.

Procedure: Do the fluid balance test first (appendix 6), then work through each of the following calculations. There are two optional calculations for fluid and carbohydrate requirements: per aid station and per time interval. If you are not a single-sport athlete you may need to do the calculations for each discipline.

Race estimates

1 Number of aid stations in race ....
  (e.g. 10) (Can you assume that they are approximately evenly spaced?)
2 Expected race time .... (e.g. 180 min)
3 Race distance .... (e.g. 42 km)
4 Expected race speed .... (e.g. 14 kph)
Calculations for race speed:
race distance (km) ÷ expected race time (min) × 60 = race speed (kph)
e.g. 42 km ÷ 180 min x 60 – 14 kph

Fluids (per aid station)

5 Hourly fluid requirement based on fluid balance test .... (e.g. 600 ml)
6 Fluid required per minute .... (e.g. 10 ml)
Calculation:
Hourly fluid requirement ÷ 60 = fluid required per minute e.g. 600 ml ÷ 60 min = 10 ml

7 Total fluid requirement for race ....
  (e.g. 1800 ml)
Calculation:
Expected race time (min) × fluid required per minute = total fluids for race
e.g. 180 min × 10 ml = 1800 ml

8 Requirement per aid station ....
  (e.g. 210 ml)
Calculation:
Total fluid requirement for race ÷ no. of aid stations = requirement per aid station
e.g. 1800 ml ÷ 10 = 210 ml

Carbohydrates (per aid station)

You require 60 g of carbohydrate (CHO) per hour (in fluids and/or solids; it can be a concentration of carbohydrate in the fluids we have just calculated) or 1–1.5 g per kilogram of body weight (whichever is higher). Once you have completed the calculation you will need to look on the packaging of the products you wish to consume during the race or look up their carbohydrate weight in grams in a nutritional book.

9 Hourly carbohydrate requirement = 60 g CHO or calculated range .... (e.g. 70 g)
Calculation:
1 g × body weight = hourly CHO requirement
1.5 g × body weight = hourly CHO requirement
(e.g. 1 g × 70 kg = 70 g)

10 Carbohydrate requirement per minute .... (e.g. 1.167 g)

Calculation:

Hourly CHO requirement ÷ 60 = CHO requirement per minute e.g. 70 g ÷ = 1.167 g

11 Total carbohydrate requirement for race .... (e.g. 210 g)

Calculation:

expected race time × CHO requirement per minute = total CHO requirement

e.g. 180 min × 1.167 g = 210 g

12 Requirement per aid station .... (e.g. 21 g)

Calculation:

Total CHO requirement for race ÷ no. of aid stations = requirement per aid station

e.g. 210 g ÷ 10 = 21 g

Be careful with this calculation because variables such as heat and humidity can affect the calculations. You cannot exactly determine your requirements. Take note of changing conditions. The carbohydrate information needs to be treated very carefully as too high a concentration of carbohydrate can cause stomach upsets. The tendency with these calculations is to err on the side of too much carbohydrate. You must train with your racing concentration first to make sure you can tolerate it. If not, make adjustments. This calculation is not always accurate, because of environmental conditions, but at least you can estimate your requirements.

If you do not wish to set your fluid nutritional strategies up per aid station you can use time.

Fluid (per time interval)

Fluid Rqmt per min = ... (from appendix 6 test)

Fluid Rqmt per min × time interval (e.g. 10, 15, 20 min race duration)

e.g. 16.7 mls × 10 min = 167 mls every 10 min.

Carbohydrates (per time interval)

1.5 g × body weight = hourly CHO requirement

e.g. 1.5 g × 70 kg = 105 g

CHO Rqmt per min = hourly CHO rqmt ÷ 60 = CHO rqmt per min

e.g. 105 ÷ 60 = 1.75 g per min

CHO rqmt per min × time interval (e.g. 10, 15, 20 min race duration)

e.g. 1.75 g × 10 min = 17.5 g

Using 10% CHO solution:

Fluid rqmt = 167 mls every 10 min

CHO rqmt = 17.5 g every 10 min

10% CHO solution from 167 mls of fluid = 167 mls × 10% (0.1) = 16.7 g

Difference:

17.5 – 16.7 = 0.8, therefore, you may need to use secondary CHO source every 30 min or hr.

Useful Calculations

To calculate speed and average speed

For minutes per kilometre (min/km)
time to complete workout (min) ÷ distance covered in workout (km) = speed (min/km)
e.g. 30 min ÷ 6 km = 5 min/km

For kilometres per hour (kph)
distance (km) covered in workout ÷ time (min) to complete workout × 60 = speed (kph)
e.g. 39 km ÷ 80 min × 60 = 29.3 kph

For metres per second (m/sec)
distance (m) ÷ time (sec) = speed (m/sec)
e.g. 500 m ÷ 425 sec = 1.18 m/sec
or distance (m) ÷ time (min) ÷ 60 = speed (m/sec)
e.g. 2000 m ÷ 7 min ÷ 60 = 4.76 m/sec

To calculate duration

Using min/km
distance (km) × speed (min/km) = duration (min)
e.g. 6 km × 5 min/km = 30 min

Using kph
distance (km) ÷ speed (kph) × 60 = duration (min)
e.g. 39 km ÷ 29.3 kph × 60 = 80 min

Using m/sec
distance (m) ÷ speed (m/sec) = duration (sec)
e.g. 500 m ÷ 1.18 m/sec = 425 sec
or distance (m) ÷ speed (m/sec) ÷ 60 = duration (min)
e.g. 2000 m ÷ 4.76 ÷ 60 = 7 min

To calculate distance

Using min/km
time (min) ÷ speed (min/km) = distance (km)
e.g. 30 min ÷ 5 min/km = 6 km

Using kph
time (min) × speed (kph) ÷ 60 = distance (km)
e.g. 80 min × 29.3 kph ÷ 60 = 39 km

Using m/sec
time (sec) × speed (m/sec) = distance (m)
e.g. 425 sec × 1.18 m/sec = 500 m
or time (min) × speed (m/sec) × 60 = distance (m)
e.g. 7 min × 4.76 m/sec × 60 – 2000 m

To calculate average weight, resting pulse, hours sleep, training time/distance

Total up each of the variables from each day during the week you are in, then divide by the number of days in the week. For weight, resting pulse and sleep, this will always be seven days if you are filling the log book out correctly. For training, divide by the number of days/workouts.

For example, for distance:
10 km + 16 km + 10 km + 20 km + 10 km + 30 km = 96 km
Divide by 6 for 6 workouts: 96 km ÷ 6 workouts = 16 km average

To calculate percentage increase/decrease

From total training time/distance and last week's total calculate % increase/decrease in training volume.

Total training time/distance = 96 km
Last week's total (obtained from last week's summary) = 87 km

To calculate % increase/decrease: total training time/distance for week (min/km) ÷ last week's total (min/km) × 100 - 100 = % increase or decrease
e.g. 96 km ÷ 87 km × 100 - 100 = 10.3% (increase)
e.g. 87 km ÷ 96 km × 100 - 100 = – 9.4% (decrease)

To calculate percentage field

placing in race ÷ total number of competitors × 100 = % field
e.g. 10th placing ÷ 750 competitors × 100 = 1.3%
(You came in the top 1.3% of the field.)

To calculate percentage time difference

your time for race (min or sec) ÷ 1st-place-getter's time (min or sec) × 100 - 100 = % time difference
e.g. 75 min ÷ 62 min × 100 - 100 = 21%
(You took 21% longer to complete the race.)

How to Use Your Log Book and Working Programme

The benefits of using a log book

The key to being a successful athlete is to train hard, train smart, and know what forms of training work for you. Do you know how many weeks of speedwork you need to peak? Do you know what your optimal training, resting and racing heart rates are? Do you know what weekly programme format you are best suited to? Do you know when the best times to race are to peak effectively?

There are a huge number of questions that a properly constructed and used log book will answer. It will enable you to train smarter and race faster. This log book acts as your personal coach. It asks you the questions your coach would ask to establish whether your training is working or not. Your log book will teach how to train far more effectively than ever before. Through analysis of your training you will be able to plan better and refine your training. With this you will be able to eliminate training errors and accentuate effective training. It will also provide a diary of previous build-ups to refer to, and which you can use to set up your next training build-up. Ultimately you have a better understanding of your own body, your training and the requirements for racing to your full potential. All it requires is a little time spent planning and analysing your training each week. This is the future of training.

How to use your log book

This log book is set up with extensive training data collection techniques. It is designed so that it can be used by anyone, from a world champion to a weekend warrior. You do not need to use all the facilities in the log book; use as many or as few as you like.

Daily log book usage – your working programme

Use the working programme record sheets in this appendix to complete the following.

Each morning before your workout

Note down your resting pulse (taken in bed lying down upon waking) and your morning weight. These will help act as indicators to your training. Write these in pen on the far left of the page in the 'Day' section under H.R.

After you have completed your workout

When you have completed your workout or workouts write the following information in the 'Activity' section of your log book in pen to indicate its completion. There is space to write down specifics for up to three disciplines (*see* pages 132–5 for worked examples).

Fill out daily
- Time to complete the workout
- Distance covered
- Average speed, if you wish (you may have equipment that can measure this; to calculate it refer to appendix 8)

- Average training heart rate (if you have a pulse monitor). If you are doing speed-work, you may want to note down speed-work heart rates and average training heart rate separately
- Under 'Specifics' write in any important format points about your workout. This would mainly be used to note down intervals (distance, time, reps, sets) during speedwork
- Under the 'Specifics' fill out the total time for your workouts if you have completed more than one workout in the day. Also fill out the Gym, Stretching/Injury/Illness questions by circling them if they apply. If they do not apply, ignore them
- Next answer all the questions in the 'Performance Analysis' section by circling the word that most suits you. Be honest with yourself. The only person you are going to be fooling is you!
- In the 'Comments' area in the Performance Analysis section note down anything that you felt may not have been covered by the questions but that is of relevance
- 'Post Exercise Weight' is also available in the Performance Analysis section to aid in determining correct hydration techniques. If you weigh yourself immediately before and after you exercise, the weight differ-ence is due to lack of adequate hydration. Drink 500 ml of fluid for every 500 g of weight lost. Remember that a 2 per cent weight loss due to dehydration (1.4 kg in a 70 kg athlete) will seriously decrease performance and recovery.

Notes on working programme record sheet
- 'Hills 1 2 3' and 'Sprint 1 2 3: 1, 2 and 3 are measures of load. 1 means very, very hilly or maximum sprinting (<1 min); 2 is hilly or longer endurance sprints (1–4 min), and 3 means small hills or maximum steady state pace speedwork (i.e. the fastest you can go without sprinting – 4 min+).

- 'Sleep' is in hours.

This may look like a lot to do but you will find that you can complete each day's entry in about two minutes. Not much work for the amazing amount of specific practical informa-tion logged.

At the end of the week
Fill in the 'Weekly Summary' in the same way as you have filled out the daily summary. You will find that because of the set-up of the working programme it is easy to identify training errors and strengths. The working programme is set up as part of the log book so that you are looking for patterns in the circling of information rather than having to read the whole week's notes. It will take you about five minutes to fill out your weekly summary.

To fill out the Weekly Summary
- Note down the week number (number of weeks into your build-up).
- Work out averages for weight, resting pulse, sleep, and training time/distance. Refer to appendix 8 if you are not sure how to calculate this.
- Estimate the percentage increase or decrease in training volume using total training time/distance and last week's total. Note this down as % increase/decrease. Refer to appendix 8 if you are not sure how to calculate this. This is useful for determining whether you are increasing your training volumes too quickly. Fill out the other questions by circling the word that is most appropriate.

Training Notes
Make any other relevant notes on your train-ing under 'Training Notes'.

Racing

Answer each of the questions in the 'Racing Analysis' pages of the log book (*see* below). Rate your personal performance on a scale of one to five. One means that you were very happy with your performance and five means that you were very unhappy with your performance. See appendix 8 for determining average speed and % field. This is useful for determining your performance on different courses against different numbers of competitors. It does help to standardise your results if it is difficult to check this any other way.

RACE: _____ PERFORMANCE: 1 2 3 4 5 PLACE:_____% FIELD _____
TOTAL FIELD _____ AV SPEED: _____ COURSE: hilly 1 2 3 / flat
DISTS: 1_____ 2 _____ 3 _____ 4 _____
       1_____ TRAN 2 _____ TRAN _____
       3_____ TRAN 4 _____ TOTAL_____
WEATHER: hot / cold / wet / windy / moderate / calm
WATER: calm / moderate / rough   AV H.R. _____
EQUIPMENT SET-UP: _____

RACE: _____ PERFORMANCE: 1 2 3 4 5 PLACE:_____% FIELD _____
TOTAL FIELD _____ AV SPEED: _____ COURSE: hilly 1 2 3 / flat
DISTS: 1_____ 2 _____ 3 _____ 4 _____
       1_____ TRAN 2 _____ TRAN _____
       3_____ TRAN 4 _____ TOTAL_____
WEATHER: hot / cold / wet / windy / moderate / calm
WATER: calm / moderate / rough   AV H.R. _____
EQUIPMENT SET-UP: _____

RACE: _____ PERFORMANCE: 1 2 3 4 5 PLACE:_____% FIELD _____
TOTAL FIELD _____ AV SPEED: _____ COURSE: hilly 1 2 3 / flat
DISTS: 1_____ 2 _____ 3 _____ 4 _____
       1_____ TRAN 2 _____ TRAN _____
       3_____ TRAN 4 _____ TOTAL_____
WEATHER: hot / cold / wet / windy / moderate / calm
WATER: calm / moderate / rough   AV H.R. _____
EQUIPMENT SET-UP: _____

RACE: _____ PERFORMANCE: 1 2 3 4 5 PLACE:_____% FIELD _____
TOTAL FIELD _____ AV SPEED: _____ COURSE: hilly 1 2 3 / flat
DISTS: 1_____ 2 _____ 3 _____ 4 _____
       1_____ TRAN 2 _____ TRAN _____
       3_____ TRAN 4 _____ TOTAL_____
WEATHER: hot / cold / wet / windy / moderate / calm
WATER: calm / moderate / rough   AV H.R. _____
EQUIPMENT SET-UP: _____

Racing analysis

DAY	ACTIVITY			PERFORMANCE ANALYSIS	
MON **DATE** **H.R.** **WGHT**	SPORT TIME: DIST: AV SPEED: AV H.R. SPECIFICS: TOTAL TIME: _____	SPORT TIME: DIST: AV SPEED: AV H.R. SPECIFICS: Stretching/Injury/Illness	SPORT TIME: DIST: AV SPEED: AV H.R. SPECIFICS:	FELT: STRESS: BENEFIT: SLEEP: NUTRITION: AIM: INTENSITY: WEATHER: WATER: COMMENTS:	Excellent/Good/Average/Tired/V.Tired Mellow/Moderate/High/V.High Excellent/Good/Average/Poor/☺☹ 11,10,9,8,7,6,5,4,3 Good/Average/Broken Good/Average/Poor/Binge Day Base – Long/Hills 1 2 3/Easy/Technique Speed – Race/Time Trial/Intervals/Sprint 1 2 3 >100%,100%,90%,80%,70%,60%,50% Calm/Moderate/Windy/Wet/Cold/Hot Calm/Moderate/Rough
	GYM: Weights–	Strength/Circuit	Aerobics/Flex	Post Exercise Weight:	
TUES **DATE** **H.R.** **WGHT**	SPORT TIME: DIST: AV SPEED: AV H.R. SPECIFICS: TOTAL TIME: _____	SPORT TIME: DIST: AV SPEED: AV H.R. SPECIFICS: Stretching/Injury/Illness	SPORT TIME: DIST: AV SPEED: AV H.R. SPECIFICS:	FELT: STRESS: BENEFIT: SLEEP: NUTRITION: AIM: INTENSITY: WEATHER: WATER: COMMENTS:	Excellent/Good/Average/Tired/V.Tired Mellow/Moderate/High/V.High Excellent/Good/Average/Poor/☺☹ 11,10,9,8,7,6,5,4,3 Good/Average/Broken Good/Average/Poor/Binge Day Base – Long/Hills 1 2 3/Easy/Technique Speed – Race/Time Trial/Intervals/Sprint 1 2 3 >100%,100%,90%,80%,70%,60%,50% Calm/Moderate/Windy/Wet/Cold/Hot Calm/Moderate/Rough
	GYM: Weights–	Strength/Circuit	Aerobics/Flex	Post Exercise Weight:	
WED **DATE** **H.R.** **WGHT**	SPORT TIME: DIST: AV SPEED: AV H.R. SPECIFICS: TOTAL TIME: _____	SPORT TIME: DIST: AV SPEED: AV H.R. SPECIFICS: Stretching/Injury/Illness	SPORT TIME: DIST: AV SPEED: AV H.R. SPECIFICS:	FELT: STRESS: BENEFIT: SLEEP: NUTRITION: AIM: INTENSITY: WEATHER: WATER: COMMENTS:	Excellent/Good/Average/Tired/V.Tired Mellow/Moderate/High/V.High Excellent/Good/Average/Poor/☺☹ 11,10,9,8,7,6,5,4,3 Good/Average/Broken Good/Average/Poor/Binge Day Base – Long/Hills 1 2 3/Easy/Technique Speed – Race/Time Trial/Intervals/Sprint 1 2 3 >100%,100%,90%,80%,70%,60%,50% Calm/Moderate/Windy/Wet/Cold/Hot Calm/Moderate/Rough
	GYM: Weights–	Strength/Circuit	Aerobics/Flex	Post Exercise Weight:	
THUR **DATE** **H.R.** **WGHT**	SPORT TIME: DIST: AV SPEED: AV H.R. SPECIFICS: TOTAL TIME: _____	SPORT TIME: DIST: AV SPEED: AV H.R. SPECIFICS: Stretching/Injury/Illness	SPORT TIME: DIST: AV SPEED: AV H.R. SPECIFICS:	FELT: STRESS: BENEFIT: SLEEP: NUTRITION: AIM: INTENSITY: WEATHER: WATER: COMMENTS:	Excellent/Good/Average/Tired/V.Tired Mellow/Moderate/High/V.High Excellent/Good/Average/Poor/☺☹ 11,10,9,8,7,6,5,4,3 Good/Average/Broken Good/Average/Poor/Binge Day Base – Long/Hills 1 2 3/Easy/Technique Speed – Race/Time Trial/Intervals/Sprint 1 2 3 >100%,100%,90%,80%,70%,60%,50% Calm/Moderate/Windy/Wet/Cold/Hot Calm/Moderate/Rough
	GYM: Weights–	Strength/Circuit	Aerobics/Flex	Post Exercise Weight:	

Working Programme Record Sheets

ACTIVITY			**PERFORMANCE ANALYSIS**	**DAY**

FRI

SPORT	SPORT	SPORT
TIME:	TIME:	TIME:
DIST:	DIST:	DIST:
AV SPEED:	AV SPEED:	AV SPEED:
AV H.R.	AV H.R.	AV H.R.
SPECIFICS:	SPECIFICS:	SPECIFICS:

TOTAL TIME: _____ Stretching/Injury/Illness
GYM: Weights– Strength/Circuit Aerobics/Flex

FELT: Excellent/Good/Average/Tired/V.Tired
STRESS: Mellow/Moderate/High/V.High
BENEFIT: Excellent/Good/Average/Poor/☺☹
SLEEP: 11,10,9,8,7,6,5,4,3 Good/Average/Broken
NUTRITION: Good/Average/Poor/Binge Day
AIM: Base – Long/Hills 1 2 3/Easy/Technique
Speed – Race/Time Trial/Intervals/Sprint 1 2 3
INTENSITY: >100%,100%,90%,80%,70%,60%,50%
WEATHER: Calm/Moderate/Windy/Wet/Cold/Hot
WATER: Calm/Moderate/Rough
COMMENTS:

Post Exercise Weight:

DATE **H.R.** **WGHT**

SAT

SPORT	SPORT	SPORT
TIME:	TIME:	TIME:
DIST:	DIST:	DIST:
AV SPEED:	AV SPEED:	AV SPEED:
AV H.R.	AV H.R.	AV H.R.
SPECIFICS:	SPECIFICS:	SPECIFICS:

TOTAL TIME: _____ Stretching/Injury/Illness
GYM: Weights– Strength/Circuit Aerobics/Flex

FELT: Excellent/Good/Average/Tired/V.Tired
STRESS: Mellow/Moderate/High/V.High
BENEFIT: Excellent/Good/Average/Poor/☺☹
SLEEP: 11,10,9,8,7,6,5,4,3 Good/Average/Broken
NUTRITION: Good/Average/Poor/Binge Day
AIM: Base – Long/Hills 1 2 3/Easy/Technique
Speed – Race/Time Trial/Intervals/Sprint 1 2 3
INTENSITY: >100%,100%,90%,80%,70%,60%,50%
WEATHER: Calm/Moderate/Windy/Wet/Cold/Hot
WATER: Calm/Moderate/Rough
COMMENTS:

Post Exercise Weight:

DATE **H.R.** **WGHT**

SUN

SPORT	SPORT	SPORT
TIME:	TIME:	TIME:
DIST:	DIST:	DIST:
AV SPEED:	AV SPEED:	AV SPEED:
AV H.R.	AV H.R.	AV H.R.
SPECIFICS:	SPECIFICS:	SPECIFICS:

TOTAL TIME: _____ Stretching/Injury/Illness
GYM: Weights– Strength/Circuit Aerobics/Flex

FELT: Excellent/Good/Average/Tired/V.Tired
STRESS: Mellow/Moderate/High/V.High
BENEFIT: Excellent/Good/Average/Poor/☺☹
SLEEP: 11,10,9,8,7,6,5,4,3 Good/Average/Broken
NUTRITION: Good/Average/Poor/Binge Day
AIM: Base – Long/Hills 1 2 3/Easy/Technique
Speed – Race/Time Trial/Intervals/Sprint 1 2 3
INTENSITY: >100%,100%,90%,80%,70%,60%,50%
WEATHER: Calm/Moderate/Windy/Wet/Cold/Hot
WATER: Calm/Moderate/Rough
COMMENTS:

Post Exercise Weight:

DATE **H.R.** **WGHT**

WEEKLY SUMMARY

WEEK NO: _____
WEIGHT (AV): _____
REST PULSE (AV): _____
SLEEP (AV): _____
TRAINING TIME/DIST (AV): _____
TOTAL TRAINING TIME/DIST: _____
LAST WEEK'S TOTAL: _____
% INCREASE/DECREASE: _____
PHYSICAL CONDITION: Excellent/Good/Average/Groan!
STRESS: Mellow/Moderate/High
EFFECTIVENESS: Excellent/Good/Average/☺☹
NUTRITION: Good/Moderate/Poor

TRAINING NOTES

_____
_____
_____
_____
_____
_____
_____
_____
_____
_____
_____
_____

Appendix 10
Training Graph

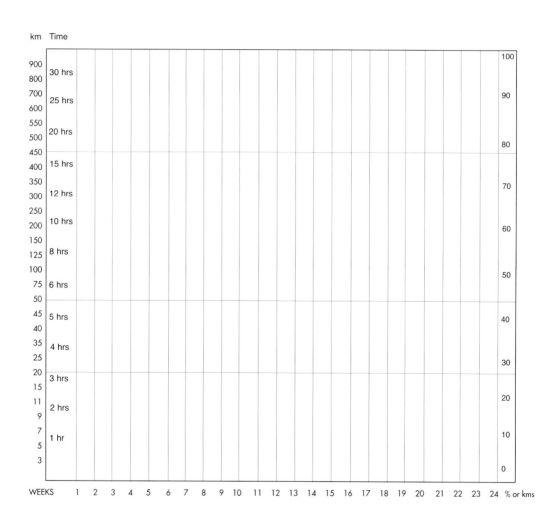

Flexibility and Stretching

Always do a warm-up and warm-down. Move slowly into all stretches and be sensitive to the tension being placed on the stretched muscle. You should slowly move into the stretch until you feel the first sign of a comfortable mild tension in the muscle and hold this for ten or fifteen seconds. Don't overstretch (stretching to pain); it will only lead to injury and will negatively affect your flexibility.

Recommendations:
1 rep each side = very flexible
2 reps each side = average flexibility
3 reps each side = below average flexibility
4–6 reps each side = poor flexibility or problem area (e.g injury)

In the case of flexibility imbalance, more reps should be used on the tighter muscle or limb.

Key:
D = duathlon   M = multisport
C = cycle and mountain bike   R = rowing
T = triathlon   RN = running

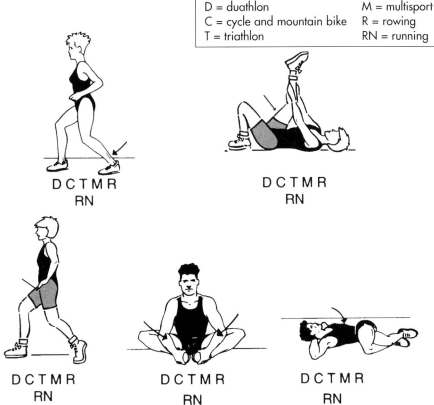

D C T M R
RN

D C T M R
RN

D C T M R
RN

D C T M R
RN

D C T M R
RN

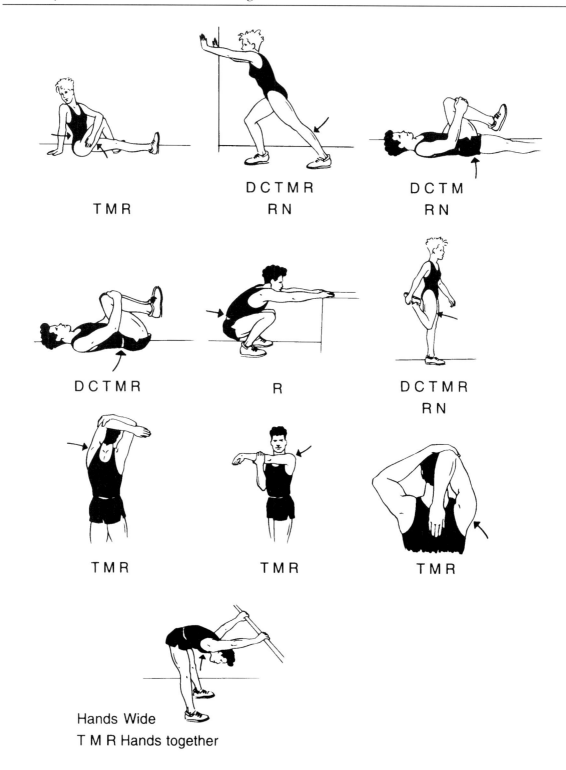

TMR

DCTMR
RN

DCTM
RN

DCTMR

R

DCTMR
RN

TMR

TMR

TMR

Hands Wide
T M R Hands together

Cycling – subphases

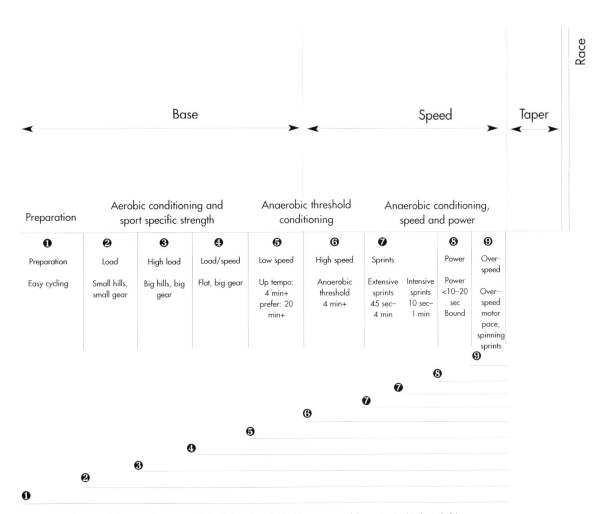

Note: Once you begin a subphase you do not stop it. Each subphase is emphasised in sequence and then maintained to the end of the programme.

Seasonal Programme Planner (Template 1)

Graph of yearly plan

Months

Set up your training seasons on this table. (Off-season, pre-season and in-season)

Peak-mileage Week Programme Planner (Template 2)

Standard weekly training format

Sport	Mon	Tues	Wed	Thurs	Fri	Sat	Sun	Total

Set up your standard training week format using this table (e.g. what workout, on what day, and what type of workout: hills/long/speed/easy).

Weekly Build-up Programme Planner (Template 3)

Build-up – week-to-week mileages

week	1	2	3	4	5	6	7	8	9	10	11	12	13	14	15	16	17	18	19	20	21	22	23	24	R A C E
date																									
meso-cycle																									
%																									
Sport 1																									
Sport 2																									
Sport 3																									

Set up your week-to-week training mileages and periodisation (base/speed/taper) using this table. Work backwards from your goal race, and include lower priority races that you will use as training races.

Weekly and Daily Build-up Programme Planner
(Template 4)

Name:
Race:
Race date:

mileage profile

Maximum distance for 100% week
Sport 1:
Sport 2:
Sport 3:

R
A
C
E

week	1	2	3	4	5	6	7	8	9	10	11	12	13	14	15	16	17	18	19	20	21	22	23	24
date b/spd meso																								
%																								
sport																								
	km/min	km/min	km/min	km/min	km/min	km/min	km/min	km/min	km/min	km/min	km/min	km/min	km/min	km/min	km/min	km/min	km/min	km/min	km/min	km/min	km/min	km/min	km/min	km/min
mon																								
tues																								
wed																								
thurs																								
fri																								
sat																								
sun																								

Bibliography

Brooks, G. A. and Fahey, D.F. *Fundamentals of Human Performance*, Macmillan Publishing, 1984**

Brotherhood, J.R. 'Nutrition and Sports Performance', *Sports Medicine*, 1984*

Burke, E.R. *Science of Cycling*, Human Kinetics, 1986**

Burke, E.R. *Medical and Scientific Aspects of Cycling*, Human Kinetics**

Burke, L. and Read, R. 'Sports Nutrition, Approaching the Nineties', *Sports Medicain*, 1989

Burlingame et. al. *The Concise NZ Food Composition Tables*, NZ Institute for Crop and Food Research Ltd, 1993

Coleman, E. *Eating for Endurance*, Bull Publishing Co., 1988*

Edwards, S. *The Heart Rate Monitor Book*, Fleet Feet Press, 1992 *

Food for Health, Report of the Nutrition Taskforce, New Zealand Department of Health, New Zealand, 1991

Foods, Nutrition and Sports Performance,. Statement from International Conference, Feb, 1991

Gisolfi, C. and Duchman, S. 'Guidelines for Optimal Replacement Beverages for Different Athletic Events', *Medicine & Science in Sports and Exercise*, Vol. 24, No. 6, 1992

Hahn, A. G. *State of the Art Review, no. 31: The Physiological Rationale for Altitude Training*, National Sports Research Centre, Australian Sports Commission, 1992

Haymes, E. M. and Wells, C. L. *Environment and Human Performance*, Human Kinetics 1986

Hellemans, I. 'Nutritional Considerations for Physically Active Adults and Athletes in New Zealand', New Zealand Dietetic Association Position Paper, Nov, 1991

Hellemans, J. *Triathlon: A Complete Guide to Training and Racing*, Reed Publishing, 1993*

Hinault, B. and Genzling, C. *Road Racing: Technique and Training*, Vitesse Press, 1988*

Howley, E. T and Franks, B. D. *Health Fitness Instructors Handbook*, second edition, Human Kinetics, 1992**

Inge, K. and Brukner, P. *Food for Sport*, William Heineman, 1986*

Janssen, P. G. J. M. *Training Lactate Pulse Rate*, Polar Electro Oy Publishers, 1987**

Lemond, G. and Gordis, K. *Greg Lemond's Complete Book of Bicycling*, The Putnam Publishing Group, 1990*

Longhurst, K. and Blundell, N. *State of the Art Review, no 9: Anaerobic Threshold and Endurance Performance*, National Sports Research Centre, Australian Sports Commission, 1986

MacKinnon, L. T. and Hooper, S. *State of the Art Review, no. 26: Overtraining*, National Sports Research Centre, Australian Sports Commission, 1991

MacKinnon, L. and Hooper, S. *Training Logs: An Effective Method of Monitoring Overtraining and Tapering – Coaches' Report*, National Sports Research Centre, Australian Sports Commission, 1991

Maffetone, P. and Mantell, M. E. *The High Performance Heart*, Bicycle Books Inc. 1991*

McArdle, W. D. Katch, F. I. and Katch, V. L. *Exercise Physiology,* Led & Febiger, 1986**

Pearce, J. *Eat to Compete,* Heinemann Reed, Auckland, 1990*

Sharkey, B. J. *Physiology of Fitness,* third edition, Human Kinetics, 1990**

Sleamaker, R. *Serious Training for Serious Athletes,* Leisure Press*

Sports Nutrition, Sports & Cardiovascular Nutritionists (SCAN). The American Dietetic Association, 1988

Wootton, S. *Nutrition for Sport.* Simon & Schuster Ltd, 1989*

Thanks to all the athletes and coaches that I've talked to over the last 10 or so years. Thanks for the explanations on why, how and when. Without your help I could never have written this book. You people are the ultimate resource on training information.

For those of you interested I have graded this bibliograpy if you wish to follow up for further reading.

Novice to intermediate athlete/new coach: *
Intermediate to experienced athlete/intermediate coach: ** and *
Experienced coach: all references

Recommended Reading

Food for Fitness by Anita Bean (A & C Black, London, 1998)

Hi-Tech Cycling by Edmund Burke (Human Kinetics, Champaign, Illinois, 1996)

Keep on Running by Eric Newsholme, Tony Leech and Glenda Duester (John Wiley & Sons, Chichester, 1994)

Serious Cycling by Edmund Burke (Human Kinetics, Champaign, Illinois, 1996)

Sports Training Principles (third edition) by Frank Dick (A & C Black, London, 1997)

The Complete Guide to Cross Training by Fiona Hayes (A & C Black, London, 1998)

The Complete Guide to Sports Nutrition (second edition) by Anita Bean (A & C Black, London, 1996)

The Complete Guide to Strength Training by Anita Bean (A & C Black, London, 1997)

The Complete Guide to Stretching by Christopher M. Norris (A & C Black, London, 1999)

Index